Contemporary Perspectives on Freud's Seduction Theory and Psychotherapy

This edited collection brings together the perspectives of a broad spectrum of experts who reflect on Freud's Seduction Theory, psychoanalysis, and the reality of child abuse through the work of Jeffrey Masson.

Jeffrey Masson's *The Assault on Truth: Freud's Suppression of the Seduction Theory* (1984) is arguably the most controversial book on psychoanalysis in the last century. It provoked a furore from mainstream psychoanalysis, yet was well-received by the emerging international trauma field and became a bestseller. Four decades on, a group of international scholars and professionals revisit Masson's original work and reflect on the lessons that can be taken from the saga. Was the reaction of Masson's peers tied to the fact that he had accused Freud of being less than heroic, or was it that he confronted psychoanalysis with a very uncomfortable truth? This book examines how *The Assault on Truth* came to be written, why it sparked such an extreme reaction, and the issues Masson was grappling with.

Complete with an extended Foreword by John Briere, a luminary of the modern trauma field, this book will be essential reading for practitioners, students, and researchers involved in contemporary psychoanalysis, psychotherapy, psychology and especially trauma care, women's mental health, child safety and the study of memory.

Warwick Middleton has been the Foundation Director of the Trauma and Dissociation Unit, Belmont Hospital, for over 25 years. He is a pioneer researcher in the area of ongoing incest during adulthood; he chairs the Cannan Institute and is a past president of the International Society for the Study of Trauma and Dissociation. He currently holds professorial appointments with the University of Queensland, Australia, and the University of Canterbury, New Zealand.

Martin J. Dorahy is Professor of Clinical Psychology at the University of Canterbury, Christchurch, New Zealand, and a past president of the International Society for the Study of Trauma and Dissociation. His published work has primarily explored cognitive and emotional underpinnings of dissociation and dissociative disorders. His clinical work is focused on the adult outcomes of abuse and neglect.

Contemporary Perspectives on Freud's Seduction Theory and Psychotherapy

Revisiting Masson's '*The Assault on Truth*'

Edited by Warwick Middleton and Martin J. Dorahy

Routledge
Taylor & Francis Group
LONDON AND NEW YORK

Front cover image: Warwick Middleton

First published 2024
by Routledge
4 Park Square, Milton Park, Abingdon, Oxon OX14 4RN

and by Routledge
605 Third Avenue, New York, NY 10158

Routledge is an imprint of the Taylor & Francis Group, an informa business

British Library Cataloguing-in-Publication Data
A catalogue record for this book is available from the British Library

ISBN: 978-1-032-55522-5 (hbk)
ISBN: 978-1-032-55634-5 (pbk)
ISBN: 978-1-003-43146-6 (ebk)

DOI: 10.4324/9781003431466

Typeset in Times New Roman
by Newgen Publishing UK

Note on cover picture taken by Warwick Middleton, in close consultation with Martin J. Dorahy, December 2023.

This picture is a photographic montage of sorts. It includes the slim volume, *Sexual Accusations and Social Turmoil* by Jules Masserman MD, published in 1994.

For those intrepid enough to track down the details underlying Masserman's book, they will find that he had training as a psychoanalyst, was a highly prolific writer on psychotherapy, the author of at least 18 books and over 400 papers, that he was an ex-President of the American Psychiatric Association (1978–79), that he had been described as the world's most famous living psychiatrist, and that he was successfully civilly sued by at least four women for sexual abuse in therapy. These included singer/composer Barbara Noel who documented being drugged during her "therapy" and being sexually assaulted by Masserman. Ms Noel filed a complaint with the Illinois Psychiatric Society, which voted to suspend Dr Masserman's membership in the Society for five years. Dr Masserman agreed to sign a consent order surrendering his license to practice. Following this, the American Psychiatric Association Appeals Board voted to suspend Dr Masserman for five years rather than expel him, effectively protecting him against unfavourable publicity. He remained on the APA board of trustees. In his late eighties he, with his wife, wrote this hastily produced book, on "false memories", which espoused an epidemic of sexual accusations against notable people. Shortly after the publication of the book in 1994, it was rumoured that Masserman suicided. Yet rapidly any reference to suicide disappeared from the official story, and duly obituaries appeared which avoided mentioning the cause of death. Masserman's book was included in the cover picture to capture the tension around sexual abuse disclosures and the reality that abusers often hide in plain sight.

We would like to dedicate this book to Robert Fliess and Florence Rush, two courageous defenders of truth.

Warwick Middleton and Martin J. Dorahy

Contents

Contributors

John Briere, Ph.D., is Professor Emeritus of Psychiatry at the Keck School of Medicine, University of Southern California. A past president of the International Society for Traumatic Stress Studies, he is recipient of the *Award for Outstanding Contributions to the Science of Trauma Psychology* from the American Psychological Association. He is author or co-author of over 140 articles and chapters, 15 books, and 9 trauma-related psychological tests.

Bruce M. Z. Cohen, Ph.D., is an associate professor and critical sociologist of mental health at the University of Auckland, Aotearoa, New Zealand. With research focusing on the expanding realms of psychiatric discourse and psy-professional power in neoliberal society, his books include *Mental Health User Narratives: New Perspectives on Illness and Recovery* (Palgrave Macmillan, 2008) and *Psychiatric Hegemony: A Marxist Theory of Mental Illness* (Palgrave Macmillan, 2016).

Christine A. Courtois, Ph.D., ABPP, a board-certified counselling psychologist, retired from clinical practice in Washington, DC, is now an author and consultant/trainer on trauma psychology and treatment. Dr Courtois was Chair of the Clinical Practice Guideline for the Treatment of PTSD in Adults for the American Psychological Association and is past president of APA Division 56 (Trauma Psychology). She co-founded and was Clinical and Training Director of a specialized inpatient and day treatment program, The CENTER: Posttraumatic Disorders Program. She has received professional recognition for her work.

Lynn Crook, M.Ed., is an investigative journalist in Seattle, Washington. She recalled sexual abuse by her father and sued her parents. Following the judge's decision in her favour she read the deposition of her parents' expert, Elizabeth Loftus, Ph.D., who testified she dropped the first six mall study subjects. Lynn's decision to find out why led to a decades-long investigation of false memory claims and a book titled *False Memories.*

Martin J. Dorahy, Ph.D., DClinPsych is a professor of clinical psychology at the University of Canterbury, Christchurch, New Zealand, and he also operates a practice working with people experiencing complex trauma disorders. He has a theoretical and research interest in the cognitive and emotional correlates of trauma and dissociative disorders. He is a past president and fellow of the International Society for the Study of Trauma and Dissociation.

Orit Badouk Epstein is a UKCP attachment-based psychoanalytic psychotherapist and supervisor based in London, UK. She is a teacher, a published writer, and the past editor of the journal, *Attachment New Directions in Psychotherapy and Relational Psychoanalysis*. Orit specialises in attachment theory, complex trauma and working with clients who have been diagnosed with DID. Her book *Shame Matters* (Routledge, 2022) won the Gradiva award 2022.

Jennifer J. Freyd, Ph.D., is Professor Emerit of Psychology at the University of Oregon and Founder and President of the Center for Institutional Courage. Freyd introduced the concepts of "institutional courage", "institutional betrayal", "DARVO", and "betrayal trauma".

Richard P. Kluft, M.D., Ph.D., is Clinical Professor of Psychiatry at the Lewis Katz School of Medicine at Temple University. He teaches at the Psychoanalytic Center of Philadelphia and the China America Psychoanalytic Alliance. A co-founder of the ISST&D, his interests include the treatment of trauma and the dissociative disorders, psychoanalysis, hypnosis, and their interface historical, conceptual, and clinical. He practices psychiatry, psychoanalysis, and medical hypnosis.

Richard J. Loewenstein, M.D., is Adjunct Professor of Psychiatry at the University of Maryland School of Medicine, Baltimore, MD. From 1987 to 2020, he was the founder and Medical Director of The Trauma Disorders Program, Sheppard Pratt, Baltimore, MD. He is Section Editor, Dissociative Disorders in the American Psychiatric Association (APA), DSM-5 Text Revision (DSM-5-TR). He is co-editor of the 4th Revision (in preparation) of the International Society for the Study of Trauma and Dissociation (ISSTD) Guidelines for Treatment of Dissociative Identity Disorder in Adults. He is a distinguished life fellow of the APA and has received the Lifetime Achievement Award of the ISSTD.

Henry Zvi Lothane, M.D., is Clinical Professor of Psychiatry at Icahn School of Medicine at Mount Sinai, New York City, USA, and in private practice, member of the American Psychoanalytic and the International Psychoanalytical Associations, historian of psychiatry and psychoanalysis and author of *In Defense of Schreber Soul Murder and Psychiatry* and *The Untold Story of Sabina Spielrein Healed and Haunted by Love, Unpublished Russian Diary and Letters*.

Jeffrey Masson was Professor of Sanskrit at the University of Toronto. He has published 31 books in various fields, ranging from Sanskrit poetics, to autobiography, to living in New Zealand, to psychoanalysis, to animal emotions. He is best known for three books: *The Assault on Truth; When Elephants Weep* and *Dogs Never Lie About Love* (which is actually true!); the last two books each sold over one million copies internationally. He lives with his wife, Leila, a paediatrician, in Sydney, Australia.

Kate McMaugh is a psychologist with a practice primarily focused on the assessment and treatment of complex trauma and dissociative disorders. She also provides training, case consultation and supervision to therapists working in this field. She has published articles on the history of the false memory movement, trauma and disability, DID, and childbirth trauma. Kate has recently completed research into incestuous abuse which has continued into adulthood.

Warwick Middleton, M.D., past-President and fellow, ISSTD, holds professorial appointments with the University of Queensland, and the University of Canterbury et al. Since 1996 he has directed the Trauma and Dissociation Unit, Belmont Hospital, Brisbane, and is the first researcher to publish a series outlining the abuse histories of Australian patients with dissociative identity disorder, as well as being the first researcher to systematically examine ongoing incestuous abuse during adulthood.

Arnold Wm. Rachman, Ph.D., F.A.G.P.A., is a psychoanalyst in private practice specializing in the treatment of sexual trauma. He is Training and Supervising Analyst, Postgraduate Institute for Psychoanalysis, NYC. He is considered a pioneer in the rediscovery, research, and publication of the work of Sándor Ferenczi and his famous analysand Elizabeth Severn. He is a Board Member, Sándor Ferenczi Center, New School University, NYC, and Honorary Member, Sándor Ferenczi Society, Budapest, Hungary.

John Read is Professor of Clinical psychology at the University of East and Chair of the International Institute for Psychiatric Drug withdrawal. His research includes the role of childhood adversities in causing psychosis, and whether mental health staff enquire about abuse and neglect. He is Editor of the scientific journal *Psychosis*. John's books include *Models of Madness* and *A Straight-Talking Introduction to the Causes of Mental Health Problems*.

Foreword

John Briere

Jeffrey Masson's publication of *'The Assault on Truth': Freud's Suppression of the Seduction Theory* in 1984 unleashed a virtual tsunami of reviews and reactions from psychoanalysts, therapists, book critics, the media, false memory proponents, feminist and anti-feminists, and readers from across the world. Some of these were very positive, but many were critical, sometimes involving ad hominem attacks on his personality, scholarliness, truthfulness, personal motives, and his temerity to question established psychoanalytic authority. Clearly, some nerves were hit, and intellectual fiefdoms threatened. Not many people in established fields cherish upstarts, especially if those upstarts might be right.

At the same time, the book was relatively adversarial in tone and highly critical of Freud and the analytic establishment, and Masson can be outspoken when so motivated. However, it may not matter whether or not Masson had an axe to grind when writing *The Assault on Truth*, nor does it really matter what other, often highly invested people – who also carried sharp implements – said about him or his book. Neutrality is unhelpful in the context of ongoing oppression and harm, and not everyone who takes a strong stand is acting inappropriately. More important is whether those who confront the status quo can back their statements with facts.

The central questions for *The Assault on Truth*, I believe, are as follows:

- *What was Masson's central message;*
- *How accurate was he when he challenged Western culture for its epidemic sexual abuse of children, and psychoanalysis for its paternalism and (literal) mistreatment of female sexual abuse survivors;*
- *Why were many of his critics' reactions so confrontational, if not hyperbolic; and*
- *What should we make of Masson's eventual total rejection of psychotherapy, introduced in "The Assault on Truth", and more fully developed in his later book, "Against Therapy"?*

Fortunately, Drs Middleton and Dorahy have assembled an excellent collection of chapters addressing these issues. No doubt in part reflecting the controversy triggered by Masson's writing, the chapter authors, themselves, disagree at times, leaving the reader to wend their own way through this fascinating volume. I have been asked to make a few comments and perhaps offer an analysis before the reader enters this story of social and personal injustice; an influential physician in the late

1800s who wrote about the reality and repercussions of childhood sexual abuse, and then changed his mind; an author who activated a maelstrom by challenging entrenched beliefs and authority; and the reactions of a culture and profession that, perhaps by virtue of their own complicity, responded with a firestorm.

I should mention here that I am an older White male academic. This is the condition of many people involved in the Masson dialogue, including (I assume) most, but not all, of the chapter authors and editors of this book. Yet, we have increasingly become aware of the small hegemony of mainstream academics, whose gender, race, and social position sometimes seem to entitle us to hold forth on issues beyond our actual qualifications (e.g., White men "explaining" women and people of colour). The issues Masson discusses in *The Assault on Truth* are deeply rooted in a social context in which European-stock men with outsized power and privilege were and are able to define reality across so many domains, including (strangely) the intricacies of female sexuality, the prevalence of crimes committed by others of their own social position and demographics, and the way in which treatment of those maltreated by others should be conducted. Given this embeddedness, issues of identity and power are very relevant to this discussion and must not be overlooked.

I am also not a psychoanalyst. In fact, like many other academic psychologists, I never really felt (until my own contemporary analytic therapy) that psychoanalysis had all that much to say about psychological suffering and evidence-based ways to approach it. This may bear emphasizing: Although much of Masson's first books and this volume focus on traditional psychoanalysis, most clinicians would not necessarily endorse Freudian psychology as the sine qua non or defining source of information on psychological difficulties and their treatment, especially vis-à-vis the notion of an Oedipal complex. As discussed later, this means that accurate criticisms of traditional psychoanalysis (the version mostly discussed in Masson's books and by his readers) may not bear tremendously on the validity and benefits of modern psychological treatment.

So, back to the questions.

What was the central message of *The Assault on Truth*?

Per Masson, Sigmund Freud discovered early in his career that the "hysterical" symptoms of his female patients were due to childhood sexual abuse and that, in fact, such victimization was common among the (primarily) female children of Viennese society. Freud later reversed his "seduction theory", deciding instead those who reported childhood sexual abuse were in the thralls of an Oedipal complex, wherein women supposedly confused their innate sexual desire for their fathers with pseudomemories of actual sexual abuse by them. In doing so, he was able to preemptively defang potential allegations of rampant child sexual assault by men and, instead, implicate supposedly fantasy-prone, inevitably Oedipally driven, girls and women in their own suffering.

Versions of Freud's seduction theory (sans the telling notion that sexual abuse was supposedly equivalent to "seduction") had been presented previously by writers like Florence Rush (1980) and Judith Herman (1981). However, Masson cited as further evidence materials he encountered as director of the Sigmund Freud Archives, including his correspondence with Wilhelm Fliess, Freud's friend, and close collaborator. Based on these papers, Masson asserted that Freud's turnabout from his initial abuse hypothesis was in part due to negative reactions to *The Aetiology of Hysteria* (Freud, 1896) by his peers, including Richard von Krafft-Ebing, who derided his theory as a "scientific fairytale" (Freud, 1954). Under pressure from his psychiatrist colleagues and influenced by the patriarchal environment that pervaded Vienna in the late 1800s and early 1900s, Freud subsequently concluded that it was unlikely that so many children could have been sexually abused by parental figures.[1] In contrast, the notion that women's sexual abuse disclosures were fantasy-based was considerably more palatable.

How accurate was Freud's seduction theory?

Despite Freud's recantation, later research, especially over the last several decades, has demonstrated the wide prevalence of childhood sexual abuse in North America. Researchers like Finkelhor (1994) and others report that at least 20% of women in the general population, and about half as many men, when asked, described childhood sexual victimization, including within their families. Although Freud was first reluctant to identify fathers as perpetrators of such abuse, we now know that this form of incest is common and often very harmful (Courtois, 2010).

Modern research also finds that those who have been sexual abused often report resultant psychological difficulties, even many years later. These impacts involve not only symptoms that were thought to represent hysteria in Freud's time (e.g., dissociation, somatization, and emotional dysregulation), but also, anxiety, depression, posttraumatic stress, substance abuse, relationship problems, suicidality, and sexual disturbance (e.g., Briere, 1996; Hailes et al., 2019; Paolucci et al., 2001).

Although we now know that sexual abuse is only one etiologic pathway to psychological dysfunction, overall Freud appears to have been right vis-à-vis his abuse hypothesis. He was also correct, in broad strokes, about the way that such impacts can be remediated, i.e., by revisiting memories of childhood trauma in the safety of a supportive therapeutic relationship. In fact, it is not much of a stretch to suggest that Freud, during his seduction theory phase, was a major contributor to modern trauma psychology, albeit from the perspective of early 1900's psychology. Of course, he changed his mind, to the detriment of generations of sexual abuse survivors. Ultimately, this redirection was a function of his and society's psychosocial difficulties, not those of his patients. This was a tragedy of significant proportion. Had Freud been raised in a less paternalistic and antifemale society, had psychiatrists in his day been less invested in male privilege, he might not have repudiated his abuse theory and psychoanalysis might not have developed a systematic delusion that persisted for over a century and significantly harmed untold women and children.

Why were many of the reactions to *The Assault on Truth* so hyperbolic?

Given the culture and time in which Freud's abuse theory was developed, it was nearly preordained that he would face massive resistance. In the early 1900s women were devalued, and their life options and entitlements were harshly constrained. With some exceptions, they were viewed as the weaker sex, intellectually inferior, and best suited to their roles as mothers and wives. Although this situation has improved in significant ways, women still suffer gender-based discrimination, frequent sexual and domestic trauma, fewer opportunities for career advancement and political leadership, and adverse gender socialization, all of which have been linked to higher rates of various psychiatric disorders and difficulties (Briere et al., 2024; Rees et al., 2011; Silove et al., 2017).

In this context, those in power in Freud's era had something to lose if women's "hysteria" and social status were linked to sexual and social maltreatment by men, as opposed to women's own supposed failings. This is especially the case if, as described in this book, some of Freud's critical colleagues were sexual abusers themselves. Freud's coerced renunciation directly turned the tables on reality, much as did the False Memory movement more recently (see Crook, Chapter 7): women who disclosed sexual abuse were now lying and men alleged to have been sexually abusive were falsely accused. To borrow an analytic term, Freud and his analytic peers seemingly were involved in a version of reaction formation: they were not maltreating or devaluing female patients – they were caring treaters of disturbed women caught in the thralls of the Oedipal complex.

Unfortunately, although things have changed, they have not changed enough. Especially at the time of *The Assault on Truth's* publication, but to this day, women experience significant sexism and social marginalization, sometimes including how they are viewed and treated in therapy. The same forces at work in Freud's time were prevalent when Masson published his book, no doubt fuelling much of the same antipathy. Freud in his early years, and Masson many years later, both faced versions of the same enemy; a culture and profession that devalued — and continues to devalue — women and those who support them.

What should we make of Masson's total rejection of psychotherapy?

In *The Assault on Truth*, Masson first argued that psychoanalysis was unlikely to be helpful in treating childhood trauma. Later, he wrote *Against Therapy: Emotional Tyranny and the Myth of Psychological Healing* (Masson, 1988), which extended this conclusion to all of psychotherapy. Reactions to *Against Therapy* were seemingly even more negative than to *The Assault on Truth*, perhaps because even many of those who agreed with his criticisms of psychoanalysis were not comfortable with a wholesale dismissal of all forms of psychotherapy. Among Masson's assertions in *Against Therapy*, implied in *The Assault on Truth*, was that "abuse of one form or another is built into the very fabric of psychotherapy" (Masson, 1988, p. 210).

Those who are committed to therapy as a way to aid human suffering, sensitive to social maltreatment, and familiar with the trauma treatment outcome literature tend to view Masson's generalizations as a bridge too far, one that potentially decreases the power of his work in *The Assault on Truth*. Among other concerns, Masson seemed to overlook the work of feminist psychotherapists like Judith Herman (1992), Christine Courtois (2010), Laura Brown (2008), and others, who are well aware of the patriarchy and the ongoing maltreatment of women, but who nevertheless assert that carefully applied trauma-focused therapy can be a liberating and healing force.

Masson's anti-therapy position notwithstanding, *The Assault on Truth* actually supports a growing movement to provide anti-sexist/-racist/-homophobic psychotherapy to socially maltreated people (e.g., Brown, 2008; Bryant-Davis, 2019; Comas-Diaz, 2012). As Herman (1992) and others have noted, psychological treatment of trauma survivors, nearly by definition, should include a social justice perspective, not only because such victimization is embedded in a prejudicial social context, but also because social maltreatment, itself, often leads to psychological distress and disorder. Apropos of this, many of those who suffer psychological symptoms are of colour, lesbian, gay, bisexual, transgender, queer, or some other sexual and/or gender identity (LGBTQ+), and often experience economic insecurity. Yet, when treated with traditional psychoanalysis, they undergo a methodology developed in the early 1900s on White, European, seemingly cis-gendered and heterosexual (although, some, no doubt, were secretly nonheteronormative in their orientation or identity) people. As reflected in relatively recent attempts to modify contemporary psychoanalysis to include increased diversity (Foster, 2003; Tummala-Narra, 2013), Masson's concerns regarding social inequity are highly relevant to any modern psychotherapeutic approach to the extent that they honour and validate those who are not necessarily similar to Freud's caseload.

Conclusions

The Assault on Truth was a cogent and important challenge to the traditional psychoanalytic model of infantile sexuality and Oedipal dynamics, irrespective of whether Masson's studies turned him against other, more socially informed, and evidence-based psychotherapies. For that, Jeffrey Masson deserves a book such as this, honouring him as a major, corrective voice in the history of psychoanalysis. The largely negative responses to *The Assault on Truth* can be seen as an indirect validation of his work rather than a cogent criticism of his thesis. Just as Freud likely would have experienced earlier celebrity had he begun his career championing the so-called Oedipal complex, Masson would have had an easier time of it had he overlooked what was ultimately a form of psychotherapeutic malpractice.

Note

1 Although perhaps farfetched, it is possible that Freud made a "Freudian slip" and acknowledged this pressure when he stated in his *New Introductory Lectures on Psychoanalysis* (Freud, 1933) that "*I was driven* [italicization mine] to recognize in the end that these reports were untrue" (p. 120).

References

Briere, J. (1996). *Therapy for adults molested as children* (2nd ed.). Springer.

Briere, J., Runtz, M., & Rodd, K. (2024). Social maltreatment as trauma: Posttraumatic correlates of a new measure of exposure to sexism, racism, and cisheterosexism. *Psychological Trauma: Theory, Research, Practice and Policy*. Advance online publication. https://doi.org/10.1037/tra0001636.

Brown, L. S. (2008). *Cultural competence in trauma therapy: Beyond the flashback*. American Psychological Association.

Bryant-Davis, T. (2019). The cultural context of trauma recovery: Considering the post-traumatic stress disorder practice guideline and intersectionality. *Psychotherapy, 56*(3), 400–408. https://doi.org/10.1037/pst0000241

Comas-Diaz, L. (2012). *Multicultural care: A clinician's guide to cultural competence*. American Psychological Association.

Courtois, C. A. (2010). *Healing the incest wound: Adult survivors in therapy* (2nd ed.). W. W.Norton & Company.

Finkelhor, D. (1994). Current information on the scope and nature of child sexual abuse. *The Future of Children, 4*(2), 31–53.

Foster, R. P. (2003). Considering a multicultural perspective for psychoanalysis. In A. Roland, B. Ulanov, & C. Barbre (Eds.), *Creative dissent: Psychoanalysis in evolution* (pp. 173–185). Praeger Publishers/Greenwood Publishing Group.

Freud, S. (1896). The aetiology of hysteria. *The standard edition of the complete psychological works of Sigmund Freud, III*, 189–221.

Freud, S. (1933). *New introductory lectures on psychoanalysis*. Norton.

Freud, S. (1954). *The origins of psychoanalysis: Sigmund Freud's letters*. Basic Books.

Hailes, H. P., Yu, R., Danese, A., & Fazel, S. (2019). Long-term outcomes of childhood sexual abuse: An umbrella review. *The Lancet. Psychiatry, 6*(10), 830–839. https://doi.org/10.1016/S2215-0366(19)30286-X

Herman, J. L. (1981). *Father-daughter incest*. Harvard University Press.

Herman, J. L. (1992). *Trauma and recovery: The aftermath of violence—From domestic abuse to political terror*. Basic Books.

Masson, J. M. (1984). *The assault on truth: Freud's suppression of the seduction theory*. Farrar, Strauss & Giroux.

Masson, J. M. (1988). *Against therapy: Emotional tyranny and the myth of psychological healing*. Atheneum Publishers.

Paolucci, E. O., Genuis, M. L., & Violato, C. (2001). A meta-analysis of the published research on the effects of child sexual abuse. *The Journal of Psychology, 135*(1), 17–36. https://doi.org/10.1080/00223980109603677

Rees, S., Silove, D., Chey, T., Ivancic, L., Steel, Z., Creamer, M., Teesson, M., Bryant, R., McFarlane, A. C., Mills, K. L., Slade, T., Carragher, N., O'Donnell, M., & Forbes, D. (2011). Lifetime prevalence of gender-based violence in women and the relationship with mental disorders and psychosocial function. *JAMA, 306*(5), 513–521. https://doi.org/10.1001/jama.2011.1098

Rush, F. (1980). *The best kept secret: Sexual abuse of children*. Prentice Hall.

Silove, D., Baker, J. R., Mohsin, M., Teesson, M., Creamer, M., O'Donnell, M., Forbes, D., Carragher, N., Slade, T., Mills, K., Bryant, R., McFarlane, A., Steel, Z., Felmingham, K., & Rees, S. (2017). The contribution of gender-based violence and network trauma to gender differences in Post-Traumatic Stress Disorder. *PLoS ONE, 12*(2), e0171879. https://doi.org/10.1371/journal.pone.0171879

Tummala-Narra, P. (2013). Psychoanalytic applications in a diverse society. *Psychoanalytic Psychology, 30*(3), 471–487. https://doi.org/10.1037/a0031375

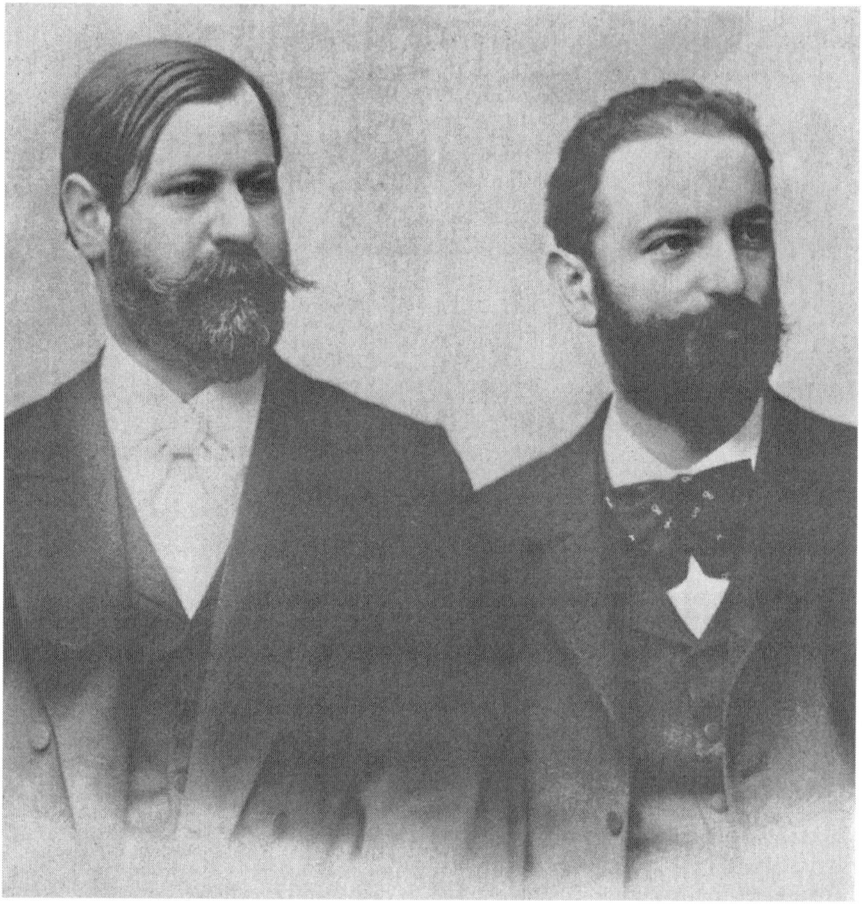

Sigmund Freud & Wilhelm Fliess, 1890.

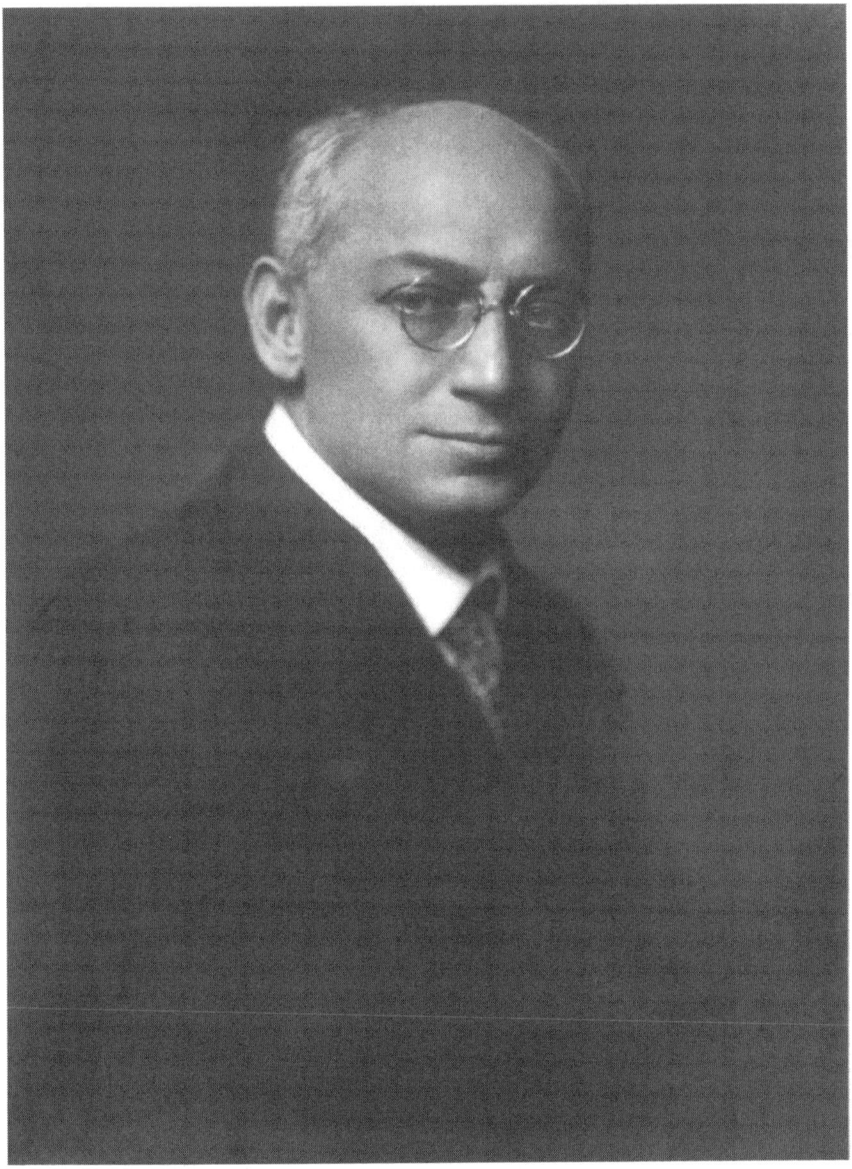

Sandor Ferenczi

Source: Copyright is held by Judith Dupont of the International Sandor Ferenczi network.

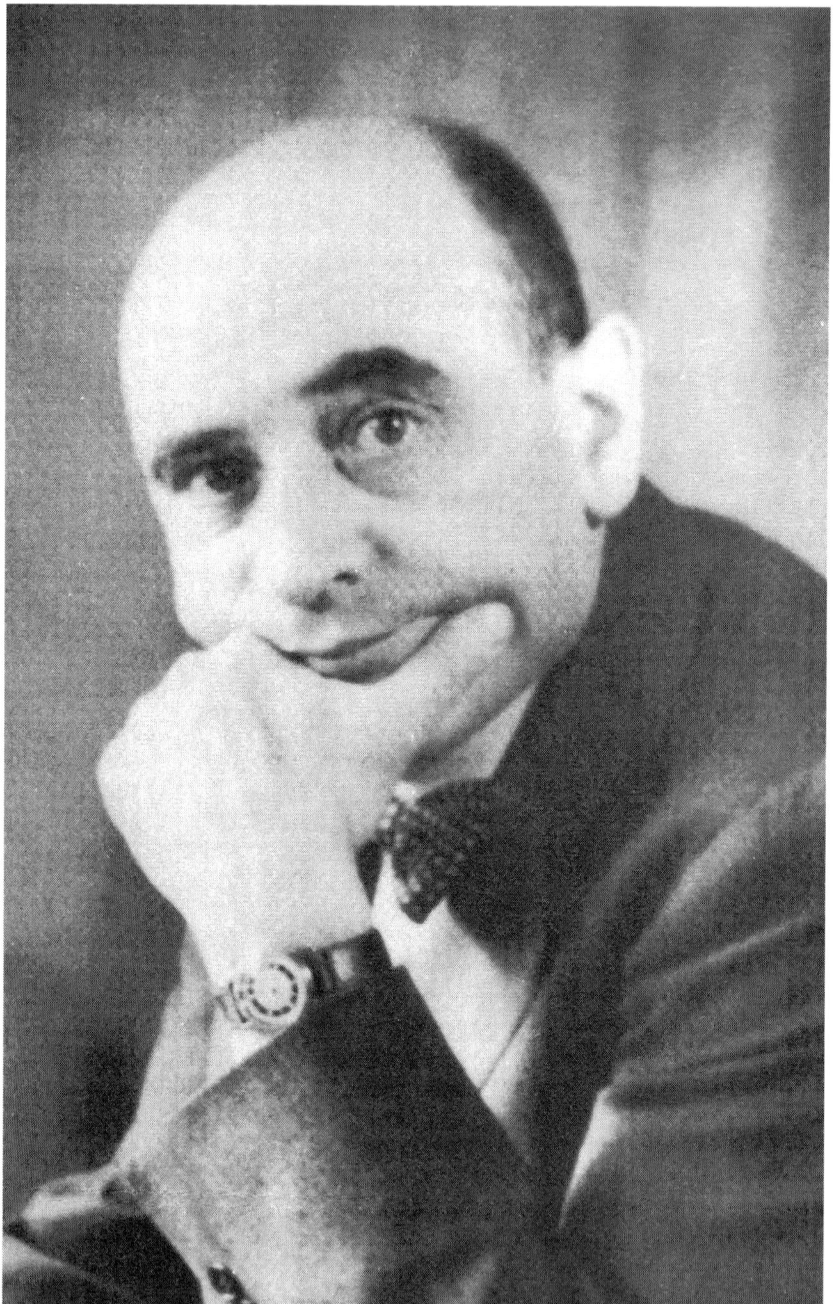

Robert Fliess – circa late 60's.

Source: The image was originally published in 1973. Fliess R. Symbol, Dream, and Psychosis with Notes on Technique – Psychoanalytic Series, Vol 3. New York: International Universities Press, 1973.

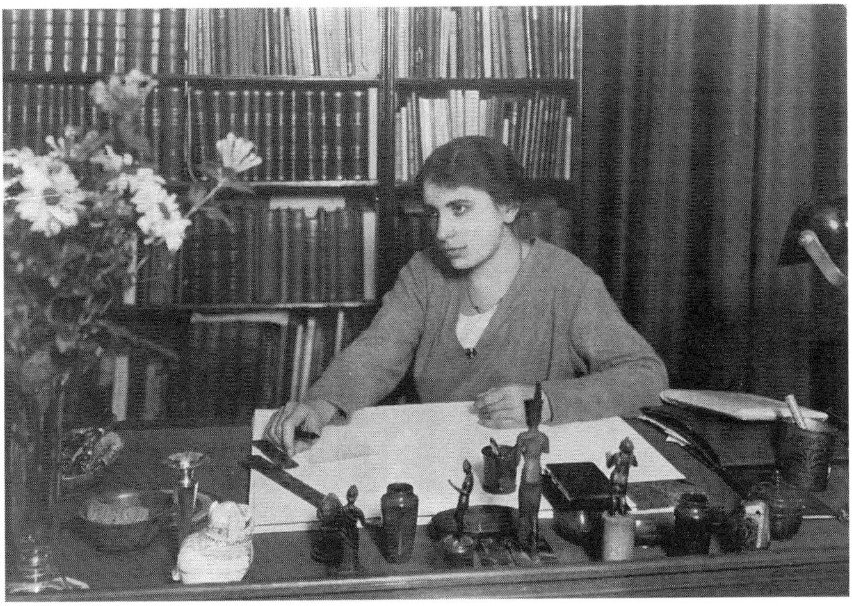

Anna Freud, seated in her study, 1920.

Source: Alamy. License C13JKW Anna Freud, 15-02-24.

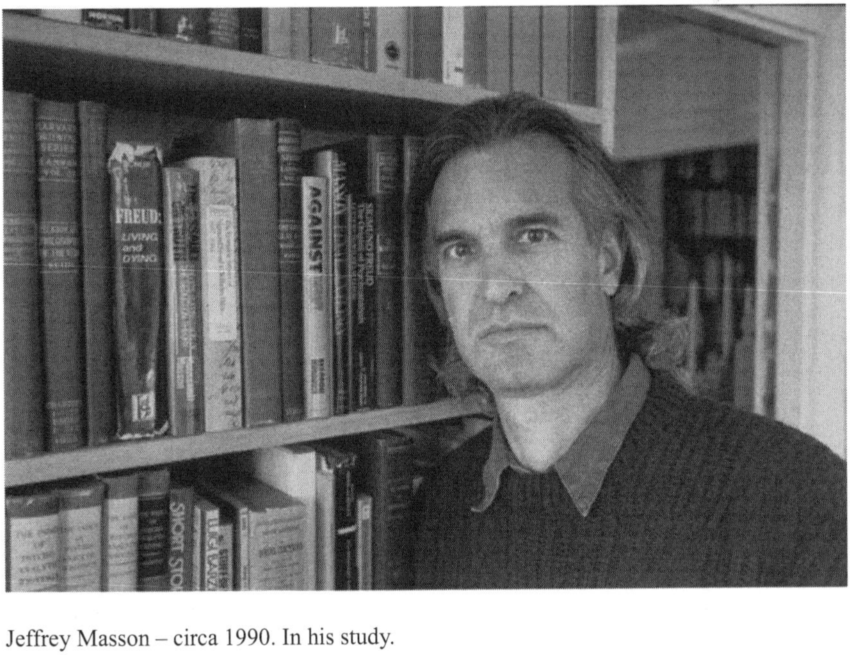

Jeffrey Masson – circa 1990. In his study.

Source: Permission to reproduce image given by the photographer, Daidie Donnelley.

Introduction

> "If liberty means anything at all it means the right to tell people what they do not want to hear."
>
> George Orwell (Unused Preface for *Animal Farm*, rediscovered in 1971)

In this volume we are discussing a book that has as its title, *The Assault on Truth*, that Jeffrey Masson unveiled to the world in 1984 and which concerned itself with the circumstances in which Freud largely abandoned his child sexual abuse theory regarding the aetiology of hysteria. On the part of victims of such abuse, having their accounts respected and validated is enormously important. While there has been controversy about how Masson framed his comments about Freud's "suppression" of his "seduction theory", the editors of this volume believe that back in 1984, no matter how gently or diplomatically the core messages of *The Assault on Truth* were communicated, or who authored them, that person was going to have a very challenging time of it. As the issue of truth, and Freud's handling of it, were central to Masson's discussion of what happened to the "seduction theory" in Freud's hands, it is helpful for us to preface the content of this volume with the inclusion of some discussion of other instances, in which Freud's truthfulness was held in question. We are aware that there are significant polarizations regarding Freud. There are some who write of him in idealized ways, and there are others who fall into the camp of what has been colloquially labelled, "Freud bashers". We believe that it is possible to take much of value from his enormous body of work, without unobjectively idealizing Freud the man and at the same time avoiding "throwing the baby out with the bathwater".

In 1920 Sigmund Freud, in a footnote to his *Three Essays on the Theory of Sexuality* (1905) made a global assertion: "With the progress of psychoanalytic studies, the importance of the Oedipus complex has become more and more clearly evident; its recognition has become the shibboleth that distinguishes the adherents of psycho-analysis from its opponents" (p. 226). When Eduardo Weiss (1889–1970) was asked what one could not doubt, and still stay on as an analyst, he "listed four central concepts of Freud's that were beyond discussion: dreams as wish-fulfillment, the instinct theory, the Oedipus complex, and the castration complex" (Roazen, 2005, p. 59).

DOI: 10.4324/9781003431466-1

In an undated interview conducted by Brad Murray and published by the International Psychoanalytic Association (IPA) in recent years, Charles Hanly, who served two terms as IPA President (2009–2013), describes forming two research groups "to do conceptual and logical research on alternative psychoanalytic theories of aggression and the Oedipus complex". As a postscript to the interview Hanly provides five references for "Further reading". Curiously, the fifth reference was "(with J. Masson) 'A Critical Examination of the New Narcissism', International Journal of Psycho-Analysis (1976)". Over 40 years ago Hanly and Masson were the closest of friends, but Hanly was one of the many analysts who piled on, in the aftermath of the publication of *The Assault on Truth: Freud's Suppression of the Seduction Theory*, to publish a scathing review of Masson's book. Hanly, as did many other analysts, severed his friendship with Masson (stating that their friendship had been based on a mutual respect of Freud) and in the International Journal of Psychoanalysis opined,

> J. M. Masson's *The Assault on Truth*, despite the sound and fury with which it appeared, has come to signify, if not nothing, then very little indeed in the estimation of its reviewers in the major English literary magazines. This review can do little to alter that critical judgment but must agree with it.
>
> (Hanly, 1986, p. 517)

In keeping with other analysts at the time, Hanly insisted that it was Masson who suppressed Freud's seduction theory. "It is Masson who, through a biased selection of textural references … suppresses for his readers the fact of Freud's continued recognition of the sexual seduction of children" (Hanly, 1986, p. 517). Yet decades later, at the age of about 90, Hanly seemingly had a need to spontaneously publicize his past collaboration with his erstwhile colleague, hinting in his advanced years, of an ambivalence about the severing of their long-distant friendship.

As with Hanly's, most published reviews of Masson's book were particularly uncomplimentary. Anthony Storr writing in *The New York Times* (1984), dismissed the book, stating, "All that it and its author deserve is oblivion". Kurt Eissler, characterized Masson's findings as "plain nonsense" and refused subsequent comment, stating, "Please do not bother me with this. It has given me so much trouble already" (Remnick, 1984). Peter Gay observed,

> Apart from publishing some hitherto unavailable pages to which he had privileged access, Masson adds nothing to our understanding of Freud and only muddies the waters with his indignant denunciation. One need not be an adorer to see *The Assault on Truth* as a grave slander on Freud's character and a severe distortion of the history of psychoanalysis.
>
> (as quoted by Remnick, 1984)

There were in fact some 40 previously unpublished passages from Freud's letters in Masson's book. At times Masson responded to the criticisms. For example, in respect to Charles Rycroft he unequivocally stated, "My point, throughout the book, was that Freud declined to give theoretical significance to sexual abuse and no longer discussed its importance in the genesis of neurosis in any of his later works". Masson (1984b) combatively concluded, "Dr. Rycroft offers no new research and cites no new literature to contradict my conclusions. In short, he attempts to refute scholarship with unenlightened indignation". Henry Lothane, a direct contemporary of Masson and a contributor to this volume, argued in 2018 that

> Freud's alleged repudiation of seduction was based solely on a letter Freud sent to Fliess in 1897: 'I no longer believe in my *neurotica*' (Masson 1985, p. 264), even though in subsequent letters and in print Freud vacillated between despair and determination.
>
> (Lothane, 2018, p. 958)

Bennett Simon, another psychoanalyst, affronted by Masson's thesis that Freud had made a major error in his abandonment of the seduction hypothesis set out to prepare a scholarly rebuttal. However, reluctantly, but honestly, Simon was led to conclude that psychoanalysis was indeed in error. In a paper, provocatively titled, "Incest – see under Oedipus Complex: The History of an Error in Psychoanalysis", he noted that the concept of the Oedipus Complex was used to virtually eclipse the reality that parents can frequently enact their sexual and aggressive impulses on their children. If Oedipal fantasy really was the shibboleth or the central underpinning of psychoanalytic theory and practice and if it was integral to the manifestations of neurotic illness seen in those treated by psychoanalysis, then Freud's writings should have revealed how during a successful psychoanalysis such a fantasy was able to be dealt with and with insights imparted and integrated no longer remained evident. The difficulty for Bennett Simon was that he could not find such an example.

> Neither Freud, nor, to my knowledge, any other analyst, publishes a case wherein a woman, not psychotic, told of an incestuous relationship with the father and then in the course of the treatment it turned out to be a fantasy!
>
> (Simon, 1992, pp. 968–969)

In 2004 noted Freud critic, Frederick Crews, was to nominate Masson's "melodramatic book *The Assault on Truth* (1984a), as "misrepresenting Freud's 'seduction' patients as self-aware incest victims rather than as the doubters that they remained". Thus, Masson was attacked from all angles by those sympathetic and unsympathetic to Freud's theorising.

Yet coming from the emerging modern trauma field, the first author of "Father – Daughter Incest" (Herman & Hirschman, 1981), Judith Herman, reported that Masson's book was well-documented, well-written, carefully reasoned, and fascinating. Noting that reviews of Masson's book were almost uniformly negative, she accused such critics of ad hominem attacks, or of criticizing Masson by focussing on issues of secondary importance. A typical example of such an ad hominem attack was that by psychiatrist Robert Coles, who offered his personalized assessment of Masson in The Boston Globe, and is quoted by Lothane (2001, p. 673): "[Masson is] a grandiose egotist—mean-spirited, self-serving, full of braggadocio, impossibly arrogant and, in the end, a self-destructive fool ... his own words reveal this psychological profile".

David Remnick's article of 19 February 1984 noted that Herman's review of Masson's book was "unique because it was favourable". "You would wish the idea that analysts pay no attention to real seductions in childhood was a caricature, but it really isn't", Herman is quoted as saying.

> The total emphasis on fantasy and such is a blind spot in the profession. There are just too many cases of women who are accused of provoking or imagining abuse rather than having the abuse itself dealt with. This is a major mental health problem for women, especially since we now know how many women have suffered abuse in childhood.
>
> (Remnick, 1984)

Masson (1992) makes the point that to the best of his knowledge there was "not a single published account of the devastating effects of incest or childhood sexual abuse before Freud's time" (p. 176), nor was there any social movement promoting acknowledgement of the issue.

Richard Webster was to reflect in 2005 that *The Assault on Truth* provoked controversy and aroused massive publicity. One is reminded of Bismarck's observation: "Never believe anything in politics until it is officially denied" (Goodreads, 2024)

Jeffrey Masson's early life is a colourful and intriguing story. He was brought up in a household that had its own live-in charlatan eastern mystic guru. He became a tenured Sanskrit scholar and then at age 29 began training in psychoanalysis, becoming in the process a close friend of the much older Kurt Eissler, the then doyen of American psychoanalysis who was a close associate of Freud's daughter, Anna. But it was about to get a whole lot more interesting.

As a young analysand Masson struggled with the advice from his analytic teachers who attributed virtually all accounts from patients about childhood sexual abuse to the realm of Oedipal fantasy. Masson, an intelligent, charismatic, and articulate free thinker, struggled with the question of why so many such patients would have a motive for speaking such mistruths and how could one be certain their accounts were factually false? Despite such questioning, he so impressed Eissler that in April 1980 he was appointed Projects Director of the Sigmund Freud Archives, giving him access to Freud's unpublished papers and allowing him to form a friendship with Anna Freud and to work on an authorized edition of the correspondence between Freud and his close friend Wilhelm Fliess (exposed after his death by his analyst son Robert as an abusive man suffering with "ambulatory psychosis", or what others might call "malignant narcissism").

Masson was puzzled as to how Freud's paper on "The Aetiology of Hysteria" based around 18 patients (12 female and 6 male) could have garnered such a frosty response. It was delivered to his neurology and psychiatric colleagues on 21 April

1896 and, in Freud's words, "[received] an icy reception by the asses" (Masson, 1984a, p. 184). One "ass" was Richard von Krafft-Ebing, who called it "a scientific fairy tale". The paper documented sexual abuse in the patients' histories and colleagues considered it an "error" to think such experiences were associated with hysteria. Yet, Freud shifted emphasis from sexual abuse to childhood sexual phantasy when he later proposed his Oedipal theory. Having access to Freud's library and as a result previously unpublished writings by Freud, Masson discovered that much had been edited out of the original edition of the Freud-Fliess correspondence (published in 1954 as *The Origins of Psychoanalysis*). The absent material, along with his research on Emma Eckstein, who almost died in 1895, and Freud's visit to the Paris morgue, lead Masson to draw the conclusion that actual childhood sexual trauma was far more significant than the revisionist Freud allowed for.

At a 1981 meeting of the Western New England Psychoanalytic Society, Masson's evolving thesis regarding Freud's suppression of his own theory attracted controversy. The *New York Times* published two articles on Masson's views as well as an interview with him. Masson (1992) has described how Eissler's rage knew no bounds, with Eissler telling him, "Just today Masud Khan called me from London and asked me to dismiss you from the Archives. The board members, all of them, or at least most of them, are asking for the same" (p. 194). This was the same Masud Khan who had boasted quite openly to Masson and others of sleeping with a patient. Masson provides the example of Khan, who "was seeing both [a woman] and her husband, and was now living with the woman, but continu[ing] to see her husband in analysis" (Masson, 1992, p. 194). Eisler, who felt betrayed by Masson, while famously agreeing that psychoanalysis was "sterile", fired Masson from the Freud Archives. Masson settled out of court for $150,000, with Masson returning numerous documents to the Archives. Janet Malcolm, a high-profile journalist, interviewed Masson at length for a two-part New Yorker article on the controversy, an article which she expanded into a book, *In the Freud Archives*. Masson filed a $13 million lawsuit for libel and the matter became a decade-long legal saga.

Psychoanalysis tried to maintain that what Masson believed was largely a fiction – that Freud had maintained a real interest in actual child sexual abuse and that actual abuse had remained a significant focus of psychoanalysis. In his 1989 book the psychoanalyst Shengold cites Ferenczi (1932) and Robert Fliess (1956, 1962, 1973) as the "most notable" of "many analysts" who had written about "the not infrequent occurrence of actual incest involving preadolescent children" (p. 160). He cites six other publications by presumably less notable analytic writers, interestingly including Masson and Masson (1978). Using Ferenczi, Robert Fliess, and Masson to bolster the case of psychoanalysis' interest in the reality of childhood sexual abuse is a tad disingenuous given the responses that Ferenczi, Fliess, and Masson endured at the hands of their psychoanalytic contemporaries for sharing their theories on the centrality of such abuse on psychological life. Thus, the most prominent papers or books cited by Shengold as evidence of psychoanalysis' interest in actual childhood sexual abuse were authored by individuals demonstrably critical of psychoanalysis' denial, neglect, or avoidance of the topic. Representative of the tenacious grip Oedipal fantasy had on psychoanalytic thinking, noted analyst and historian, Peter Gay (1989), selected 51 key Freud papers. This list included "The Aetiology of Hysteria", but not without warning one should be aware that Freud had made a "major error".

Like Ferenczi and Robert Fliess, John Bowlby was critical of psychoanalysis' concentration "on fantasy and the reluctance to examine the impact of real-life events" (1988, p. 87). Bowlby also didn't mince his words:

> Ever since Freud made his famous, and in my view disastrous, volte-face in 1897, when he decided that the childhood seductions he had believed to be etiologically important were nothing more than the products of his patients' imagination, it has been extremely unfashionable to attribute psychopathology to real-life experiences.

Despite his prodigious gifts as a theoretician and writer, one cannot ignore the reality that on many occasions Freud demonstrated less than enlightened judgement. Examples include having a very close relationship with the fairly disturbed and abusive, Wilhelm Fliess, how he was endlessly involved in what today would be seen as messy boundary transgressions (including psychoanalysing his own daughter) (Gabbard & Lester, 1996), and how his official biographer, Ernest Jones, was seemingly always a difficult man interpersonally and was credibly accused of the sexual abuse of children (Maddox, 2006; Rachman, 2022).

In 1984/2003, Masson observed that analysts were claiming, in respect to actual sexual abuse,

> [t]hat it is now and has always been a major concern within psychoanalysis. But if we look at the journals, we do not find this to be so. The cumulative index of the authoritative *Journal of the American Psychoanalytic Association*, more than 600 pages, contains the contents of the journal from its inception in 1953 through 1974 – thus the heyday of psychoanalysis and its influence – and has five columns devoted to the words Oedipus Complex. By contrast, the word abuse is not found in the index. Nor is there a single entry under sexual abuse.
>
> (p. 341)

Masson published *The Complete Letters of Sigmund Freud and Wilhelm Fliess (1887–1904)* in 1985, *A Dark Science: Women, Sexuality, and Psychiatry in the Nineteenth Century* in 1988, *Final Analysis* in 1991, *Against Therapy* in 1992, *Lost Prince: The Unsolved Mystery of Kaspar Hauser* in 1996 and *My Father's Guru* in 1998. From the mid-1990s Masson branched into writing an ongoing series of books about the emotional life of animals, including best-sellers, *When Elephants Weep* (with Susan McCarthy) and *Dogs Never Lie About Love*.

In his characteristic irrepressible style embodying self-deprecating humour, Masson explained his transition to writing about the emotional lives of animals:

> I'd written a whole series of books about psychiatry, and nobody bought them. Nobody liked them. Nobody. Psychiatrists hated them, and they were much too abstruse for the general public. It was very hard to make a living, and I thought, *as long as I'm not making a living, I may as well write about something I really love – animals.*
>
> (Welch, 2002, italics added)

But much has happened in the four decades since Masson published perhaps the most controversial book in the field of psychoanalysis in the last century. Some salient examples include the following:

- In 1988, Christine Courtois published *Healing the Incest Wound*, a detailed overview of incest (that in 2011 was to be supplanted by an encyclopaedic second edition).
- In 1989 the United Nations drafted its Convention on the Rights of the Child, the same year in which the first comprehensive texts on the diagnosis and treatment of Multiple Personality Disorder were published (Putnam, 1989; Ross, 1989).
- In 1991 the *International Journal of Psychoanalysis* published a paper by Eyre titled, "Therapy with a sexually abused woman", 95 years after Freud presented to his colleagues, "The Aetiology of Hysteria".
- In 1992 Judith Herman published the best-seller, *Trauma and Recovery* and John Briere published the highly cited, *Child Abuse Trauma: Theory and Treatment of the Lasting Effects*.
- In 1996, 300,000 Belgian citizens marched in protest at perceived cover-ups by police and compromised politicians concerning the serial killer and paedophile, Marc Dutroux, and his accomplices.
- In 2002, world-wide attention was focussed on the Boston Archdiocese and the sexual abuse of children by more than 10% of its priests.
- In 2011 – "Operation Rescue" was revealed in respect to an international police operation which destroyed the then largest online paedophile network in world history, and which had more than 70,000 members. In the following year, there was exposure of the child sex abuses perpetrated by prominent TV personality, charity supporter, and friend of (then) Prince Charles, Jimmy Savile, involving 450+ victims over a period of more than 50 years.
- In 2013 there was published the first systematic research identifying the widespread and endemic nature of ongoing incestuous abuse during adulthood (Middleton, 2013a, 2013b).
- In 2014 the Jay report concluded that an estimated 1,400 children, most of them White girls, had been sexually abused in Rotherham, UK, between 1997 and 2013 by predominantly British-Pakistani men.
- When it was shut down in February 2015 by the FBI, the darknet site, "Playpen" had over 215,000 users and hosted 23,000 sexually explicit images and videos of children as young as toddlers.
- In 2016, seven years after his death, three women made public allegations of child sexual abuse and rape by Sir Clement Freud, British politician, BBC radio

identity, and Sigmund Freud's grandson. Clement Freud's widow, Lady Jill Freud, apologized to his victims.

- The #MeToo spread virally in October 2017 as a hashtag used on social media to help demonstrate the widespread prevalence of sexual assault and harassment, especially in the workplace.
- November 2017 saw the successful conclusion of the Australian Royal Commission into Institutional Responses to Child Sexual Abuse (the most effective such national enquiry in human history). One victim of clergy sexual abuse who gave open evidence to the Australian Commission was Philip Nagle, who from the witness box held aloft his black and white grade-four St Alipius Primary School photo from 1974. Sexually abused by Christian Brother Stephen Farrell, Nagel as a child had found himself on the precipice of a cliff seriously contemplating suicide. Nagel testified that a third of the boys in his class picture were dead, believed by suicide. Metres away from St Alipius school was the St Alipius Presbytery in which resided Fr Gerald Ridsdale (the school's chaplain) and, for a time, Fr George Pell (who went on to become a Cardinal, and at one point his role at the Vatican had him third in line to the Pope), and who became the first Catholic cardinal to be the convicted and jailed for the sexual abuse of children (with the conviction belatedly quashed on appeal to the high court). Earlier police reporting by Detective Sergeant Kevin Carson in 2011 and 2012 detailed the suicides of at least 40 people sexually abused by Catholic clergy in Victoria. The report linked the 40 suicides to the sexual abuse perpetrated by a small number of paedophile clergy, including Gerald Ridsdale, Robert Best, Bryan Coffey, Paul Ryan, and Edward Dowlan. Br Gerald Fitzgerald of St Alipius died in 1987 while being investigated but was never charged. The Australian Royal Commission found that 22% of Christian Brothers since 1950 were alleged to be sexual predators (King, 2017). Among those named suicide victims were brothers Noel and Damien Walsh, and their cousin Martin Walsh. Another brother, Rob Walsh, who was also sexually abused by Ridsdale and Best, testified against them in court (McKenzie et al., 2012). It would not be hard to form the conclusion that some serial sexual abusers of children are responsible for causing more death and psychological destruction than the average serial killer!
- In 2018 more than 150 women, including Olympic gymnasts Aly Raisman and Jordyn Wieber, spoke during the sentencing hearing for Lawrence G. Nassar.
- In June 2019, writer E. Jean Carroll alleged via *New York Magazine* that President Donald Trump raped her in a department store dressing room in 1995 or 1996. In Carroll's defamation case against Trump (based on his alleged lies about her), the jury unanimously found in May 2023 that Trump had indeed sexually abused her and awarded her $5 million in damages.
- On 8 July 2019, there was the arrest in New York of billionaire Jeffrey Epstein (past friend of Donald Trump, Bill Clinton, Prince Andrew, Alan Dershowitz amongst others) for sex trafficking of minors, while 18 days later Dean Graeme Lawrence of Newcastle's Anglican cathedral became the second most senior churchman in Australia to be found guilty of child sexual abuse. Two weeks

later, on 10 August 2019, Epstein, the USA's most high-profile prisoner, died by (disputed) suicide in a Manhattan Metropolitan Correctional Centre.

- On 31 December 2019 the False Memory Syndrome Foundation (which had been founded in 1992 and who ardently attacked many therapists engaged in treating victims of childhood sexual abuse) formally dissolved (McMaugh & Middleton, 2022).
- In November 2021 the trial of Jeffrey Epstein's accomplice, Ghislaine Maxwell, began in New York. She was sentenced to 20 years in prison, but no other US citizens involved in Epstein's large-scale teenage sex trafficking operation spanning around 25 years have ever been charged.
- In March 2023 the Boy Scouts' record $2.46 billion sex abuse settlement was upheld by Judge Richard Andrews, to resolve claims by more than 80,000 men who stated that as children they were abused by troop leaders (Knauth, 2023).

While the emergent trauma field became embroiled in the late 1980s and 1990s in controversies about "false memories", alleged "Satanic Ritual Abuse", and the status of dissociative disorders, it became evident, via a series of scandals and inquiries, along with psychological research and investigative journalism, that the sexual abuse of children in family and institutional settings was unfortunately all too common. And as Robert Fliess and Sándor Ferenczi had noted, many abusers hid in clear sight, with a cultivated public image, totally at odds with how they conducted themselves in private. There are many such fairly contemporary examples of high-profile abusers – e.g., Jerry Sandusky (prominent Pen State football coach), Jimmy Savile (British television personality and charity supporter), Harvey Weinstein (wealthy and influential movie producer), Jeffrey Epstein ("billionaire" on friendly terms with two American presidents), Ghislaine Maxwell (high-profile socialite and procurer for Jeffrey Epstein), Bill Cosby (American comedian and father figure), Bob Montgomery (high-profile Australian psychologist and ex-Australian Psychological Society President), Professor Paul Wilson (who was Australia's best-known criminologist), Keith Wright (leader of the State Labor Party in Queensland, Australia, from 1982 to 1984), Cardinal Theodore McCarrick (defrocked American Catholic Cardinal), Lawrence King (most senior black Republican in the Reagan era), Fr Marcial Maciel Degollado (personal friend of Pope John Paul II and head of the order of the Legionnaires of Christ), Gary Glitter (pop star), R. Kelly (famous singer), Dr Larry Nasser (team doctor for US Olympic gymnastics team), Warren Jeffs (for a time head of the polygamous Mormons and also on the FBI's 10-most wanted list), Frank Arkell (a Lord Mayor of Wollongong, Australia), Bob Collins AO (Australian Federal Government Minister) and parliamentarian and broadcaster, Clement Freud.

Freud does not seem to have personally adhered all that closely to the psychoanalytic model of treatment that he recommended for others. Nor seemingly, did many get well under Freud's care. In a very detailed examination of 38 of Freud's personal patients, Borch-Jacobsen (admittedly a high-profile critic) concluded, "With a few ambiguous exceptions, such as the treatments of Ernst Lanzer, Bruno Walter and Albert Hirst, Freud's cures were largely ineffective, when they were not downright destructive" (2021, p. 7). Amongst the most boundaryless treatments and poorest outcomes was that of the recurrently psychotic Dr Horace Frink, who Freud had directed to become president of the New York Psychoanalytic Society (established in 1911 by AA Brill), and whom Freud encouraged to divorce his wife and to marry his patient, Angelika, an heiress and the wife of a prominent New York millionaire, Mr Abraham Bijur. Freud had written to his patient,

> Your complaint that you cannot grasp your homosexuality implies that you are not yet aware of your phantasy of making me a rich man. If matters turn out all right let us change this imaginary gift into a real contribution to the Psychoanalytic Funds.
>
> (Goleman, 1990, p. C3)

Dr Frink's daughter, Mrs Helen Frink Kraft (who died in October 2023 at the age of 103), felt that Freud tried to engineer the marriage (which rapidly failed) for money. Mr Bijur composed an open letter that he planned to run as a newspaper advertisement in New York City. Mrs Frink Kraft found it in the archives at Johns Hopkins University in 1985. In the letter the outraged Mr Bijur demanded to know how Freud could presume to break up his marriage, concluding with, "Great Doctor, are you a savant or a charlatan?" (Goleman, 1990, p. C12). In his official biography of Freud, Ernest Jones acknowledges Dr Frink's second marriage causing a scandal but gives no clue about Freud's prominent role in the matter.

Writing in 1987 Michael Specter commented,

> When Freud wired Angelika Bijur in June 1923 to say that he was sorry the marriage had fallen apart, he argued [somewhat cryptically] that 'the point where you failed was money.' Bijur was shocked by Freud's willingness to wash his hands of the marriage he had created and the man he had chosen as his apostle.

Central to the controversy regarding *The Assault on Truth* was Masson's strong perception that Freud's distancing himself from his seduction theory represented an act of dishonesty and cowardice. In Masson's challenging words,

> Freud gave up his theory, not for theoretical or clinical reasons, but because of a personal failure of courage. I do not think that Freud ever made a conscious decision to ignore his earlier experiences or that he ever recognised what he did as a failure of courage. No doubt he believed he was doing the right thing, and the difficult thing, when he shifted his attention from external trauma to internal fantasy as the causative agent in mental illness. But that does not mean it represents the truth.
>
> (Masson, 1984a, p. 189)

There has perhaps been long-term a strong tendency to imbue Freud with human qualities and capacities that he did not possess. Freud was undoubtedly a driven individual, using whatever influence he could muster to achieve public awards and carve out a place in history. While he had high intelligence and prodigious writing skills, his frailties seem typical of the human species, and for someone steeped in a process designed to bring insight and psychological relief, he seemed at times to demonstrate less than profound insight. Examples include somehow blaming Emma Eckstein for the botched life-threatening nasal surgery performed on her by his erstwhile friend Wilhelm Fliess (who believed he had discovered the cause of "neurasthenia" in the nose), psychoanalysing his own daughter Anna, setting up the messy arrangement that had Helene Deutsch analysing Victor Tausk at the same time as he was analysing Deutsch, or somehow allowing the highly controlling Ernest Jones, described by Glen Gabbard as a "rather seedy practitioner" (quoted by Rachman, 2022, p. 90) and referred to by colleagues James and Alix Strachey as "l.b." ("Little Beast") (Breger, 2000), to assume long-term the most powerful positions within psychoanalysis.

Jones, who was both a censor and a publicist for psychoanalysis, was described by Roazen (1975) as "a fiery little man, with a staccato, military manner", and who "at his worst, could be spiteful, jealous and querulous … He did not make friends easily and was much hated" (p. 354). Max Eitingon described to Freud his experience of Jones at the Tenth Psychoanalytic Congress in 1927 – "Jones was horrid, intent on causing annoyance, on needling one, while creating the impression he has more in stock, which he is keeping back to spare us … A lust for evil is unmistakable" (as quoted by Rachman, 2022, p. 69). Karl Menninger, a trained analyst and a giant in the history of 20th century psychiatry in the USA, described Jones as a "peculiar, crusty, crabbed guy" (Roazen, 2002, p. 221).

Freud was not a particularly great judge of men, and he inherited a Victorian mindset about women. Nor, despite the claims of Ernest Jones, was he unusually honest. Yet, the defence of Freud's honesty was central to the outrage of the original reviewers of *The Assault on Truth.* For example, Anthony Storr stated,

> Although Freud was often dogmatic and sometimes wrong, he was far too proud, too used to isolation and too honest to discard a theory because it was unacceptable to the medical establishment. Everything we know about his character makes Mr. Masson's accusation wildly unlikely.
>
> (1984, p. 35)

Despite the protestations associated with any questioning of Freud's forthright and genuine character, he was not immune to the human frailty of holding honesty at bay at times. As the matter has become a central theme in discussions about the claims Masson made about Freud in *The Assault on Truth,* it seems important, as a backdrop to the discussions in this book, to look in a little detail at other instances in which Freud's honesty was brought into question.

In a pamphlet published in 1906, "In Eigener Sache" ("In my own defense"), Wilhelm Fliess incorporates three letters from Freud (written 26 April, 23 July and 27 July 1904; see Masson, 1984a) that accused Freud of complicity in the plagiarism of Fliess' bisexuality theory and his theories about periodicity. In recalling their meeting at Achensee (1897), Fliess wrote, "On that occasion, Freud showed a violence toward me which was at first unintelligible to me... I thought I detected a personal animosity against me on Freud's part which sprang from envy" (Quoted in Malcolm, 1984, p. 133). The Freudian historian, Peter Swales, wrote (as quoted by Malcolm, 1984) that

> privately, to some of his family and to at least one friend, Fliess confided a much more provocative and sinister version of that meeting... According to Fliess, it was Freud's intention to lure him into a lonely mountainous region, then to push him over a precipice or into water below. While hardly a man of integrity, given the seeming treatment of his family behind closed doors, Fliess claimed he escaped because he had cause to suspect Freud's intention – he was a man of very small stature, and he could not swim.
>
> (p. 133)

They did not meet again, but in 1904, Freud replied to the letter from Fliess regarding the circumstances of how via a patient of Freud's (Herman Swoboda 1873–1963), a gifted, but very disturbed young man, Otto Weininger, had appropriated Fliess' theory on bisexuality and published it in a book, "Sex and Character" (Gay, 1988).

On 20 July 1904 Fliess had confronted Freud directly: "I have no doubt that Weininger obtained knowledge of my ideas via you and misused someone else's property. What do you know about it?" (Masson, 1985, p. 463). Freud obfuscated, covered up and lied, falsely claiming only vague knowledge, and finalizing his response by stating, "That's all I know about the matter" (Jones, 1961, p. 272). Jones commented that "It was perhaps the only occasion in Freud's life when he was for a moment not completely straightforward" (p. 272) (Masson's translation of that sentence is a little different from Jones', "Herewith everything I know about it" – see Masson, 1984a, p. 464). On 27 July 1904, Freud had written to his former friend, "The fact is that in the past few years ... you have no longer showed an interest in me or my family or my work" (Masson, 1984a, p. 467). John Kerr (1994) observed that "Freud's behaviour had been plainly indefensible" (p. 86).

At the end of 1905 Fliess got a friend to publish the pamphlet attacking Weininger, Swoboda, and Freud. Freud responded by writing to two editors, describing the pamphlet in one communication as

> a disgusting scribble, which amongst other things casts absurd aspersions on me... Actually, [this has] to do with the phantasy of an ambitious man who in his loneliness has lost the capacity to judge what is right and what is permissible..."
>
> (Jones, 1961, p. 273)

Writing to Carl Jung on 17 February 1908 Freud reflected that he had

> been in contact with a few paranoia cases in my practice and can tell you a secret ... . I have regularly encountered a detachment of libido from a homosexual component which until then had been normally and moderately cathected ...

> My one-time friend Fliess developed a dreadful case of paranoia after throwing off his affection for me, which was undoubtedly considerable.
>
> (quoted in Kerr, 1994, p. 174)

Freud's ex-patient, Swoboda, sued Fliess for defamation, but lost.

Of course, Freud, like many leaders of movements, was never quite as honest as those who idealize him would wish to believe. We now know through a dogged investigation carried out over a century after the event that Freud spent two nights with his sister-in-law Minna Bernays, having signed into one of the largest rooms of the upmarket Hotel Schweizerhaus, as man and wife on 13 August 1898 (Hirschmüller, 2007). At the same time, he was corresponding with his wife Martha that they were staying in "humble" lodgings, despite staying in the second fanciest hotel in town (Blumenthal, 2006). Writing in 2006, Franz Maciejewski, having found the sign-in register for the Hotel Schweizerhaus, somewhat triumphally declared, "The mystery surrounding the precise nature of the relationship between Freud and Minna Bernays was finally resolved in an unexpected and even altogether serendipitous manner" (p. 499).

In a public lecture on 18 November 1987, the Freudian scholar Peter Swales had previously expanded on his thesis that Freud and Minna Bernays had been lovers and that during a trip to Italy he had made her pregnant and had thus arranged an abortion under the cover of taking her to a spa for the treatment of tuberculosis. The rumour of an affair had started with Carl Jung, who told an interviewer, John Billinsky, in 1957, that Minna had taken him aside and confided to him the secret that her relationship with Freud was "very intimate" (see Malcolm, 1984; Gay, 1989a,b). Masson's erstwhile friend, Kurt Eissler, had interviewed Jung in Zurich in 1953 and had raised the issue of Freud's relationship with Minna. Eissler then, potentially to protect an idealized image of Freud as a figure beyond reproach, sealed the 61-page transcript in the Freud archives (Gale, 2016), not to be accessed for 50 years, with an additional embargo of a further 10 years then imposed. The Freudian historian, Peter Gay, writing in 1989, concluded that the rumour launched by Carl Jung lacked convincing evidence but in the light of the recently uncovered documentary evidence revised his opinion (Blumenthal, 2006).

Jung had maintained that on his first visit with Freud in March 1907, Minna had told him of her sexual intimacy with Freud. Jung recalled that Minna

> was very much bothered by her relationship with Freud and felt guilty about it. From her I learned that Freud was in love with her and that their relationship was indeed very intimate. It was a shocking discovery for me, and even now (May 1957) I can recall the agony I felt at the time.
>
> (Billinsky, 1969, p. 42)

Jung recalled that in the mutual dream analyses Freud and Jung conducted during their voyage to USA in August 1909,

> Freud had some dreams that bothered him very much. The dreams were about the triangle – Freud, his wife and wife's younger sister. Freud had no idea I knew about the triangle and his intimate relationship with his sister-in-law. And so when Freud told me about the dream… I asked (him) to tell me some of his personal associations… He looked at me with bitterness and said, "I could tell you more, but I cannot risk my authority!"
>
> (Billinsky, 1969, p. 42)

Ernest Jones, Freud's biographer, himself associated with multiple personal sexual scandals (Gabbard & Lester, 1996; Maddox, 2006), was the first to take up his pen and deny "the malicious and entirely untrue legend that [Minna] displaced his wife in his affections" (Jones, 1961, p. 153). Yet clearly several people had already been whispering concerns about the nature of Freud's relationship with his younger sister-in-law. For example, Judith Heller, Freud's niece, was aware of "lots of gossip within the family", regarding Freud's "second wife" (see Gale, 2016). Freud himself mentioned the rumours to a patient, Eva Rosenfeld, a close friend of his daughter, Anna. Gale (2016) reminds us of the stakes for Freud if an affair at the time became public knowledge,

> Revelations of an affair would have been devastating, particularly because of the special emphasis Freud placed on sexuality in his theories, for which he was already being severely criticized. Remember, at the time people were not only sceptical of Freud, they were sneering at him, even laughing at him.
>
> (p. 86)

Both the Fliess plagiarism allegation and Freud's alleged affair have attracted unending discussion – indeed Gale has written an entire book on "The Sigmund Freud – Minna Bernays Affair". Lothane (2016) adds to the discussion about whether evidence that Freud and Minna signed in as man and wife implies what it seems to imply, by drawing attention to Swiss cohabitation laws at the time which forbade an innkeeper providing accommodations to an unmarried couple. But of course, for this to represent a plausible way of preserving Freud's reputation in this matter, we still have to go with the assumption that Jung, not exactly blameless in sexual matters, made up the entire account of how Minna Bernays had approached him, never spoke of it around the time, and then long after Minna Bernays and Freud were dead, spoke of the matter privately twice. The first time was in 1953 to Kurt Eissler, and the second time in 1957 to John Billinsky, who 12 years later, long after Jung too was dead, and stimulated by a Time Magazine article on 5 September 1969, then published what Jung had told him. Lothane and others, contrary to the conclusions reached by Maciejewski, Gale, Swales, Gay et al., must posit that (1) Jung lied to Billinsky, and that (2) Billinsky's account is anyways, inaccurate. It is hard to identify an innocent explanation as to why Freud in his contemporaneous card to Martha demonstrably misled her about the nature of the accommodation he booked himself and Minna into on 13 August 1898.

Masson followed to some degree a path attempted previously by Sándor Ferenczi, Robert Fliess, and Florence Rush in trying to bring the topic of child sexual abuse back into psychoanalytic focus, but he was much younger than any of them. Whether psychologically prepared for it or not, he took on a "whistle-blower" role and wrapped his thesis in a title that included the unambiguous words, "assault on truth". While there has been debate about whether psychoanalysis maintained some interest in actual sexual abuse, it is hard to deny that when in September 1932 Ferenczi wanted to give a Congress paper about it, the reception from Freud, Ernest Jones, and others of the inner circle, was hostile. Ferenczi insisted on reading to Freud his paper as Freud was unable to attend the Congress: Freud in a letter to his daughter Anna very clearly outlined his position on his "seduction theory" when he unambiguously stated, "… I listened, shocked. He has completely regressed to etiological views I believed in, and gave up, thirty-five years ago: that the regular cause of neuroses is sexual traumas in childhood…" (cited by Gay, 1988, pp. 583–584). For the remainder of his life Ferenczi was subjected to Totschweigen or "death by silence" (Rachman, 2022) with Freud's official biographer, Ernest Jones, writing Ferenczi into history as "psychotic", despite there being no evidence to support such an extreme claim.

Ferenczi, in his famous, but at the time ignored 1932 Congress paper, returned psychoanalysis to its origins – traumatized dissociative individuals. He provides a very cogent description of dissociative identity disorder (DID) when he states,

> If traumatic events accumulate during the life of the growing person, the number and variety of personality splits increase, and soon it will be rather difficult to maintain contact without confusion with all the fragments, which all act as separate personalities but mostly do not know each other.
>
> (in Masson, 1984a, p. 293)

Anticipating the concept of polyfragmented or extremely complex DID (Kluft, 1991), he goes on; "In the end, one might reach a state which one need not hesitate to call *atomization*, to continue the metaphor of *fragmentation*" (p. 293).

Robert Fliess, around half a century ago, found strong corroboration of his analytic findings in Leontine Young's unpublished doctoral thesis (*Parents Who Neglect and Abuse Children*, New York School for Social Work, 1958), dealing with her analysis of 120 case reports of child neglect and abuse. By the time of his death Robert Fliess was writing in "isolation" from the mainstream analytic "movement" upon which he had "turned" his "back" (Fliess, 1973, p. 411). Given the challenges faced by whistle blowers and given what had happened to Ferenczi and then to Robert Fliess in pursuing a similar goal, it is not hard to appreciate that Masson was going to have a very challenging time.

Comments by Richard (Rich) J. Loewenstein, M.D.

In finalising the manuscript for this book, we had some detailed conversations with Richard (Rich) J. Loewenstein, M.D., one of the pioneers of the modern dissociative disorders/complex trauma field. He is an "adult child of psychoanalysts" who grew up among European psychoanalysts who fled the Holocaust in the 1940s. Rich offered pertinent observations about psychiatry, psychoanalysis, areas in their respective histories where they merged, and the challenges of using a contemporary lens to assess earlier theories or historical figures. We share here in summary form some of these, as they represent thought-provoking perspectives through which to conceptualize why the "seduction theory", in Freud's hands (or in anyone else's for that matter), was always going to attract extreme resistance.

He writes:

> We cannot talk about "psychoanalysis" as a unitary construct. Psychoanalysis is a clinical theory whose basic concepts (e.g., transference, countertransference, therapeutic alliance, introjection, unconscious mind, intrapsychic conflict, and intrapsychic defences) are central to the treatment of DID and related disorders (Kluft, 2000; Loewenstein & Brand, 2023; Simeon & Abugel, 2023). Psychoanalysis is a theory of the mind, and a social movement. Organized psychoanalysis is a quasi-religious institution with an intransigent hagiography. In the USA, organized psychoanalysis[1] was linked to psychiatry, with the general requirement that US psychoanalysts be physicians and psychiatrists. From the 1950s until the late 1970s, training as a psychoanalyst was a necessary credential to advance in psychiatric professional organizations, and in some of the most prestigious US academic psychiatry departments (e.g., in New York, San Francisco, Boston, Chicago, New Haven, etc.), including advancement to department chair. Many psychiatrists went into analytic training because their department chairs, teachers, and professors were analysts, without any real interest in the field. Starting in the early1980s, US psychoanalysts were increasingly supplanted in academic departments by behaviourally oriented psychologists and biological psychiatrists. Insurance companies would no longer pay for long-term dynamic psychotherapy – which harmed DID patients. American interest in psychoanalysis declined and it was attacked as fustian, meritless, and without empirical foundation.
>
> It is a symptom of our time that we tend to judge historical figures as if they are our contemporaries, rather than recognize that they lived in radically different cultural, social, and political worlds, and in whose minds we cannot put ourselves. (Even the word "seduction" tells you what a different view of incest and child rape these people had). Freud was born in 1856, eight years before the abolition of slavery in the USA. He was a citizen of the Austro-Hungarian Empire, a constitutional monarchy where, compared to many European countries, Jews were treated relatively well. However, there were Austrian antisemitic political parties, and one of these won the 1895 election for mayor of Vienna, remaining in power until 1911. Kluft (2018a, 2018b, 2018c, 2019; Chapter 4) proposed that Freud was undoubtedly acutely aware of anti-Semitism, and he was treating the children of wealthy, bourgeois, "assimilated", Austrian Jews. To promulgate that they were routinely raping

their daughters (and sons) would have fit with the stereotype of Jews with horns eating babies in bloody rituals. Jews were routinely killed throughout Europe for less at those times.

None of us rțeally can know what would have happened had Freud persevered with the seduction theory. Many seem to implicitly think that, had Freud persisted, psychoanalytic history would have been exactly the same, but with a different etiological view. However, if Freud had continued, I doubt we would have ever heard of him. He likely would have been buried in the lost history of people who said this sort of thing in the late 19th century. We would have said, "How interesting that he said that then. No wonder he was never heard from again." In his writings, Masson discusses the work of Auguste Tardieu, a mid-19th century French medical forensic scientist who wrote works on rape, child rape, child torture, and murder of children in the context of rape. Masson speculates that Freud had read Tardieu's writing and seen his lectures on these topics. If so, Freud would likely have gleaned that these works were mostly suppressed and ignored by the medical establishment. In contrast, to this day the works of Kraft-Ebbing – who demeaned Freud's child rape/hysteria lecture – are well known.

The "icy rejection" of Freud's theories of child rape and maltreatment as the etiology of hysteria, and the withdrawal by those he considered (or he hoped would become) colleagues, tells us that it is unlikely these ideas were going to be accepted. The notion that women and children lie about sexual crimes was not only a psychological theory. Until recently, this has been a dominant legal theory that protected "upstanding men". Judy Herman's most recent book "Truth and Repair" (2023) reviews how difficult it still is for sexual assault survivors to get justice in the American legal system. In the US, adoption of mandated reporting of child abuse did not reach all 50 states until the mid-1980s. No such system existed in 1890s Vienna or Paris.

In "Trauma and Recovery" (1992), Herman articulates the many negative implications of Freud's recantation of the "seduction theory". However, she points out that Freud had no professional community, social, or political group to support him. Richard Kluft (Chapter 4) criticizes Freud and his earlier followers for the pernicious errors that have been described at length. He observes that subsequent generations of psychoanalysts could have attempted to change the dogma as more modern data emerged but most unquestioningly persisted with these beliefs.

The issues around child rape are *still* controversial, notwithstanding how different the times are. And probably always will be. Mainstream academic views of sexual violence against children, adolescents, and adults only began to change with the rise of feminist psychiatry/psychology in the late 60s-70s, and there is still a long way to go.

Also, I wonder, assuming our species survives for another 100 years, what the scholars of that time will say of us! How crude and primitive they were, what terrible things they did in the name of therapy; but some of them were insightful and thoughtful, at least for their times. How interesting what they understood

> back then; how if they only had followed this one other pathway, we would laud them now as our contemporaries. Maybe future scholars will discover some of our writings and be amazed what some of us understood "back then" – albeit primitive and head-scratchingly, prejudicially obtuse.

We need to be historically humble and not project our current understanding of social and psychological matters onto historical figures and then criticize them for not knowing what we know. And we can also see throughout history the challenges human beings have had coming face-to-face for any length of time with the reality and impact of child abuse and violence against women. There is greater acceptance in some parts of modern society of the devastating effects of child maltreatment. Yet, the dissociative disorders field itself is still relatively marginalized, ignored, and denigrated, even among those who have promulgated the ICD-11 diagnosis of complex PTSD. It has not been incorporated systematically into psychoanalysis (Loewenstein & Brand, 2023; Kluft, Postscript). These truths are still assaulted in various ways from many directions today just as they were in Freud's era.

Insights and perspectives

The chapters ahead represent a set of insights and perspectives, from a range of well-informed professionals on what *The Assault on Truth* was about, how its central theses have held up, and what, 40 years on from the publication of that book, we now know about child sexual, physical, emotional, and related abuses, as well as the capacity for endless perpetrators to hide in plain sight.

Warwick Middleton and Martin J. Dorahy

Note

1 One problem is that psychoanalysis in the USA fractured into different "schools" (Horneyan, Sullivanian, et al.) that opposed, to varying extents, many of the tenets of what, for simplicity, might be termed "orthodox" psychoanalysis: the group that was most "faithful to Freud" (note the religious language) and that attacked, excommunicated, and shunned Jeffrey Masson. There were splits within institutes with older analysts viewing ego psychology as heresy, and later ego psychologists questioning self-psychology, etc.

References

Billinsky, J. M. (1969). Jung and Freud (the end of a romance). *Andover Newton Quarterly*, *10*, 39–43.

Blumenthal, R. (2006, December 24). Hotel log hints at desire that Freud didn't repress. *The New York Times*. Retrieved from http://tiny.cc/frh0q

Bonaparte, M., Freud, A., & Kris, E. (Eds.). (1954). *The origins of psychoanalysis: Letters to Wilhelm Fliess, 1887–1902*. Basic Books.

Borch-Jacobsen, M. (2021). *Freud's patients: A book of lives*. Reaktion Books.

Bowlby, J. (1998). *A secure base*. Routledge.

Breger, L. (2000). *Freud, darkness in the midst of vision.* John Wiley.
Crews, F. (2004, March 11). The trauma trap. *The New York Review.* Retrieved from http://tinyurl.com/3j8p6j9v
Eyre, D. P. (1991). Therapy with a sexually abused woman. *International Journal of Psycho-Analysis, 72*(3), 403–415.
Ferenczi, S. (1932/1984). Confusion of tongues between adults and the child. In J. M. Masson (Ed.). *The assault on truth: Freud's suppression of the seduction theory* (pp. 283–295). Faber and Faber, .
Fliess, R. (1956). *Erogeneity and libido: Addenda to the theory of the psychosexual development of the human* – Psychoanalytic series (Vol. 1). International Universities Press.
Fliess, R. (1962). *Ego and body Ego: Contributions to their psychoanalytic psychology* – Psychoanalytic series (Vol. 2). International Universities Press.
Fliess, R. (1973). *Symbol, dream, and psychosis with notes on technique* – Psychoanalytic series (Vol. 3). International Universities Press.
Fliess, W. (2006). *In Eigener Sache: Gegen Otto Weininger und Herman Swoboda.* E. Goldschmidt.
Freud, S. (1905/1920, 2001). Three essays on the theory of sexuality. (J. Strachey Ed, Standard ed., Vol. 7, pp. 123–246). Vintage Arrow.
Gabbard, G. O., & Lester, E. P. (1996). *Boundaries and boundary violations in psychoanalysis.* Basic Books.
Gale, B. G. (2016). *Love in Vienna: The Sigmund Freud – Minna Bernays affair.* Bloomsbury Publishing.
Gay, P. (1988). *A life in our time.* J. M. Dent & Sons Ltd.
Gay, P. (1989a). *The Freud reader.* W.W. Norton & Company.
Gay, P. (1989b, January 29) Sigmund and Minna? The biographer as voyeur. *The New York Times.* Retrieved from https://tinyurl.com/d4ajmfvy
Goleman, D. (1990, March 6). Therapist, Freud fell short, scholars find. *New York Times.* C1 & C12.
Goodreads. (2024). *Otto von Bismarck quotes.* Retrieved from http://tinyurl.com/4a768c3d
Hanly, C. (1986). Review of Masson and Malcolm. *International Journal of Psychoanalysis, 67*, 517–519.
Hanly, C., & Murray, B. (undated). An interview with Charles Hanly. *International Psychoanalytic Association.* Retrieved from https://tinyurl.com/33vx9v9x
Herman, J. L. (1984, March 10). The analyst analyzed. *The Nation.* 293–296.
Herman, J. L. (1992). *Trauma and recovery.* Basic Books.
Herman, J. L. (2023). *Truth and repair: How trauma survivors envision justice.* Basic Books.
Herman, J. L., & Hirschman, L. (1981). *Father–daughter incest.* Harvard University Press.
Hirschmüller, A. (2007). Evidence for a sexual relationship between Sigmund Freud and Minna Bernays? *American Imago, 64*(1), 125–129. https://doi.org/10.1353/aim.2007.0013
Jones, E. (1961). *The life and work of Sigmund Freud* (L. Trilling & S. Marcus, Ed. & Abr.) Penguin.
Kerr, J. (1994). *A most dangerous method.* Sinclair-Stevenson.
King, C. (2017). Violent and sexually 'defective': What the royal commission taught us about the Christian Brothers. *ABC News.* Retrieved from http://tinyurl.com/36698h64
Kluft, R. P. (1991). Clinical presentations of multiple personality disorder. *Psychiatric Clinics of North America, 14*(3), 605–629.
Kluft, R. P. (2000). The psychoanalytic psychotherapy of dissociative identity disorder in the context of trauma therapy. *Psychoanalytic Inquiry, 20*(2), 259–286. https://doi.org/10.1080/07351692009348887

Kluft, R. P. (2018a). Freud's rejection of hypnosis, Part I: The gnesis of a rift. *American Journal of Clinical Hypnosis*, *60*(4), 307–323. https://doi.org/10.1080/00029157.2018.1426321

Kluft, R. P. (2018b). Freud's rejection of hypnosis, Part II: The perpetuation of a rift. *American Journal of Clinical Hypnosis*, *60*(4), 324–347. https://doi.org/10.1080/00029157.2018.1426326

Kluft, R. P. (2018c). Reconsidering hypnosis and psychoanalysis: Toward creating a context for understanding. *American Journal of Clinical Hypnosis*, *60*(3), 201–215. https://doi.org/10.1080/00029157.2018.1400810

Kluft, R. P. (2019). Freud's rejection of hypnosis: Perspectives old and new: Part III of III – Toward healing the rift: Enriching both hypnosis and psychoanalysis. *American Journal of Clinical Hypnosis*, *61*(3), 208–226. https://doi.org/10.1080/00029157.2018.1544432

Knauth, D. (2023). Boy Scouts' record $2.46 bln sex abuse settlement upheld by judge. *Reuters*. Retrieved from https://tinyurl.com/32cyuhf3

Loewenstein, R. J., & Brand, B. (2023). Dissociative identity disorder: A disorder of diagnostic and therapeutic paradoxes. *Psychoanalytic Psychotherapy*, *37*(4), 339–380. https://doi.org/10.1080/02668734.2023.2272771

Lothane, Z. (2001). Freud's alleged repudiation of the seduction theory revisited: Facts and fallacies. *Psychoanalytic Review, 88*(5), 673–723. https://doi.org/10.1521/prev.88.5.673.17712

Lothane, Z. (2016). Freud and Minna: Facts and fictions. *Journal of the American Psychoanalytic Association, 64*(6), 1237–1254. https://doi.org/10.1177/0003065116680568

Lothane, Z. (2018). Freud bashers: Facts, fictions and fallacies. *Journal of the American Psychoanalytic Association*, *66*(5), 953–969. https://doi.org/10.1177/0003065118807932

Maddox, B. (2006). *Freud's wizard: The enigma of Ernest Jones*. Da Capo Press.

Malcolm, J. (1984). *In the Freud archives*. Jonathan Cape.

Marshall, K. (2015, May 20). Suicide common among clergy sex abuse victims in Ballarat. *The Age*. Retrieved from http://tinyurl.com/t4tescun

Masson, J. M. (1984a). *The assault on truth: Freud's suppression of the seduction theory*. Faber and Faber.

Massonn, J. M. (1985) The complete letters of Sigmund Freud to Wilhelm Fliess, 1887–1904. Harvard University Press.

Masson, J. M. (1992). *Final analysis: The making and unmaking of a psychoanalyst*. Fontana.

Masson, J. M. (1984/2003). *The assault on truth: Freud's suppression of the seduction theory*. Ballantine Books.

Masson, J., & Masson, T. (1978). *The navel of neurosis: Trauma, memory and denial*. Unpublished manuscript.

McKenzie, N., Baker, R., & Lee, J. (2012, April 13). Church's suicide victims. *The Age*. Retrieved from http://tinyurl.com/479w5fea

McMaugh, K., & Middleton, W. (2022). The history and politics of 'false memories': The Australian experience. *Journal of Trauma and Dissociation*, *23*(2), 177–190. https://doi.org/10.1080/15299732.2022.2028223

Middleton, W. (2013a). Parent-child incest that extends into adulthood: A survey of international press reports, 2007–2011. *Journal of Trauma and Dissociation*, *14*, 184–197. https://doi.org/10.1080/15299732.2013.724341

Middleton, W. (2013b). Ongoing incestuous abuse during adulthood. *Journal of Trauma and Dissociation, 14*(3), 251–272. https://doi.org/10.1080/15299732.2012.736932

Putnam, F. W. (1989). *Diagnosis and treatment of multiple personality disorder*. Guilford Press.

Rachman, A. W. (2022). *Psychoanalysis and society's neglect of the sexual abuse of children, youth and adults: Re-addressing Freud's original theory of sexual abuse and trauma*. Routledge.

Remnick, D. (1984, February 19). *The assault on Freud*. The Washington Post. Retrieved from http://tinyurl.com/5ah2xhj9

Roazen, P. (1975). *Freud and his followers*. Alfred A. Knopf.

Roazen P. (2002). *The trauma of Freud: Controversies in psychoanalysis*. Routledge.

Roazen P. (2005). *Edoardo Weiss: The house that Freud built*. Transaction Publishers.

Ross, C. A. (1989). *Multiple personality disorder: Diagnosis, clinical features, and treatment*. John Wiley & Sons.

Rush, F. (1977). The Freudian cover-up. *Chrysalis*, *1*, 31–45.

Shengold, L. (1989). *Soul murder*. Yale University Press.

Simeon, D., & Abugel, J. (2023). *Feeling unreal: Depersonalization disorder and the loss of self* (2nd ed.). Oxford

Simon, B. (1992). Incest – See under Oedipus complex: The history of an error in psychoanalysis. *Journal of the American Psychoanalytic Association*, *40*, 955–988. https://doi.org/10.1177/000306519204000401

Specter, M. (1987, November 8). Sigmund Freud and a family torn asunder. *The Washington Post*. Retrieved from http://tinyurl.com/ek6arazk

Storr, A. (1984, February 12). Did Freud have feet of clay? *New York Times*, 3 & 35.

Webster, R. (2005). *Why Freud was wrong: Sin, science and psychoanalysis*. The Orwell Press.

Weininger, O. (1906, original work published 1903). *Sex and character*. W. Heinemann.

Welch, D. (2002, November 14) Walking on the beach with Jeffrey Masson's cats. *Powell's books – Author interview*. Retrieved from https://tinyurl.com/88u9bapw

1 Background to *The Assault on Truth*

Jeffrey Masson

I played a part in finding unusual documents relating to the sexual abuse of children. The documents were unusual because their existence should have been known but was not. I should amend this comment: *Somebody* knew about them before I found them, but we will probably never know who that person was.

I am referring to communications in Freud's desk in London. In the top right-hand drawer of that famous desk, I found a series of approximately 15 typed letters between Freud and his psychoanalytic colleagues, including Max Eitingon, A.A. Brill, and others, written in everyday German script (some were originally sent as typewritten letters, others possibly transcribed from an original handwritten copy) about a brewing crisis involving the much-beloved Hungarian analyst, Sándor Ferenczi, who had been slated to become the president of the International Psychoanalytical Association (IPA). But there was a problem: he had just shown Freud the paper he intended to read at the 12th (1932) IPA Congress. The paper was about the sexual abuse of children by adults, an apostasy, if that is what you want to call it. There was a clear reference to Freud's "seduction theory" (when for some years he articulated the belief that the symptoms presented by many of his patients, both men and women, had their origin in childhood sexual abuse). Freud and his colleagues were incensed that Ferenczi continued to believe in what Freud called his "initial error," namely that child sexual abuse was real, was frequent, and had terrible consequences for the lives of those who experienced it. The letters collected in that drawer, portions of which Anna Freud allowed me to translate at the time, showed that Freud was appalled by Ferenczi's thesis (so much for historians who claim that Freud never abandoned the seduction theory but only modified it) and wanted to prevent him from giving this paper. These letters had never been published, nor, as far as I could ascertain, been seen by anyone except the person who put them there. Their historical importance cannot be exaggerated. (Ferenczi's paper itself has since gone on to become one of the most profound and influential papers ever written on the topic – and we are talking 1932!)

So, let me ask: who collected those letters and who placed them in Freud's desk, where he sat daily? I remember asking Anna Freud, who simply shook her head, indicating she had no idea. So, it could not have been her. Not many people have had access to that desk since Freud died in 1939 (three weeks after the beginning of

DOI: 10.4324/9781003431466-2

the Second World War). Perhaps Ernest Jones, Freud's biographer? But he showed little interest in this topic (for good reasons, it turns out, given that he himself was accused of sexually abusing children – for discussion, see Middleton, 2018). I would have to presume it was Freud himself. And therein lies the core of our mystery.

In 1984 I published *The Assault on Truth: Freud's Suppression of the Seduction Theory*, in which I argued that Freud was right the first time (1896) when he realized the extent of child sexual abuse in the patients he was seeing in analysis. He was led to this belief in the reality of child sexual abuse, and its importance in explaining what he called "hysteria" (which today would cover presentations like complex trauma disorders, dissociative disorders, somatoform disorders, and some personality disorders) by the accounts of his patients which he had no reason to doubt. It was only when his colleagues mocked him that he came to understand that this was an issue about which everyone had strong feelings. This was especially true of his male colleagues (psychiatrists and neurologists) who accused Freud of believing in fairy tales (i.e., the accounts, primarily by women, of their childhood abuse, including incest). Freud was at first adamant that he was correct. I was able to show that he was encouraged in his beliefs by a trip to the Paris Morgue, where he saw children who had been raped and murdered (this visit had not been previously picked up by historians). He also had in his possession a book about childhood abuse written by a French forensic physician, Ambroise Tardieu, that I conjecture would have also encouraged his belief that he was right. But when Freud realized that his colleagues (all men) were not willing to entertain even the possibility of real abuse, and were not going to send him patients, he slowly began to backtrack.

I remember Kurt Eissler, the powerful New York psychoanalyst, defending Freud's honour. He obviously thought I was attacking that, but I was not, I was simply trying to find historical documents that could clarify what happened between 1896 and 1903 that led Freud to give up his initial theory about abuse. Yes, I personally believed he made a serious error, but I was trying to keep myself out of this debate: "Here," I said, "are the documents that nobody has seen until now. Make up your own mind how important they are." Well, Eissler and his defenders did precisely that: they were not important, and I was wrong to think they were. I believe even analysts today would take a different view. Eissler did make one point that was valid: he said that there was no evidence that Freud had read the book by Tardieu. That is true, but the fact that he purchased the book, and that it remained in his library until his death, is surely some evidence that he knew the book. It was not, I must admit, annotated, but then many of Freud's books were not. As for the Paris Morgue, I just don't see how this could not have influenced Freud at the time.

I had refrained from speculating about Freud's motives for renouncing his "seduction theory." (By the way, what Freud meant by this term is what today we would call sexual abuse, including rape, incest, and not infrequently, sadism.) It is so difficult to enter another person's head when they are about to make a decision that would have far-reaching consequences for them, and in this case, for the entire world. Had Freud stuck by his original "theory," many thousands, or perhaps even millions, of women would have been believed rather than belittled, especially by the very profession they turned to for help (e.g., psychiatry and psychology influenced by virtually *all* schools of analytic thought). You might as well try to determine what is in Vladimir Putin's mind now that he is destroying Ukraine. It is impossible to know, and in any event, it really doesn't matter: it is wrong. Period. And Freud was wrong too. But in the case of Putin, millions know this to be the case. In the case of Freud, at the time nobody knew, and it would be more than a hundred years before people saw what a colossal error he had made.

In my 1984 book, I claimed it was a "failure of courage." I still believe that, but there must be more to it. Did Freud really believe that his colleagues were right in dismissing his abuse theory, and that what his patients told him were "fairy tales"? I cannot see how this could be. Yes, it stung Freud that he was rejected by all his peers (with the exception of Wilhelm Fliess, hence the intense friendship between the two men that was a unique part of Freud's life). On 26 April 1896 Freud wrote to Fliess,

> A lecture on the etiology of hysteria at the psychiatric society was given an icy reception by the asses and a strange evaluation by Krafft-Ebing: "It sounds like a scientific fairy tale." And this, after one has demonstrated to them the solution of a more-than-a-thousand-year-old problem, a caput Nili [source of the Nile]! They can go to hell, euphemistically expressed.
>
> (Masson, 1985, p. 184)

Yes, he had become, as he described in an important letter that Marie Bonaparte, Anna Freud, and Ernst Kris in 1954 had left out of their edition of the Freud/ Fliess letters, effectively, a pariah (a state of existence that would in time be visited upon, Sándor Ferenczi, Robert Fliess, and me). Freud had written to Fliess on 4 May 1896,

> I am as isolated as you would wish me to be. Word was given out to abandon me, for a void is forming all around me. So far, I bear it with equanimity. I find it more troublesome that this year for the first time my consulting room is empty, that for weeks on end I see no new faces, cannot begin any new treatments, and that none of the old ones are completed. Things are so difficult and trying that it requires, on the whole, a strong constitution to deal with them.
>
> (Masson, 1985, p. 185)

In translating the existing Freud–Fliess letters, it became apparent that Marie Bonaparte et al., in their abridged translation of the letters, had excised all case histories written after September 1897 that concerned themselves with the sexual abuse of children. One such passage dates from 12 December 1897, and references Freud's patient and newly practising analyst, Emma Eckstein:

> My confidence in paternal etiology has risen greatly. Eckstein deliberately treated her patient in such a manner as not to give her the slightest hint of what

> would emerge from the unconscious and in the process obtained from her, among other things, the identical scenes with the father. Incidentally, the young girl is doing very well.
>
> (Masson, 1985, p. 286)

Ten days later on 22 December 1897 in another letter to Fliess, Freud had included a detailed account of extreme abuse, an excerpt of which appears below (Masson, 1985, p. 288):

> When she was two years old, he brutally deflowered her and infected her with gonorrhea, as a consequence of which she became ill, and her life was endangered by the loss of blood and vaginitis. The mother now stands in the room and shouts: "Rotten criminal, what do you want from me? I will have no part of that. Just whom do you think you have in front of you."

I remember showing Anna Freud this letter her father had written to Fliess as we discussed why Freud backtracked about abuse, and I asked her why she omitted this crucial letter from *The Origins of Psycho-Analysis* (1954). "Well," she told me, "It makes my father look paranoid." I answered that he was not, that he was prescient! He got it then, and only under the pressure of all his colleagues did he do an about-face! She looked at me, and shook her head, as if I were a recalcitrant child.

Freud was correct: his colleagues ridiculed him. He had a relatively new practice, so their opinion would be very important to his success. This was another reason he caved in. Also, consider the fact that many of his patients were from affluent families that included medical colleagues (Borch-Jacobsen, 2021). It would be very embarrassing for them if Freud knew about any possible incest. There were few people in Vienna at that time who even believed such a thing was possible (for that matter, this was true probably over the entire world). Freud may well have come to doubt himself: "Could I be right, and everyone else I know, wrong?" That is a difficult position to take. Ferenczi did and look what happened to him. Robert Fliess, the son of Wilhelm Fliess, did and he too was banished. I did as well, but the difference was that by the early 1980s there were many feminists who would back me up and who had already recognized how important and how common the sexual abuse of children was. Yet I too had to pay a price.

You may wonder "Is it possible that Freud really believed he had made a major clinical mistake?" much as does a surgeon who operates on the wrong side of the brain or amputates the wrong limb (it does happen). I suppose we will never know the answer to that question unless new documents become available. The mystery of the right-hand drawer in Freud's desk may never be solved but I am sure it will intrigue researchers for years to come.

I was in training in a Freudian institute to become a psychoanalyst when I first encountered Freud's initial belief in the power of sexual abuse in childhood to profoundly impact adult psychological functioning. I was told that Freud eventually realized he had made a major mistake: either the patients were engaging in fantasy (out of Oedipal longing) or they had been encouraged by Freud to invent a story they thought would please him. However, some selected letters that Anna Freud allowed me to read, unpublished letters from Freud to Fliess, showed clearly that this "history" was incorrect, or at the very least, incomplete. For in those letters that Miss Freud allowed me to see, translate, and eventually publish in full, Freud comes back to his belief in the reality of abuse based on further clinical experience. Also, Emma Eckstein, one of his patients, who had suffered the long-term effects of a botched operation by Freud's friend Wilhelm Fliess (it would be considered malpractice then and now), was beginning to see patients herself, under Freud's guidance, and she too had found real sexual abuse. In discussing this with Anna Freud, it became clear to me that she hated any mention of Emma Eckstein. The saga of her nose operation, carried out by Wilhelm Fliess, reflected badly on her father. The story becomes even more intriguing when we add in Freud's favourite disciple, Sándor Ferenczi, who *also* concluded that abuse was real and frequently found in psychiatric patients. In fact, the abuse *explained* why they were patients in the first place. (See my book for more details on that story.)

Let me back up a bit to explain. How did I come to be in Freud's study, next to his desk and opening the drawers, with Anna Freud by my side? It is a complex story that I have told many times (see *Final Analysis: The Making and Unmaking of a Psychoanalyst,* Masson, 1991), but each time I tell it, I seem to stumble upon new puzzles. I don't believe anyone has tried to unravel the mystery of those letters in the top right-hand drawer. Sometimes it feels like sheer luck that I came upon them. I was in the Freud House, 20 Maresfield Gardens, London, because Kurt Eissler, the formidable director of the Freud Archives (housed in the Library of Congress, Washington, DC), had made me his successor. This too requires a back-story which I will not give here. Suffice it to say this was an immense honour for someone who had just recently graduated as a psychoanalyst from the Toronto Institute (in 1979). Anna Freud herself was at first sceptical of me but came to admire the fact that I was putting so much effort into learning German and showed such zeal for historical research. We also bonded over a love of dogs! Anna Freud was professionally close to Eissler and respected him enormously. Muriel Gardiner, another close friend of Anna Freud and the Freud family, vouched for me as well.

And why was I so interested in the sexual abuse of children? There are any number of answers (such as shouldn't everyone?), but for a psychoanalyst, sexual abuse stood as the main watershed in the history of Freud's theoretical developments and the creation of psychoanalysis itself. Freud came to believe that he was mistaken in thinking that child sexual abuse was a major etiological factor in his patients' symptoms. Instead, these events had in fact not taken place and patients imagined (fantasized) them to gain protection from their own incestuous desires (he called these memories "screen memories" to indicate that they screened their real purpose – fantasies of abuse or desire for sexual contact). These ideas prompted the formulation of the Oedipus complex, and theories about infantile sexuality and the nature of memory (i.e., a memory of abuse, for example, "screened" the impulses of the child by inventing a scene that was not real). All analysts in their training were taught the historical details of this momentous shift in direction. But when I was first exposed to this view, I balked. "Wait a minute," I remember saying in the seminar where we candidates were being taught the fundamentals of psychoanalytic theory, "Exactly how do you determine that something a patient says happened, did *not*, in fact, happen?" I did not receive a good answer then, and I still cannot imagine today what it would be: even in the rare case where a patient withdraws the abuse claim, there could be other explanations for so doing. (No doubt there are cases of claimed abuse that turn out to have been untrue, but these don't appear to be common.)

Learning that memories of abuse were fantasies was hardly a trivial matter. We were, all of us candidates, about to see our first patient in analysis. We were warned that some of them would tell us that they were abused and that we were not to believe them. They were suffering from what our teachers called "hysterical mendacity," that is, they were lying about the abuse because of their own sexual desires, a view consistent with Freud's re-working of his initial explanation. To put it mildly, I did not feel comfortable with this explanation. I found it hard to understand Freud's change of heart, and I determined then, in my very first year of being a candidate to become a psychoanalyst, that I would delve into this in further depth as soon as I was able.

The reason I was sceptical had to do with my belief, very early on, that real events had real consequences. I had married Thérèse (Terri) Claire Alter (later Masson), who was born in Warsaw in 1937 and had spent her childhood in the Warsaw Ghetto (see her remarkable book, posthumously published by the Holocaust Museum in Sydney, *My Kaddish*, Masson, 2019). She and I had a mutual interest in psychoanalysis, but we both believed that it was primarily a means of exploring childhood trauma. I am not sure where I got that idea: perhaps from reading the influential 1946 book by Otto Fenichel, *The Psychoanalytic Theory of Neuroses*. I did not know it at the time, but Fenichel was a socialist (with communist leanings) and very involved in anti-Fascist activities. I only recently learned that in 1934 he spent a year in Oslo meeting leftist intellectuals who were later prominent in the Norwegian resistance. In that book, he spoke of psychoanalysis being a "traumatogenic theory of the neuroses," that is, neuroses were produced by trauma. Precisely what I believed.

I admit that at the time I was somewhat contemptuous of my teachers in Toronto and much looked forward to hearing what people better informed would tell me. And so, I arranged, in 1973, to meet Anna Freud in London, along with my wife Terri. Terri only left Poland at the end of the war (to move to Paris) in 1945 after a severely traumatic childhood in the Warsaw Ghetto. Anna Freud was arrested by the Gestapo on 22 March 1938, and interrogated for an entire afternoon. (This was the final straw for Freud, and he and his family left Vienna for London two months later.) I don't believe Anna Freud ever told anyone (except, perhaps, her father) what happened during that questioning, but she, of all people, would know how traumatic such a visit would be, and how difficult it would be to be living in Vienna as a Jew from 1933 on (if not before). So, I believed that Terri and Anna had much in common, and I looked forward to a lively discussion. The meeting, however, was not what I had hoped for. Anna Freud was cold and abrupt: "Why have you come to see me?" I plunged right in and told her who my wife was, and that we were both interested in traumatic events, such as fascism, war, child abuse, and I, for one, wondered why there was not more written about it in the psychoanalytic literature. Especially, I said, the Second World War. After all, so many Jewish analysts had come from Germany and Austria where they had direct experience of fascism. Her response was something like, "Psychoanalysis is concerned with the inner life so it's not surprising that there is so little written about these topics that you are interested in." And that was it. She showed no interest in Terri's past, did not ask her a single question and we left, both deeply disappointed.

When I next met Anna Freud, the situation was very different, but my interests were not so different. I made no attempt to hide them from her, and she still maintained her position that "my father" (as she liked to say, which always gave me chills!) was right to abandon the seduction theory. She thought I was wrong to want to investigate this, and that I would be wasting my time. There was nothing to be found. She was wrong. And I do believe now that Anna Freud slowly began to see that this was hardly a trivial historical issue. Otherwise, it is hard to explain why she would allow me to read the unpublished Freud/Fliess letters (some 163 of them). She told me there would be no point in publishing these letters, as they contained nothing of any scientific interest. I can still remember how excited I was to show her the letter, from 22 December 1897, where Freud recounts a terrible case of father/daughter incest (the young child almost died from loss of blood), and Freud then famously shared with Fliess, "a new motto" for his new science: "Poor child, what have they done to you?" (Masson, 1985, p. 288.). I remember saying to Anna Freud that this was the most beautiful thing I had ever seen Freud say. And then I asked, perhaps unaware of how tactless this was, "Miss Freud, how can you possibly say that this letter is of no scientific interest?" "Because," she answered, "he was wrong." Moving right along in my obliviousness, I said: "Why not let people decide for themselves, by having the entire correspondence published?" I cannot explain why she allowed me to go ahead with this publication of the complete letters between Sigmund Freud and Wilhelm Fliess (Masson, 1985), even though she had warned me somewhat darkly, "You may come to regret it." What was she thinking? Perhaps how Freud himself had suffered near ostracism from his colleagues when he gave a lecture to the Vienna Psychiatric Society in 1896 about the prevalence and seriousness of sexual child abuse. Or was she thinking about her beloved Ferenczi (everyone seemed to love Ferenczi – he evidently had an open and warm nature that attracted patients and analysts alike), who suffered complete disgrace when he gave his paper in 1932 about the reality of child abuse? Freud turned away from him, as did his analysand Ernest Jones, and all of Freud's colleagues, and he died a few months later, at 59, a broken and lonely man.

In short: These were not merely minor squabbles about the history of psychoanalysis. We are talking about the very fundamentals of human society.

I found it difficult to understand why so many people who heard me speak about these matters before my book was published were so eager to attack me personally. I remember in particular, one incident in Munich. A friend (!) who was a child psychiatrist asked me to give a paper to the Department of Psychiatry at the University of Munich. I chose to speak about Ferenczi. This was the first time that

I would be quoting the unpublished letters, and I assumed there would be great interest. After all, here was new information about Ferenczi, his relationship with Freud, his views about child abuse, and his death. There was also new information about many of the analysts close to Freud, Ernest Jones, Max Eitingon, and about the Berlin psychoanalysts. This was not about *me*. I made it clear that it was not my research diligence that had turned up these letters: Anna Freud presented them to me as a gift, as it were. I was just lucky, and in the right place at the right time, asking the right questions. But that was all irrelevant. The importance was that here were new letters, letters of striking historical *and* current importance, about the reality of child sexual abuse, and how hard it was for even psychiatrists (*especially psychiatrists* I now believe) to accept this reality and to adjust their own practices accordingly. There might well be differences of opinion on these matters, but it would be impossible to overlook the importance of the documents themselves, the previously unknown even unsuspected letters. I expected a lively discussion.

Instead, my "friend" in the chair, who I had gone skiing with in the Austrian Alps the week before, was nearly apoplectic with rage. He openly accused me of being paranoid (for what? I guess for believing the women who accused the men), and of disgracing psychoanalysis. Or rather, *I* was the disgrace. He reminded the audience that in Germany, a person could be incarcerated in a mental hospital if two psychiatrists insisted that he was a danger to himself and to others. I was such a person. He asked for another psychiatrist in the audience to join him in having me committed. When I understood that he was not joking, it was a terrible experience for me, and completely beyond my understanding. Embarrassed by his outburst, nobody supported him. I never saw him again or spoke with him. I am sorry because I would love to know what he thinks today. I was so naive as to believe that this was a completely personal matter, it was a one-off and unlikely to be repeated. Maybe, I thought, it had something to do with me being Jewish and this being Germany.

I was wrong. I had, to varying degrees, the same experience whenever I came to speak about the letters Anna Freud had given me access to and the research I had been doing as a result. I should not entirely accuse myself of having found nothing new on my own. I did track down the reason why Freud had stated that he saw things in the Paris morgue "of which science preferred to take no notice" (Masson, 1984, p. 33). I had asked Anna Freud what her father meant by this comment, and she could throw no light on it. So, I visited the Paris morgue and looked at the records for the day that Freud visited, and discovered that a case had been presented, with Freud present, of a child who had been raped and murdered. *That* is what Freud was referring to. I believe Anna Freud believed this was possible. Certainly, no other explanation has come to light.

I met Bruno Bettelheim quite by accident in the hills of Palo Alto, next to Stanford University. I was walking with an elderly German woman friend, and we had lost our way, when a man came along. As soon as he spoke, we both realized it must be Bruno Bettelheim (I had heard him lecture). We introduced ourselves, and he indicated that he knew something about me, and would I tell him about the unpublished Freud/Fliess letters that Anna Freud had given me to translate and publish. Yes, I replied, and knowing that he was familiar with German literature, I told him that one of the letters contained a remarkable quote from the great German poet Goethe and read: "Poor child, what have they done to you?" Freud told Fliess that this quote should be the motto of psychoanalysis. "Is that not interesting?" I asked Bettelheim. "Not at all," he said and continued on his way.

A very similar incident happened to me when I met Erik Erikson. I had criticized a paper he had written about Gandhi, but I don't believe he would have remembered this, although it is never a good idea to underestimate a writer's ego. I quoted the same passage I had to Bettelheim, for the very same reasons, and this time he answered: "You will no doubt use this quote as the title of your book, merely in order to wound poor Anna Freud." As you can see, it still feels troubling to this day that these two prominent analysts (actually there is considerable doubt about Bettelheim's credentials) would reject me out of hand as being a mean-spirited upstart. They would not engage with the ideas, only with me, of whom they seriously disapproved.

Some reviewers were critical that the first edition of "The Assault on Truth" did not acknowledge the writings of relevant feminist authors, such as Florence Rush, Diana Russell, and Judith Herman. (In later editions, I corrected this.) But my contribution was different: I was bringing to the argument *new* documents, mostly in the form of letters from Freud, that gave us a completely different and deeper sense of what was happening at the time. The feminists were not wrong, but they were arguing from a theoretical and clinical point of view, which was fine. I was looking at documents and historical moments. Our views and strategies are complementary. I was not trying to usurp their work and claim priority. I was delighted with their work, as I was with Ferenczi, and Robert Fliess, and anyone else who told the truth.

In attempting to understand why Anna Freud allowed me to see all the unpublished Freud/Fliess letters, I think that one incident stands out. Ernest Jones, Freud's biographer, wrote that Freud was deeply disappointed in his mentor, the popular Viennese physician Josef Breuer. To prove this, Jones (1953) quoted one of the unpublished letters that Anna Freud allowed him to see. In "The Life and Work of Sigmund Freud," Vol. 1, p. 255, Jones states,

> In February [1896] he wrote to the latter [Fliess] that it was impossible to get on any longer with Breuer, though only a week later he admitted that it was painful to think that Breuer was so entirely out of his life. A year later he was glad he saw no more of him; the very sight would make him inclined to emigrate.

As Jones noted: "These are strong words." They are indeed, but they were not written by Freud. Somehow, and I do not know how it came about, Jones completely misunderstood the words that Freud wrote about Breuer. He wrote on 29 March 1897, "How fortunate that I no longer see Breuer. He would surely have advised me to emigrate" (Masson, 1985, p. 233) (Here is the German original: Welch ein Gluck dass ich Breuer nicht mehr sehe; er haette mir schon geraten auszuwandern). When I showed Anna Freud the German original letter and Jones' mistranslation, she was very upset. But she did thank me for finding the error.

I think she then realized that there could be other matters in those letters that would provide a deeper understanding of the early Freud.

The larger question is this: were the new letters and documents I was presenting to psychoanalysts the source of the antagonism to me on a personal level? Was it that I was simply not the right messenger? Was it the message? Was it the sense that they had been wrong about child abuse all those years? I think there can be no doubt that many analysts (I cannot say all, but I know of very few exceptions) dismissed their female patients' accounts of sexual abuse as fantasy. They believed they were following Freud's historical progress. He had believed them in the beginning and soon claimed to realize he had made a serious error. Correcting that error, he wrote, allowed him to see the power of unconscious fantasies, the universality of the Oedipus complex, and even penis envy and castration anxiety, all pillars of psychoanalytic theory then and possibly even in many psychoanalytic schools now.

I was suggesting that the existence of these new letters called all that into question. Maybe it was the fact that I did not really have skin in the game. After all, I had not yet begun my analytic practice, so I had no embarrassing retractions to make to my female patients. They did. Who wants that? I know that Kurt Eissler, the director of the Freud Archives, and dear friend of Anna Freud, to whom I owed my career up to that point, felt betrayed at a deeply personal level. It was almost like an omerta issue within the Mafia. I had turned. I was on the other side. I was a traitor. This was a view widely shared by analysts, even my closest friends. It came as a shock to me. My closest friend at the time, Charles Hanly (later to become president of the IPA), would no longer speak to me, explaining: "Our friendship was based on a mutual respect for Sigmund Freud." Other friends were quick to announce their distrust of me. Some would even cross the street so as not to be seen in my presence. It was a very odd experience. Many senior analysts, who had previously supported me, fell away: Victor Calef and Edward Weinshel in San Francisco would no longer speak with me. Even to this day, I find this difficult to understand. After all, I would tell myself, it is not as if psychoanalysis is a church, with Freud as the pope, and me a heretic. But I suppose that to many in the field, I was the Anti-Christ. It felt weird then. It still does now.

Perhaps if I had simply published all the letters I had been given without any explanation or analysis, the intellectual storm would not have overtaken me. Possibly I should have asked Anna Freud herself to be the co-author of anything I would write about the letters. But I could not see how I could publish these letters without comment when they were of such electrifying significance to anyone who had been traumatized as a child. It would have been intellectual dereliction. Mind you, when it came to publishing the complete letters of Freud to Fliess, that is exactly what I did. They were published by Harvard University Press, and I made certain that it was a scholarly publication, with minimum personal comments by me, except for the text of the letters themselves. But even that was not enough: the letters were hardly reviewed, even within psychoanalysis. The original edition of the letters by Marie Bonaparte, Anna Freud, and Ernst Kris published in 1950 in German, and in 1954 in English, did not contain the 163 letters that she deemed "purely personal in nature and without historical or scientific interest." But there were still reviews that claimed they preferred the earlier edition, *without* the new letters. The new letters were simply a distraction.

They were not.

The Truth-Teller's "Fate?"

When he delivered his paper about child abuse to his male colleagues on 21 April 1896, Freud was met with disbelief, derision, and contempt. In 1932, when Sandor Ferenczi attempted to convince Freud and other analysts that the sexual abuse of children was common and hardly a fantasy, he was dismissed as mentally unstable by his colleagues, and even by his own analysands, such as Freud's biographer Ernest Jones, and the paper was ridiculed. Robert Fliess, the son of Freud's erstwhile closest friend, Wilhelm Fliess, was basically hounded out of the prestigious New York Psychoanalytic Institute and forced to move to Upstate New York, for writing about the abuse he experienced from his father, and arguing that fantasies cannot create illness, that is reserved for memories, especially memories of traumatic abuse that have been forced into repression. Warwick Middleton asked me how I could be so certain that I would not meet the same fate that befell each of these men for sharing ideas about the importance of child maltreatment for psychological distress?

My answer is that I was naive. I was not nearly as important as these three psychoanalysts, and I did not see how anyone could direct blame onto me for providing letters that Anna Freud made available to me. She not only made them available, but she also gave me permission to translate *and* publish them. She went further: she agreed to my being one of the three directors of the Freud Copyright (along with the late Masud Khan, an analyst in London, and the late Mark Paterson, an English lawyer). Yet a further step: she agreed that I could move into her house in London, in Maresfield Gardens, after her death, and turn it into a research centre.

Of course, I was aware of the fate of the first two analysts who dared to speak about child sexual abuse. But I don't believe I knew the whole story of Robert Fliess until I met his widow after my book was published. But even had I known all this, and even had I known that I would soon lose my directorship of the Freud Copyright; be fired as the Projects Director of the Sigmund Freud Archives; lose my access to the Freud House, and further, have my membership in the Toronto, the Canadian, and the international psychoanalytic institutes cancelled, I *still* would have published the material. I cannot see how I could do otherwise: the letters Anna Freud gave me access to were of enormous importance to women. They shed completely new light on the origins of trauma. How could I hold back that information, merely because it would affect my personal career? Would I do the same thing today? The answer is a resounding Yes!

I do admit that I was naive in the sense that I could not believe that such a torrent of abuse would come down on my head, given that Anna Freud herself allowed me to publish these letters. She knew what was in them. She knew the effect that publishing them would have on the analytic community. She knew that I did not share her belief or the belief of almost all analysts at the time (the 1970s and 1980s) that abuse was in the minds of patients and not in their reality. But she also believed that I should be allowed to make my case in publishing my book and the letters. At no point did she ask me *not* to publish. She did not believe that what I did was a betrayal either of her personally or of the wider analytic community. That belief was held by Eissler, Masud Khan, and other senior analysts around the world (especially, it would seem, in France). I am not sure why Eissler was so upset, since he too, like Anna Freud, knew what I found and what I thought about the material I had found. We may have disagreed, but he too never asked me not to publish. He told me that he felt I had betrayed "the family," but this argument did not impress me. For me, a family is your own, not an institution. I had no obligation to hold back documents that *might* reflect badly on early analysts (even on Freud) if by so doing I distorted the historical psychoanalytic record. I still believe I told the truth and that the truth was important and could not be covered up. I have no regrets.

References

Bonaparte, M., Freud, A. & Kris, E. (Eds) (1954). *The origins of psycho-analysis: Letters to Wilhelm Fliess, drafts and notes: 1887–1902 by Sigmund Freud.* Basic Books.

Borch-Jacobsen, M. (2021). *Freud's patients: A book of lives*. Reaktion Books.

Fenichel, O. (1946). *The psychoanalytic theory of neuroses.* Routledge.

Ferenczi, S. (1932/1984). Confusion of tongues between adults and the child. In J. Masson (translated by Masson, J. & Loring, M.) *The assault on truth: Freud's suppression of the seduction theory* (283–295). Farrar, Straus & Giroux.

Jones, E. (1953). *The life and work of Sigmund Freud.* Vol. 1, Basic Books.

Masson, J. (1984). *The assault on truth: Freud's suppression of the seduction theory*. Farrar, Straus & Giroux.

Masson, J. (1985). *The complete letters of Sigmund Freud to Wilhelm Fliess*, 1887–1904. Harvard University Press.

Masson, J. (1991). *Final analysis: The making and unmaking of a psychoanalyst.* Addison-Wesley.

Masson, T. C. (2019). *My Kaddish: Memoir of a childhood in the Warsaw Ghetto*. Holocaust Museum in Sydney.

Middleton, W. (2018). Robert Fliess, Wilhelm Fliess, Ernest Jones, Sándor Ferenczi and Sigmund Freud – ISSTD President's editorial, In W. Middleton, A. Sachs, & M. J. Dorahy (Eds.), *The abused and the abuser: Victim – perpetrator dynamics* (234–250). Routledge.

2 Sándor Ferenczi, Robert Fliess, Florence Rush, and Jeffrey Masson

Warwick Middleton

I started training in psychiatry in 1980. Two significant books were published that year: the *DSM-III* and the third edition of the *Comprehensive Textbook of Psychiatry*. The *DSM-III* provided operationalized criteria for diagnosing post-traumatic stress disorder (PTSD) and multiple personality disorder, which advanced our understanding of interpersonal trauma. The *Comprehensive Textbook of Psychiatry* assigned incest, as with the previous edition, a prevalence in the order of one in a million (Henderson, 1980), which thus spectacularly undermined our understanding of interpersonal trauma. In my training in psychiatry, it was apparent that prevailing paradigms stretched the concepts of schizophrenia, bipolar disorder, depression, and borderline personality disorder to cover most functional psychiatric illness. Yet, even back then, I had the troubling sense that I was not understanding much about the presentations of individuals who displayed rapid changes in their mental state, and even in those unenlightened days, seemed to have been heavily traumatized.

Nothing was taught in my psychiatry training about dissociation, yet on reflection I was repeatedly encountering it – never more graphically than on an occasion in 1982 in the acute admission ward of the asylum-style hospital in which I trained. This incident involved "Stella", a young woman with a diagnosis of "schizophrenia" and even in an era where such matters were not routinely focussed on, a history of extensive sexual abuse. "Jim" was a male nurse, friendly, mild-mannered, hard-working, professional, and likeable. On this particular afternoon, I was nearby when "Stella" was passing "Jim" in the corridor. Suddenly she screamed, "I don't fuck dogs!" as she deeply scratched "Jim" across his face with her fingernails, drawing blood. He leapt at her, wrapping both his hands around her throat, and brought her crashing down. His grip on her throat was unrelenting and his expression glazed. "Jim!", I yelled. There was no response. I knelt beside them. "Jim! Jim!" "Stella" was speechless, unable to breathe and looking alarmed. I pulled his hands from her throat as he slowly began to reorientate, though for a time remained dazed and uncommunicative. Looking back, I would now say that the most likely explanation for what happened was that both individuals were overtaken by a dissociative switch, occurring seconds apart.

DOI: 10.4324/9781003431466-3

Towards the end of my training, as a 29-year-old registrar, I became what I subsequently learned was a "whistle-blower", when I sent to my Regional Director of Health, a 120-page submission detailing extensive abuse, incompetence, and corruption within the hospital in which I trained, which ultimately lead to the medical superintendent and director of nursing being dismissed. Around the same time in late 1983, I chanced upon a two-instalment *New Yorker* article written by Janet Malcolm titled, *Trouble in the Archives: The rise and fall of an unorthodox Freud scholar* which were subsequently published in book form titled, *In the Freud Archives* (1984). In a racy, readable, extended piece of journalism, Malcolm traced the origins of the unusual relationship between Kurt Eissler, the doyen of American psychoanalysis, and the much younger Sanskrit scholar and trainee analyst, Jeffrey Masson.

In keeping with the engaging style of the article, Malcolm, who would subsequently become embroiled long-term in litigation that was initiated by Masson, characterized things by observing,

> In contrast to the gradually and cautiously developing, and never totally satisfying, friendship of Anna Freud and Eissler, the friendship of Jeffrey Masson and Eissler took off like a rocket. When they met in Denver in 1974, the sixty-six-year-old analyst and the thirty-three-year-old candidate immediately hit it off.

She explored their personalities and their relationship, observing,

> Eissler, incredibly, held back no part of himself, refused Masson nothing, loved him quite beyond all expectation. He gave him the greatest gift that it was in his power to bestow, he arranged to make him his successor as Secretary of the Freud Archives. And Masson, in return, fitted himself to the image that Eissler had formed of him. That things should have ended so badly between them was probably inevitable.
>
> (Malcolm, 1983, p. 13)

On October 11, 1984, having read Malcolm's extended article, I bought a first edition copy of Masson's book, *The Assault on Truth* for $26.95.

No doubt Masson, in his appointment to the Archives, had been the focus of professional envy and resentment, with one senior analyst confronting him publicly with:

> I just want to ask one question. Why you? Who's ever heard of you? We never heard of you. You're not famous. You haven't written much. You're a nobody. Why should you get all these privileges and we get nothing?
>
> (Malcolm, 1984, p. 20)

Masson's contemporaries at the time saw little positive in his motives for re-examining Freud's relationship with the "seduction theory". They then piled on, to denounce him in print, once he openly became one of a small group, dating from Sándor Ferenczi in the 30s, Robert Fliess in the 50s and 60s, and Florence Rush in the 70s, who had publicly questioned the basis Freud had for rejecting his original theory regarding a childhood sexual abuse aetiology for hysteria (Freud, 1896b).

These four leading critics of Freud's essential abandonment of what in time became known as his "seduction theory" are a diverse grouping, but no one can doubt that each had "skin in the game".

Sándor Ferenczi, himself abused as a child, was an analyst and ex-President of the International Psycho-Analytic Association (IPA). He had the largest correspondence with Freud (their correspondence extended to some 1,250 letters), and one who, like a younger Freud, sought to corroborate the accounts of childhood sexual abuse of his patients. Like many of the early analysts, he became messily embroiled in substantial sexual boundary transgressions, exemplified by being emotionally involved with a psychologically unstable young woman, Elma, his patient, who was the daughter of a woman (Gizella Pálos) with whom he had been conducting an affair and whom he ultimately married in 1919, after referring Elma to Freud, and subsequent to this short analysis, taking Elma back into analysis himself (Gabbard & Lester, 1996).

Robert Fliess' father, Wilhelm, was outwardly a successful doctor and respectable member of his community, albeit one with some unusual ideas about a male periodic cycle equivalent to the female menstrual cycle and what he called the "nasal reflex neurosis", a condition he believed curable by nasal surgery. He was for 15 years Freud's closest friend. His son, Robert Fliess, served in World War I (earning an Iron Cross), completed his medical and psychoanalyst training in Berlin, and in 1933 moved to the USA where he practised as a psychoanalyst in New York (Fliess, 1982). Sexually abused, it is likely by his own father, a man who was Freud's closest professional confidant during the years in which he developed both his seduction theory and his theory of Oedipal fantasy, Robert Fliess worked extensively with abused patients who had suffered childhood physical and sexual abuse, and he became increasingly combatively direct in confronting the theories of his father's erstwhile friend, Sigmund Freud.

Florence Rush was a clear-thinking social worker assisting abused women and girls and was herself sexually abused as a child. What is striking about Rush is how well, in the absence of the additional Freud documents that Masson had access to, she makes an articulate case, which ultimately Freud, himself a product of misogynist Victorian society, fell in line with a general societal dynamic of disbelieving sexually abused women and girls, and silencing them with shame. Put simply, she argued that Freud's rationale for abandoning the "seduction theory", analysed from the level of basic logic, wasn't credible (Rush, 1977).

Jeffrey Masson, who was brought up in a household with a live-in charlatan mystic, was clearly talented, and not someone to unquestioningly accept dogma. He was a language scholar, and a prolific writer, with lived experience of debunking false narratives. He was given a unique opportunity – access to Freud's unpublished letters to Wilhelm Fliess, written in German.

I am struck by how much we don't allow ourselves to see. Ferenczi in 1932 observed,

> Even children of highly respected, high-minded puritanical families fall victim to real rape much more frequently than one had dared to suspect. Either the parents themselves seek substitution for their lack of [sexual] satisfaction in this pathological manner, or else trusted persons such as relatives (uncles, aunts, grandparents), tutors, servants, abuse the ignorance and innocence of children. The obvious objection that we are dealing with sexual fantasies of the child himself, that is, with hysterical lies, unfortunately is weakened by the multitude of confessions of this kind, on the part of patients in analysis, to assaults on children.
>
> (Masson, 1984 p. 227)

Congruent with Ferenczi's observations, Robert Fliess in 1956 observed that,

> amnesia removal uncovers much more frequently than Freud's writings lead one to expect, memories of which there can be no doubt as to their authenticity, yet which are of so bizarre a nature that, if one followed the general trend in these writings, one would declare them – erroneously – as fantasies of the polymorphously perverse child. Finding this, I found also the cause. It lies in the unbelievable frequency of the (undiagnosed) ambulatory psychosis. When one is able to diagnose it, one sees relatively few families of one's patients that are entirely free of it; and one recognises that the patient in need of a long and thorough analysis would appear to be, by and large, someone who had been damaged by and has identified with a psychotic parent… I can therefore say only in passing that the child of such a parent becomes the object of substantially defused aggression (maltreated and beaten almost to within an inch of his life), and of a perverse sexuality that hardly knows an incest barrier (is seduced in the most bizarre ways by the parent and, at his instigation, by others.
>
> (p. xvii)

In his last book Robert Fliess (1973) observed,

> If you remove the amnesia for early traumata in your patients who come from different walks of life and have never so much as seen each other, you are told over and over by each of them, to the point of tragic monotony, of their abuse as a child.
>
> (p. 224)

What Robert Fliess meant by "ambulatory psychosis" was a person like his father. He observed that the ambulatory psychotic "*is distinguished by such an excellent contact with reality that he is able to keep secret his psychotic life*" (1973, p. 221, italics added). Robert Fliess had an extended conversation with Freud himself about his onetime friend. Robert's wife, Elenore, described her father-in-law as a man "who however charming to patients and acquaintances was a tyrant at home. His children were second-class citizens, from diet to schooling" (E. Fliess, 1974, p. 10).

Psychoanalyst Bennett Simon, initially affronted by Masson's thesis that Freud had made a major error in abandoning his seduction hypothesis, reviewed all the relevant psychoanalytic literature and concluded,

> Neither Freud, nor, to my knowledge, any other analyst, publishes a case wherein a woman, not psychotic, told of an incestuous relationship with the father and then in the course of the treatment it turned out to be a fantasy!
>
> (Simon, 1992, pp. 968–969)

It has become increasingly apparent that there are many like Freud's close friend, Wilhelm Fliess and Freud's grandson, Clement Freud (exposed as a child sex offender after his death in 2009), in our world: charming, talented, personable, affluent, well-connected, and closely associated with at least several of our most powerful institutions and frequently on good terms with our national leaders. And there are not-so-charming examples of extremely narcissistic individuals who capture disturbing and violent populist followings, proclaiming ahead of time what they will do when they seize the levers of power. Some of the population cling to the rationalization, that once in office, such individuals (whether they be Adolf Hitler or Donald Trump) will ameliorate their extreme ambitions. Some practise appeasement, others do not.

Ferenczi and Robert Fliess seem to have tellingly developed an appreciation of something missed by so many of their peers, and that is the frequency with which seemingly respectable members of society, conduct their abuses in plain sight, aided by an unwillingness on the part of society to know. Both Ferenczi and Robert Fliess were seriously marginalized. Ferenczi was incorrectly portrayed by Ernest Jones, his previous analysand, as declining into a regressed paranoid delusional state prior to his death (Jones, 1961), while Robert Fliess was effectively forced out of the New York Psychoanalytic Society. His widow would write to Dr. Milton Klein that because of his views, Fliess, who ended his career in professional isolation, was relieved of teaching a course at the New York Psychoanalytic Institute (see Lothane, 2001). Ernest Jones, who had a very problematic history on matters relating to sexual boundaries, had himself in 1906 been credibly charged after four disabled children (three girls and a boy) attending Edward St School, in southeast London, accused him of sexual abuse (Maddox, 2006).

Freud's seduction theory

Florence Rush (1977), in a clearly articulated paper, made the very salient point that in addition to her own case evidence,

> Freud certainly realized that his Victorian world was notorious for its sexual license, particularly in the sexual abuse of children. He could not have avoided

> news scandals exposing the existence of large numbers of children in the brothels of Europe, the active international white-slave traffic in children, or the available statistics on increased sex crimes against children.
>
> (p. 266)

Josef Breuer's famous patient, Bertha Pappenheim, was to establish a national reputation as a campaigner against the sex trafficking of women and girls.

In Freud's retraction of his "seduction" theory it is particularly puzzling, and implausible, that all 18 (12 female, 6 male) of the individuals he described in The Aetiology of Hysteria (1896) required very lengthy psychoanalytic assessments to uncover the childhood sexual abuse origins of their "hysteria", yet in other of his accounts, patients with no substantial difficulty simply told him of similar such abuses in response to gentle enquiry.

In his earlier 1896 paper, "Further Remarks on the Neuro-Psychosis of Defence", Freud includes a preliminary analysis of 13 cases of individuals with hysteria, all with what he describes as a "severe" illness of many years' duration. Amidst his report, he states,

> In one of my cases a brother, a sister, and a somewhat older male cousin were all of them ill. From the analysis which I carried out on the brother, I learned that he was suffering from self-reproaches for being the cause of his sister's illness. He himself had been seduced by his cousin, and the latter, it was known in the family, had been the victim of his nursemaid.
>
> (p. 165)

So confronting was directly mentioning the issue of paternal incest, that despite taking on the role of the singular enlightened discoverer, Freud used editorial licence on occasions to change the descriptor of the abuser.

Close to this passage by Freud, the editor of the 1962 Standard Edition, James Strachey, feels compelled in a footnote to paraphrase a version of the prevailing psychoanalytic doctrine of the time:

> I myself am inclined to think that the stories of being assaulted which hysterics so frequently invent may be obsessional fictions which arise from the memory trace of a childhood trauma.
>
> (p. 164)

One is obliged to ask – "What is an *obsessional fiction*? What is a *memory trace of a childhood trauma* that isn't related to a trauma?"

The disparaging way in which Strachey describes individuals suffering with "hysteria" takes one back to a 29-year-old Freud who with feeling stated,

> During the last few decades a hysterical woman would have been almost as certain to be treated as a malingerer, as in earlier centuries she would have been certain to be judged and condemned as a witch or as possessed by the devil …In

> the out-patient department in Berlin, however, I found that ... when a diagnosis of "hysteria" had been made, all inclination to take any further notice of the patient seemed to be suppressed.
>
> (Freud, 1886/2001, pp. 11–12)

Before Masson had made Freud's paper, The Aetiology of Hysteria a cornerstone of his 1984 book, Herman and Hirschman in their 1981 landmark book observed:

> At the origin of every case of hysteria, Freud asserted, was a childhood sexual trauma. But Freud was never comfortable with this discovery, because of what it implied about the behavior of respectable family men. If his patients' reports were true, incest was not a rare abuse, confined to the poor and the mentally defective, but was endemic to the patriarchal family. Recognizing the implicit challenge to patriarchal values, Freud refused to identify fathers publicly as sexual aggressors. Though in his private correspondence he cited "seduction by the father" as the "essential point" in hysteria, he was never able to bring himself to make this statement in public. Scrupulously honest and courageous in other respects, Freud falsified his incest cases. In "The Aetiology of Hysteria", Freud implausibly identified governesses, nurses, maids, and children of both sexes as the offenders. In Studies in Hysteria, he managed to name an uncle as the seducer in two cases. Many years later, Freud acknowledged that the "uncles" who had molested [his patients] Rosalia and Katharina were in fact their fathers.
>
> (p. 9)

Rush noted Freud's need to protect fathers and had congruently wondered at Freud categorizing similar-aged siblings as most frequently being responsible for creating sexual trauma, along with contributions from nurses, maids, governesses, and teachers. She observed multiple inconsistencies.

> This large category of predominantly female offenders did not fit the illness in question. Hysteria was primarily a female affliction (a "male hysteric" was hard to find), and the sexual assaults Freud mentioned were heterosexual. Furthermore, in general discussion of sexual assault and hysteria, he always referred to the abuse of children by adults. Suddenly to claim that the largest number of offenders came from among children of the same age was a contradiction.
>
> (p. 267)

Freud (1896b) observed that in 2 of his 13 hysteria cases the sexual abuse had started in the child's second year. He also stated,

> The commonest in my observation is the fourth or fifth year. It may be somewhat by accident, but I have formed an impression from this that a passive sexual experience occurring only after the age of eight to ten is no longer able to serve as the foundation of the neurosis.
>
> (pp. 152–153)

Freud is right on the money. Putnam (1997) quoted Bronfenbrenner Life Course Centre research indicating that the highest risk for sexual abuse to females occurs at about three to four years of age. Writing in 2007, Julian Sher in his book, *Caught in the Web* stated, "Nowadays, almost half – 39% – of the victims of child porn identified by the National Centre for Missing and Exploited Children (NCMEC) are under the age of five" (p. 270). The clinical consensus in the dissociative disorders field is that the ongoing sexual or other trauma that occasion dissociative identity disorder must have started before around the age of eight.

In presenting his paper, "The Aetiology of Hysteria", on April 21, 1896, Freud advanced his thesis

> that at the bottom of every case of hysteria there are *one or more occurrences of premature sexual experience*, occurrences which belong to the earliest years of childhood, but which can be reproduced through the work of psychoanalysis in spite of the intervening decades.
>
> (p. 203)

It seems that in all 18 cases of hysteria subjected to Freud's investigation and treatment, his patients reportedly initially had amnesia for their sexual abuse. But progressively in every case, over a period of what might have been more than 100 hours of analytic therapy, the patient recovered memories of their childhood sexual abuse. Freud, leading up to this time, was mostly employing the technique of applying pressure with his hands on the patient's forehead to somehow overcome their resistance to producing the required memories (Schimek, 1986). This technique overlapped with his gradual introduction of free association. In two cases, Freud was able to obtain objective confirmation of the abuse memories that had presented themselves. To quote Freud:

> In one instance, it was the brother (who had remained well) who of his own accord confirmed – not, it is true, his earliest sexual experience with his sister (who was the patient) – but at least scenes of that kind from later childhood, and the fact that there had been sexual relations dating further back. In the other instance, it happened that two women whom I was treating had as children sexual relations with the same man, in the course of which certain scenes had taken place à trois. A particular symptom, which was derived from these childhood events, had developed in both women, as evidence of what they had experienced in common.
>
> (p. 206)

Freud withdrew from his "seduction" theory, at first privately in his letter to Wilhelm Fliess on September 21, 1897, and then publicly on subsequent occasions, in what taken together, represent a somewhat contradictory set of utterances up to 1933. But on December 22, 1897, he famously had second thoughts about abandoning his seduction theory when confronted with the account of a patient who as a three-year-old experienced a sadistic rape (Masson, 1984, pp. 116–117).

Yet, Freud never once offered an alternative explanation for those particular cases of child sexual abuse that he described in 1896, which he had presented with substantive corroboration that he himself had assembled. Five months prior to his retraction, and just a week after presenting "The Aetiology of Hysteria", on April 28, 1897, Freud in a letter to Wilhelm Fliess stated that,

> a lucky chance this morning brought confirmation of my theory of paternal aetiology. Yesterday I started treatment of a new case, a young woman whom for lack of time I should have liked to have frightened off. She had a brother who died insane and her chief symptom – insomnia – dates from the time she heard the carriage driving away from the house taking him to the asylum. Since then, she had been terrified of carriage drives and convinced that an accident was going to happen. Years later, while she was out driving, the horses shied, and she took the opportunity to jump from the carriage and break a leg. To-day she came and said she had been thinking over the treatment and had found an obstacle. "What is it?" "I can paint myself as black as necessary, but I must spare other people. You must allow me to mention no names." "What you mean is your relationship with the people concerned. We can't draw a veil over that." "What I mean is that earlier in the treatment would have been easier for me than now, earlier I didn't suspect it, but now the criminal nature of certain things has become clear to me, and I can't make up my mind to talk about them." "On the contrary, I should say that a mature woman becomes more tolerant in sexual matters." "Yes, there you're right. When I consider that the most excellent and high-principled men are guilty of these things, I'm compelled to think it's an illness, a kind of madness and I have to excuse them." "Then let's speak plainly. In my analyses I find it's the closest relatives, fathers, or brothers, who are the guilty men." "It has nothing to do with my brother." "So, it was your father, then".
>
> Then it came out that when she was between the ages of eight and twelve her allegedly otherwise admirable and high-principled father used to regularly take her into his bed and practice external ejaculation (making wet) with her. Even at the time she felt anxiety. A six-year-older sister to whom she talked about it later admitted that she had had the same experiences with her father. A cousin told her that at the age of fifteen she had had to resist the advances of her grandfather. Naturally she did not find it incredible when I told her that similar and worse things must have happened to her in infancy. In other respects, hers is a quite ordinary hysteria with usual symptoms.
>
> (Freud, 1897/1954, pp. 195–196)

In reading this account (which pre-dated Masson's more comprehensive translation in 1985), we find that Freud had laid out for him within two sessions, salient details of the activities of an incestuous father, an incestuous grandfather, and three female victims. This was quite unlike the many hours of psychoanalysis invested in his earlier hysteria patients before he appreciated the impact of abuse on psychic functioning (e.g., with the 18 patients described in "The Aetiology of Hysteria", he claimed his "laborious individual examination" [p. 220] in most cases had taken up 100 or more hours of work). Yet in this case where no particular effort is made with memory recovery, he describes the woman as having "quite ordinary hysteria". In this patient's account we see evidence of the shame and self-hate so commonly seen in victims of incestuous abuse and a focus on self-blame, while her father's abuse is excused as an "illness" in an otherwise high-principled man. Freud seemingly did nothing more than sympathetically and intuitively respond when his patient spontaneously brought up for discussion her "obstacle". He didn't hypnotize her, have her free-associate or press forcibly on her forehead. Her account seems to have flowed quite readily as soon as she deduced that her listener understood the nature of her sensitivity and was very familiar with the origins of the sorts of trauma she reported. Freud clearly believed that the nature of symptomatology indicated additional sexual trauma dating from infancy, a proposition his patient, even at that early stage, took seriously. To turn this patient's account into fiction, a product of "Oedipal fantasy", would as Rush points out (1977), require "mental acrobatics".

There was nothing remotely vague about the way Katharina's story was assembled and indeed the account of her incestuous abuse involving her father (initially described in Freud's account as her "uncle"). The history was elicited in a single impromptu consultation with Freud on a mountain top in August 1893. There was simply no time in which to cultivate a transference-laden therapeutic relationship, or the progressive elicitation of vague early childhood memories created by the active progression of Oedipal fantasy. Detective work by Peter Swales, Gerhart Fichtner, and Albrecht Hirschmüller (see Appignanesi & Forrester, 1993) established Katharina to be Aurelia Kronich. As recounted to Freud, Katharina's mother did believe her daughter's account of her father establishing a sexual relationship with Katharina's young cousin and did move with her children to a new lodge across the valley from the one her husband then occupied with Katharina's cousin, with whom he had two children born in 1896 and 1897. In 1919 or 1920 Katharina's war-traumatized son had a consultation with Freud.

Freud had been the first person in history to publicly proclaim a child sexual abuse theory for hysteria and by extension draw attention to the high frequency with which incest occurs in contemporary society. Then, in the absence of any new data to justify his change of stance, and without reference to cases he himself had corroborated, he announced in that now famous letter to Wilhelm Fliess on September 21, 1897 that he no longer believed in his "neurotica (theory of neuroses)" (Freud, 2001, p. 259). This occurred within 28 months of the publication of "Studies on Hysteria" and 17 months since publicly giving his paper on "The Aetiology of Hysteria" in Vienna to the Society for Psychiatry and Neurology. Freud's reasoning to Fliess was that the prevalence of incestuous abuse by fathers would have to be "widespread" and much more frequent than the prevalence of hysteria, given that hysteria would only arise in susceptible individuals where there had been "an accumulation of events" (Freud, quoted in Masson 1985 p. 264)

Freud baulked at the idea that if his patients' accounts of sexual abuse by the father were to be believed, then such abuse would have to be widespread and well-represented in the middle-class environment in which he practised. Sacco

(2009) discovered that 19th-century Americans were familiar with allegations of father-daughter incest. She located more than 500 reports of father-daughter incest, published in more than 900 newspaper articles across the country, mostly between 1817 and 1899, which indicates that at the time Freud was examining the aetiology of hysteria, such matters, while not subjected to systematic study, existed in public and legal awareness. Masson (1984) also showed that Freud's time at the Paris morgue had made him intimately familiar with such abuse. The frequency of press reports suggested that father-daughter incest was not rare. Until the last quarter of the 19th century, such news reports most often identified "incest fiends" as respectable, even prominent white men, clergymen, local officials, etc. After the turn of the 20th century however the number of reports of father-daughter incest abruptly declined and Sacco was only able to locate 136 cases of father-daughter incest reported between 1900 and 1940, with more than half of this number occurring in the first decade of the 20th century.

The reason for the decline in such reports Sacco (2009) argues was due to a reversal in the aetiological understanding of how gonorrhoea was contracted. With improved medical technology gonorrhoea could be diagnosed with unprecedented accuracy, which uncomfortably led to the observation that gonorrhoea vulvovaginitis was "epidemic" among girls, including the daughters of white middle and upper classes. Even though knowledge about how gonorrhoea was contracted (i.e., via sexual contact) had been known for centuries, doctors baulked at concluding that respectable white Americans, even ones infected with gonorrhoea at the same time as their daughters could have spread their infection to them "in the usual manner". Finding that gonorrhoea, a sexually transmitted disease, was "epidemic" among all classes of girls – not just girls from socially marginalized families – healthcare professionals revised their views about gonorrhoea, not incest.

Mainstream psychoanalysis and psychiatry largely did not register the evidence before them. Even as late as the 60s there was a failure to appreciate how widespread severe child abuse was. When Leontine Young's book "Wednesday's Children: A Study of Child Neglect and Abuse" was published in 1964, the original data set of 120 families was supplemented by a second set of 180 families selected from seven different localities. Young found that viewing child neglect simply in terms of physical and psychological well-being was too general. She classified parental misconduct in terms of "severe neglect", "moderate neglect", "severe abuse", and "moderate abuse". As an example of these categories, according to Dr. Young, children who were starved, chained to a bed, or who were found in a cellar, caged like animals, and covered with insects would be considered "severely neglected".

Young's research began almost by accident, when on another project she read a cross section of case records in the public child welfare department of a small midwestern city and "discovered this nightmare world within a world" (p. 4). Young includes Robert Fliess in her bibliography. Given how low a profile child abuse had in the professional literature when Young was doing her research over half a century ago, it is interesting to see her quote the frequency with which child abuse surfaced in the lay press. She cites a then recent report of the Children's Division of the American Humane Association which found that there were 662 cases of child abuse reported in US newspapers from January through December of 1962. These 662 children came from 557 families. While they ranged in age from infancy through 17 years, barely 10% of them were over 10 years of age. Over 55% of the children were under four years of age. Of the 662 children, one in every four, or a total of 178, died because of parent-inflicted injuries. Over 80% of those killed were children under four.

Although not systemically explored, incest appeared common in Young's original group of 120 families. For example,

> [I]n another case the mother reported that the father had been sleeping with his pre-adolescent daughter for some time, and as she aptly pointed out, "it doesn't look nice." In this case the father defended himself by pointing out that the mother had been sleeping with the son.
>
> (Quoted in Fliess, 1962, p. 14)

Freud's free association technique developed very gradually between 1892 and 1895 (Jones, 1961). Though I have never heard it put this way, it seems to me that Freud, who discussed his findings regarding 18 patients with hysteria at the Vienna Society for Psychiatry and Neurology on April 21, 1896, was endeavouring to do by way of applying forehead pressure or "free association", what modern practitioners in the dissociative disorders field endeavour to do by identifying and speaking with "the voices" or alters. That is, they both work to allow the patient to access compartmentalized material, including trauma-based compulsions, and process their trauma in a safe environment that addresses shame, fear, and internal conflict, including tangled and trauma-laden attachments to familial abusers. One wonders what would have happened with Freud's early hysteria patients who clearly had been substantially unwell over an extended period of time, if instead of having them hypnotized, having pressure applied to their foreheads, or having them free associate for many sessions, once a workable therapeutic alliance had been established, he had simply, but empathically, asked them in a settled state, if they experienced gaps in their memory, heard voices or self-harmed, and if so, was there a part of them that could provide information about the various ailments, compulsions, emotions, intrusive images, or memory gaps that formed elements of their presentations?

The presentations of many contemporary patients fall in the complex trauma/dissociative identity disorder spectrum, and they frequently manifest the multiple somatic complaints associated with what used to be known as "hysteria" (Middleton & Butler, 1998). Occasionally such patients may have unusually broad amnesia, but most at the time of presentation have a fair bit of accessible information about their traumas, and a sense of what the gaps in their memory signify.

In their preliminary communications (1893), Breuer and Freud observed that:

> the splitting of consciousness which is so striking in the well-known classical cases under the form of "double conscience" is present to a rudimentary degree in every hysteria, and that a tendency to such a dissociation, and with it the

> emergence of abnormal states of consciousness (which we shall bring together under the term "hypnoid") is the basic phenomenon of this neurosis.
>
> (p. 12)

We know from Hirschmüller (1989) that Bertha Pappenheim, the subject of the first psychoanalytic case ever published, slashed herself with broken glass. We know from her physician, Josef Breuer, that she switched regularly between defined identity states. In 1895 Breuer wrote,

> Throughout the entire illness her two states of consciousness persisted side by side; the primary one in which she was quite normal physically, and the secondary one which may well be likened to a dream in view of its wealth of imaginative products and hallucinations, its large gaps of memory and the lack of inhibition and control in all its associations... It is hard to avoid expressing the situation by saying that the patient was split into two personalities of which one was mentally normal and the other insane... Not only did the second state intrude into the first one, but...even when she was in a very bad condition – a clear-sighted and calm observer sat, as she put it, in the corner of her brain and looked on at all the mad business.
>
> (pp. 45–46)

Breuer described his patient as "hallucinating" black snakes on occasions. He observed, "[t]he contrast between the irresponsible invalid by day, beset by hallucinations, and the perfectly lucid person at night-time, was most remarkable" (Hirschmüller, 1989, p. 285). Embracing the construct of repression, Freud had no use for Breuer's "hypnoid states", which he renounced prior to dispatching his seduction theory. In 1896 he wrote,

> For Breuer assumed – following Charcot – that even an innocuous experience can be heightened into a trauma and can develop determining force if it happens to the subject when he is in a special psychical condition – in what is described as a *hypnoid state*. I find, however, that there are often no grounds whatever for presupposing the presence of such hypnoid states.
>
> (Freud, 1896/2001, Vol. 3, pp. 194–195)

Many of Freud's early patients, who appear in his case studies, give the appearance of being highly dissociative. Freud's patient, Emmy Von N, aged around 40 when Freud began treatment in 1888 or 1889, had a history of past unsuccessful treatments. Freud noted that she complained about gaps in her memory – "especially about the most important events" (Breuer & Freud, 1895, p. 84). Freud described Emmy Von N as having experienced "numerous psychical traumas" which resulted in many years of chronic hysteria. He noted that her "remarkably well-stocked memory showed the most striking gaps" while his patient complained that it was as though her life was "chopped into pieces" (p. 70). It was noted Emmy Von N would at times alternate between states of "hysterical delirium" and normal consciousness. "The two states were separated in her memory, and she sometimes would be highly astonished to hear of the things which the delirium had introduced piecemeal into her normal conversation" (p. 97). On one occasion, the identity state encountered by Freud claimed to be a woman from the previous century. A quarter of a century after the completion of Freud's largely unsuccessful treatment, he was approached by Frau Emmy's daughter, a qualified doctor who informed Freud she was planning to take legal proceedings against her mother who she described as a cruel and ruthless tyrant who had broken off contact with both her children and had refused them financial assistance (Breuer & Freud, 1895, footnote, p. 105).

In 1925 Freud referred to his seduction theory as "an error into which I fell for a while, and which might well have had fatal consequences for the whole of my work". He goes on to conclude, "however, I was at last obliged to recognize that these scenes of seduction had never taken place, and that they were only fantasies which my patients had made up or which I myself had perhaps forced on them" (Freud, 1925, p. 31).

Freud's last summary of the seduction theory dates from 1933:

> In the period in which the main interest was directed to discovering infantile sexual traumas, almost all my women patients *told* me that they had been seduced by their *father*. I was driven to recognise in the end that these reports were untrue and so came to understand that hysterical symptoms are derived from phantasies and not real occurrences.
>
> (Freud, 1933, p. 120; italics added)

Roazen (2002) raises an important point with his observation that nowhere else in Freud's writings does Freud maintain that "almost all" his female patients had, without seemingly being subjected to some sort of truth-gathering process, simply "told" Freud of their "seduction" (as was the case with the woman he described on April 28, 1897, and as with Katharina who he met on vacation). Roazen explains that if Freud's original 1896 published account was accurate then his 1933 version was misleading. However, the contradictions do engender speculation, with Roazen (2002) noting, "[p]erhaps in 1896 he had over dramatized the resistances of his patients, in order to highlight the hypothesized underlying truth that he then wanted to propound" (p. 12). Roazen (2002) asks the question that if Freud was straightforwardly "told" about the seductions, why did he wait 37 years to finally reveal what happened? He gives an intriguing speculation:

> After repeatedly fudging matters, we are confronted with the starkly different 1933 claim… Like others with political objectives, it was for Freud to think that the end – the promotion of his "cause" – justified the means.
>
> (p. 12)

Yet, one of the biggest paradoxes regarding early psychoanalysts' relationship with Oedipal fantasy is the fact that so many of them had themselves been sexually abused as children. Included in this number are Carl Jung, who early in his relationship with Freud had revealed that as a boy he had been homosexually assaulted by a man he trusted (see McGuire, 1974), Otto Rank, abused as a seven-year-old (Breger, 2000, p. 311), Sándor Ferenczi, abused as a child by his mother and nursemaid (Goldwet, 1986; Rudnytsky, 1996), and Sigmund Freud himself, who wrote to Wilhelm Fliess (October 3 and 4, 1897) referring to his old childhood nurse, whom he termed "my teacher in sexual matters" (Masson, 1985, p. 269). (For a more complete discussion see Middleton, 2018 and Rachman, Chapter 3)

What systematic research into the largely hitherto unexplored topic of ongoing incest during adulthood has unequivocally proven is that the extreme and most traumatizing form of incest can be verified by court convictions to be a widespread international issue and that extreme paternal abusers such as Josef Fritzl are not one-off aberrations (Middleton, 2022). If many cases of such extreme forms of sadistic long-term incest can be proven without anyone invoking a defence relying on Oedipal fantasy, it indicates that we are looking at one (awful) end of the spectrum of incest-related abuse experiences. It makes no sense (leaving aside the many proven cases), that as we move to the left of the chart in the distribution of incest cases, that suddenly their cause is fantasy. (It was always perplexing in respect to Oedipal fantasy theory, that even if for some innate psychological reason, a child fantasized about having sex with the opposite sex parent, why they couldn't at least, make it a "pleasant fantasy" instead of one filled with threats, parental lies, and actual violence, including sadism directed at themselves and others.) Young adults might have sexual fantasies about pop singers, movie stars et al., but usually without incorporating a desire to be threatened, beaten, sodomized, and otherwise tortured. The prevalence of sexual abuse is hardly trivial. In a 2023 Australian survey, 37.3% of women and 18.8% of men reported they had experienced sexual abuse as children, and 12.5% of women and 4.3% of men reported penetrative abuse (Mathews et al., 2023).

Conclusions

Masson's support for the general premises of Freud's original seduction theory cut deep like that of the other three protagonists that have been focussed on in this discussion. Ferenczi was already in ill-health when he insisted on reading his paper at the 1932 IPA Congress. The following year he was dead and written into history as mentally unwell by Freud's biographer, Ernest Jones (Ferenczi's analysand), who had plenty of reasons to distance himself from validating the accounts of sexually abused children. Robert Fliess ultimately was a lone voice and despite writing substantial books relevant to the issues of outwardly respectable members of society who behind closed doors sexually and often sadistically abused children (with such traumas validated at the time by the community research of Leontine Young), nevertheless, died in professional obscurity. In a sense, the gritty writings of Florence Rush, though not particularly noticed by Masson, when he wrote *The Assault on Truth*, represented an early component of a loose grouping of individuals who were the advance wave of what was evolving into the modern trauma field. They were all very aware of the high prevalence of child abuse in its varied forms. Included in this grouping were individuals such as Judith Herman, Richard Kluft, David Finkelhor, Christine Courtois, Colin Ross, Bessel Van der Kolk, Frank Putnam, Rich Loewenstein, and John Briere.

While one can debate the pros and cons of how Masson communicated his conclusions regarding Freud abandoning his seduction theory, it is important not to lose sight of the larger picture. My conclusions?

1. Despite attempts on the part of a few beleaguered individuals, psychoanalysis, until recent years, failed to make actual child sexual abuse, a central focus.
2. There was a widespread belief in psychoanalysis for many years and repeatedly encountered by Masson in his training, that female patients speaking of childhood sexual abuse, demonstrated Oedipal fantasy.
3. After September 1897, Freud's occasional peripheral references to "seduction" occurred over a narrow range of perspectives – from any belief being an error, to such accounts occasionally being true, but representing a much less important issue than fantasy.
4. Freud's accounts of how he accessed memories of childhood sexual abuse, and who the abusers were, are simply so internally inconsistent in multiple ways that they can only be considered very unreliable.
5. Freud's concern, that if his patient's accounts were true, it would mean a substantial percentage of society's fathers were incestuous abusers, something he baulked at accepting (to the point of doctoring the facts), has unfortunately in multiple studies been demonstrated to be true.
6. Hysteria and its modern equivalent, trauma-spectrum disorders (dissociative identity disorder/PTSD/somatization disorder), all manifestly demonstrate a large amount of dissociation, but this was not a model that Freud embraced, and this would result in a less than complete understanding of his patients.
7. Freud was a middle-class male professional in the Victorian epoch and as such, was in many ways, a product of his times.
8. "Oedipal fantasy", "recovered memory therapy", and "false memories" are crude psychological entities that have been constructed and then used repeatedly to attempt to explain away the frequently valid accounts of those sexually abused as children.

References

American Psychiatric Association. (1980). *Diagnostic and statistical manuel – III*. American Psychiatric Press.

Appignanesi, L, & Forrester J. (1993). *Freud's women*. Virago Press.

Breger, L. (2000). *Freud: Darkness in the midst of vision*. Wiley.

Breuer, J., & Freud, S. (1895). *Studies in hysteria* (J. Strachey, Ed.) (Standard ed., Vol. 3). Vintage Arrow.

Fliess, E. (1974). *Robert Fliess: The making of a psychoanalyst*. Roffey & Clark.

Fliess, E. (1982). Robert Fliess: *A personality profile*. *American Imago, 39*, 195–218.

Fliess, R. (1956). *Erogeneity and libido: Addenda to the theory of the psychosexual development of the human* – Psychoanalytic series (Vol. 1). International Universities Press.

Fliess, R. (1962). Ego and body ego: Contributions to their psychoanalytic psychology – Psychoanalytic Series Vol 2. International Universities Press.
Fliess, R. (1973). *Symbol, dream, and psychosis with notes on technique* – Psychoanalytic series (Vol. 3). International Universities Press.
Freud, S. (1886/2001). *Report on my studies in Paris and Berlin* (J. Strachey, Ed.) (Standard ed., Vol. 1, pp. 1–16). Vintage Arrow.
Freud, S. (1896a/2001). *Further remarks on the neuropsychoses of defence* (J. Strachey, Ed.) (Standard ed., Vol. 3, pp. 157–186). Vintage Arrow.
Freud, S. (1896b/2001). *The aetiology of hysteria* (J. Strachey, Ed.) (Standard ed., Vol. 3, pp. 187–222). Vintage Arrow.
Freud, S. (1897/2001) Extracts from the Fliess Papers (1950 [1892–1899]) (J. Strachey, Ed.) (Standard ed., Vol 1, pp 175–279). Vintage Arrow.
Freud, S. (1897/1954). *The origins of psycho-analysis, Letters to Wilhelm Fliess, drafts and notes: 1887–1902* (M. Bonaparte, A. Freud, & E Kris, Eds.) Basic Books.
Freud, S. (1925/2001). *An autobiographical study* (J. Strachey, Ed.) (Standard ed., Vol. 20, pp. 1–70). Vintage Arrow.
Freud, S, (1933/2001). *New introductory lectures on psychoanalysis* (J. Strachey, Ed.) (Standard ed., Vol. 22, pp. 1–183). Vintage Arrow.
Gabbard, G. O., & Lester, E. P. (1996) *Boundaries and boundary violations in psychoanalysis*. Basic Books.
Goldwert, M. (1986). Childhood seduction and the spiritualization of psychology: The case of Jung and Rank. *Child Abuse & Neglect,* 10, 555–557. https://doi.org/10.1016/0145-2134(86)90062-1
Henderson, J. L. (1980). Incest. In A. M. Freedman, H. I. Kaplan, & B. Sadock (Eds.), *Comprehensive textbook of psychiatry* (3rd ed., pp. 1806–1808). Williams & Wilkins.
Herman, J. L., & Hirschman, L. (1981). *Father–daughter Incest*. Harvard University Press.
Hirschmüller A. (1989). *The life and work of Josef Breuer: Physiology and psychoanalysis*. New York University Press.
Jones, E. (1961). *The life and work of Sigmund Freud.* (L. Trilling & S. Marcus, Eds. & Abr.). Penguin.
Lothane, Z. (2001, October). Freud's alleged repudiation of the seduction theory revisited: Facts and fallacies. *Psychoanalytic Review,* 88(5). https://doi.org/ 10.1521/prev.88.5.673.17712
Maddox, B. (2006). *Freud's wizard: The enigma of Ernest Jones*. Da Capo Press.
Malcolm, J. (1983, November 27). Trouble in the archives—I. The rise and fall of an unorthodox Freud scholar. *The New Yorker*. Retrieved from https://tinyurl.com/urdzerff
Malcolm, J. (1984). *In the Freud archives*. Jonathan Cape.
Masson, J. M. (1984). *The assault on truth: Freud's suppression of the seduction theory*. Faber and Faber.
Masson, J. M. (Trans. & Ed.). (1985). *The complete letters of Sigmund Freud to Wilhelm Fliess 1887–1904*. Belknap.
Mathews, B., Pacella, R., Scott, J. G. Finkelhor, D., Meinck, F., Higgins, D. J., Erskine, H. E., Thomas, H. J., Lawrence, D. M., Haslam, D. M., Malacova, E., & Dunne, M. P. (2023). The prevalence of child maltreatment in Australia: Findings from a national survey. *Medical Journal of Australia, 218*(6suppl), S13–S18. https://onlinelibrary.wiley.com/doi/10.5694/mja2.51873
McGuire, W. (1974). *The Freud/Jung letters: The correspondence between Sigmund Freud and C.G. Jung.* Harvard University Press.

Middleton, W. (2018) Robert Fliess, Wilhelm Fliess, Ernest Jones, Sándor Ferenczi and Sigmund Freud – ISSTD president's editorial, In W. Middleton, A. Sachs, & M. J. Dorahy (Eds.), *The abused and the abuser: Victim–perpetrator dynamics* (pp. 234–250). Routledge.

Middleton, W. (2022). Beyond death: Enduring incest – The fusion of father with daughter. In M. J. Dorahy, S. N. Gold, & J. A. O'Neil (Eds.), *Dissociation and the dissociative disorders: Past, present, future* (pp. 218–232). Routledge.

Middleton, W. & Butler, J. (1998). Dissociative identity disorder: An Australian series. *Australian and New Zealand Journal of Psychiatry,* 32, 794–804. https://doi.org/ 10.3109/00048679809073868

Putnam, F. W. (1997). *Dissociation in children and adolescents: A developmental perspective*. Guilford.

Roazen, P. (2002). *The trauma of Freud: Controversies in psychoanalysis*. Transaction Publishers.

Rudnytsky, P. L. (1996). Introduction: Ferenczi's turn in psychoanalysis. In P. L. Rudnystsky, A. Bókay, & P. Giampieri-Deutsch (Eds.), *Ferenczi's turn in psychoanalysis* (pp. 1–22). New York University Press.

Rush, F. (1977). The Freudian cover-up. *Chrysalis, 1*, 31–45.

Sacco, L. (2009). *Unspeakable: Father-daughter incest in American history*. Johns Hopkins University Press.

Schimek, J. G. (1986). Fact and fantasy in the seduction theory: A historical review. *Journal of the American Psychoanalytic Association, 35*(4), 937–965. https://doi.org/10.1177/000306518703500407

Sher, J. (2007). *Caught in the web*. Carroll and Graf Publishers.

Simon, B. (1992). "Incest—see under Oedipus Complex": The history of an error in psychoanalysis. *Journal of the American Psychoanalytic Association, 40*(4), 955–988. https://doi.org/10.1177/000306519204000401

Young, L. (1964). *Wednesday's children: A study of child neglect and abuse*. McGraw-Hill.

3 Child Sexual Abuse and Psychoanalytic Theory

Sigmund Freud and Sándor Ferenczi's Childhood Seduction

Arnold Wm. Rachman

I wish to note three courageous events in psychoanalytic history that should not be neglected. We are approaching the 100-year anniversary of the courageous presentation Sándor Ferenczi made to the 12th International Psychoanalytic Congress in Wiesbaden, Germany, in September 1932, introducing his Confusions of Tongues theory (Ferenczi, 1933). Freud, along with Ernest Jones and other orthodox followers, did not want him to present it and prevented it from being published in the English language (Rachman, 1997a,b). What is more, a deliberate campaign was developed which I have called Totschweigen, "Death by Silence" (Rachman, 1999, 2016, 2018, 2022), to remove Ferenczi's theory and methods from psychoanalysis and ostracize Ferenczi from the psychoanalytic community. Freud and Jones's campaign was so mean-spirited that Paul Roazen called it, "political assassination" (Roazen, 1975). Freud and Jones also announced to the analytic community that Freud's once favorite "son" was a seriously disturbed individual who could no longer be considered a psychoanalyst in good standing (Rachman, 2016, 2018, 2022). As a result of Totschweigen, generations of psychoanalysts were trained without any appreciation of Ferenczi's pioneering contributions to psychoanalysis.

Ferenczi's intention on that September morning in Wiesbaden was to encourage the evolution of psychoanalysis to integrate Freud's original idea that sexual abuse of children by their parents and others was an important reality in the development of psychological disorder. Ferenczi had come to the same conclusion in 1932 that Freud had in 1897, through his experience during 20 years of clinical analysis with his so-called difficult cases. Freud's discovery of the importance of sexual abuse of children he called, the source of the Nile, the origin, the bedrock of neurosis, which he first reported in his pioneering paper, "The aetiology of hysteria" (Freud, 1896). This iconic paper, delivered to the Society for Psychiatry and Neurology of Vienna on April 21, 1896, described the clinical data he had collected from his clinical practice, which he presented as evidence for his discovery. He presented 18 of his cases of hysteria/neurosis, six of them were men – all of whom had been sexually abused, to which he referred to as "seduction" of children. This sexual seduction was carried out by fathers, nursemaids, relatives, siblings, and family friends. This finding contradicted the socially held idea that child abuse was the result of attacks on children by undesirable strangers.

DOI: 10.4324/9781003431466-4

Jeffrey Moussaieff Masson's book, *The Assault on Truth: Freud's Suppression of the Seduction Theory* (Masson, 1984), was a second courageous attempt to encourage psychoanalysis to accept the truth of Freud's original theory of psychoanalysis that "the sexual abuse of children was common and hardly a fantasy" (Masson, Chapter 1). Masson reported the research he had completed as Projects Director for the Sigmund Freud Archives. He uncovered 116 previously unpublished letters from Freud to his close friend Wilhelm Flies, an eccentric nose and throat specialist (Masson, 1985). In that correspondence, written between 1887 and 1902, Freud shared the disclosures of his self-analysis with Fliess which became his original theory of psychoanalysis. These disclosures both established the Seduction Theory that childhood sexual abuse was a significant factor in the origin of neurosis, but then Freud abandoned the Seduction Theory and replaced it with Oedipal Complex Theory. The reality of child sexual abuse was replaced with the idea that the origin of neurosis was the unconscious sexual drama that developed in a child's mind regarding their sexual desires for their parents, and that this drama determines the onset of psychological disorder and personality development.

The Assault on Truth was severely criticized because it was seen as a personal attack on Freud's character and as an attempt to destroy psychoanalysis. Masson also suffered the same Totschweigen campaign against himself that Ferenczi had endured when he introduced the Confusion of Tongues Theory (Masson, Chapter 1).

There have been other suggestions to explain Freud's abandonment of "The Seduction Theory" than Masson's conclusion about Freud's failure of courage and rejection by peers (Masson, 1984). Such explanations suggest personal issues for Freud were relevant. Rush (1980) suggested it was "Freud's own faltering conviction" arising from the fact that he was "extremely unhappy with the idea of father as seducer" that led to him asserting that the infantile "sexual scenes" he claimed to have uncovered were mostly fantasies (pp. 88–89). Herman (1981) asserted that the change of view "was based on Freud's own growing unwillingness to believe that licentious behavior on the part of the father could be so widespread" (p. 10). Miller's (1981) contention that Freud's "betrayal of the truth in 1897" occurred because [he] could not bring himself to confront the truth about his own childhood (p. 45). Perhaps, using Ferenczi's theory, we can state here that Freud was a victim of identification with the aggressor, blaming the child (himself) for the sexual trauma (through fantasies) and not the adult (through actual abuse).

The third courageous event in psychoanalytic history that is a contribution to the evolution of psychoanalysis is this volume. Warwick Middleton, M.D., and Martin Dorahy, Ph.D., leading scholars in trauma studies and dissociative disorders, are asking contemporary psychoanalysts and other mental health professionals to reassess Masson's *The Assault on Truth* (Masson, 1984), as a courageous attempt to examine the influence of Masson's thesis on contemporary psychoanalysis and social life more broadly, after Freud abandoned the important reality that child sexual abuse is a factor in the development of psychological disorder and influences personality development. In the last 40 years since *The Assault on Truth* was published, psychoanalysis has been considering more seriously the analysis of trauma, the theory of attachment and relationship principles. This book can help psychoanalysis end the rejection of Sándor Ferenczi and Jeffrey Moussaieff Masson (Rachman, 2022).

The Role of the Nursemaid/The "Other Mother" in Freud's Vienna at the Fin-de-Siècle

I wish to add to the issue of Sigmund Freud's abandonment of the Seduction Theory by examining the Role of the Nursemaid/The "Other Mother" in his childhood Vienna. A neglected area of child seduction has been the seduction of children by nursemaids, nannies, and household servants. In the history of psychoanalysis there is also a neglect of study on the childhood seduction of prominent psychoanalysts and the development of their theories (Middleton, 2018). The contrast in the theories of Sigmund Freud and Sándor Ferenczi regarding the integration of child seduction as a significant psychodynamic in the development of psychological disorder will be examined in the light of their childhood seduction.

Prophecy Coles's book, entitled, *The Uninvited Guest from the Unremembered Past* (Coles, 2011), brings to the psychoanalytic audience the social and psychological importance of the neglected issue of the nurse, nursemaid, and nanny in the upbringing of children from privileged upper-middle, and upper-class European families during the Fin-de-Siècle period. Coles provided descriptions about Freud's early life (since corroborated by other scholars: Breger, 2009; Brothers, 1995; Krüll, 1986; Marcel, 2005; Masson, 1985; Miller, 1981; Partridge, 2014; Vitz, 1993). Coles's (2011) research has suggested that Freud had largely been raised by a nursemaid for the first two and a half years or so of his life. He must have had other nurses after this early period because his mother was more or less continuously pregnant until he was ten. One can understand the idea of Freud having an "other mother" in his experiences with nursemaids. In our discussion, we will explore the seduction behavior and attachment trauma that Freud experienced with his nursemaid of his earliest years.

Childhood seduction of prominent psychoanalysts

The incidence of the childhood sexual seduction of prominent psychoanalysts has been reported in the literature. The childhood seductions of Carl Gustav Jung and Otto Rank were described by Goldwert (1986). Rank wrote of his

> introduction to erotic experience in my seventh year through one of my friends, for which I still curse him even today, vividly remembering … the foundation stone of my later sufferings was laid at that time; it was at the same time the gravestone of my joy.
>
> (Berger, 2009, p. 311)

Their childhood seductions were thought to have shaped their psychological perspectives, with Goldwert concluding that Jung and Rank's childhood sexual seduction is a reason why "[t]hey resisted Freud's emphasis on sexuality and adopted the spiritual stance which marks their place in the history of psychoanalysis" (Goldwert, 1986, p. 555).

The childhood seduction of Sigmund Freud has rarely been discussed, which is in keeping with traditional psychoanalysis's desire to protect Freud's personal life from examination. There is an opening in the Relational Psychoanalytic Perspective that is beginning to bring attention to Freud's childhood seduction. Partridge (2014, pp. 139–140) has said, "I hope my argument that Freud himself was also a victim of sexual abuse in his infancy will have a better chance of being taken seriously".

I wish to join the aforementioned researchers who are willing to examine the backgrounds of psychoanalytical pioneers in the search for truth and understanding. To further this aim, I wish to contribute to the examination of Sigmund Freud's childhood sexual seduction in detail, as well as to discuss the theoretical implications of his childhood seduction for the abandonment of his Seduction Theory. I wish also to add to this discussion by examining Sándor Ferenczi's childhood sexual seduction, which has been totally neglected. The comparison of Freud's and Ferenczi's childhood seduction will aid understanding about the importance of child sexual abuse in their theories of psychoanalysts.

Childhood sexual abuse in Freud's Vienna

Child sexual abuse was an issue in Vienna at the turn of the 19th century (Wolff, 1995). In fact, Vienna, the most cosmopolitan city in the world at that time, was engrossed in the disturbing event of child abuse, specifically, two cases of child murder, and two of abuse. The newspapers proclaimed the ugly reality of child abuse, but the interest in child abuse vanished quickly. Like Vienna, Freud seemed to ignore the issue of child abuse in his writings after he abandoned the Seduction Theory. A very important person has to become part of the discussion of why Freud abandoned the Seduction Theory and did not integrate childhood sexual abuse as a standard for psychoanalytic theory. We will come to her.

Perhaps we should mention that, at the end of his life, Freud did include again the pathogenic importance of real trauma in *Moses and Monotheism* (Freud, 1939). Of course, this inclusion was only considered in articulation with the Oedipal theory, the inherited and the constitutive. It was a partial inclusion, but an inclusion, nonetheless. I think this inclusion (in 1938/1939) was influenced by Ferenczi and the Confusion of Tongues Theory. But Freud does not refer to Ferenczi, as he continued the silence of Totschweigen. In *Moses and Monotheism* Freud wrote,

> All these traumas occur in early childhood up to about the fifth year. Impressions from the time at which a child is beginning to talk stand out as being of particular interest; the periods between the ages of two and four seem to be the most important [Freud's seduction trauma occurred during this period]; it cannot be determined with certainty how long after birth this period of receptivity begins, (b) the experiences in question are as a rule totally forgotten, they are not accessible to memory and fall within the period of infantile amnesia, which is usually broken into a few separate mnemic residues, what are known

> as 'screen memories', (c) they relate to impressions of a sexual and aggressive nature, and no doubt also to early injuries to the ego (narcissistic mortifications). In this connection it should be remarked that such young children make no sharp distinction between sexual and aggressive acts, as they do later. (Cf. the misunderstanding of the sexual act in a sadistic sense). The predominance of the sexual factor is, of course, most striking and calls for theoretical considerations.
>
> (Freud, 1939, p. 74)

Since psychoanalysis is built upon psychodynamic explanations for human behavior, we need to search for a psychodynamic explanation for Freud's abandonment of his Seduction Theory. Jeffrey Moussaieff Masson and Paul Roazen, iconic "psychohistorians" of psychoanalysis, have written that the controversy surrounding the Seduction Theory of Freud was one of the most important issues in the history of psychoanalysis (Masson, 1985; Roazen, 2002). The controversies that have been presented throughout the years have basically focused on the theoretical perspectives of Freud abandoning his Seduction Theory and replacing it with The Oedipal Complex Theory (Izenberg, 1991). Ferenczi's perspective reformulated the Seduction Theory into a Confusion of Tongues theory of psychological trauma whose origin was childhood sexual abuse by parents or parental surrogates (Ferenczi, 1933). When Freud abandoned the Seduction Theory, he abandoned the very important idea that children were being regularly sexually abused by adults. To this date, traditional psychoanalysis has neglected the reality of child sexual abuse and its implication for psychoanalysis and society (Rachman, 2022). There are some important exceptions to this neglect, one being Judith Herman's contributions to the reality of sexual seduction of children by parents (Herman, 1981). A discussion of Freud and Ferenczi's childhood seductions and their relevance to understanding the continued controversy is now necessary.

Freud's childhood seduction and abandonment trauma

There are two basic sources which reveal Freud's childhood seduction. First, we have Freud's own words in the letters he wrote to Wilhelm Fliess, which revealed his seduction through his self-analysis (Masson, 1985). The second source is the research conducted by Marianne Krüll, a German sociologist who did an extensive study on Freud's family and childhood (Krüll, 1986). On October 3, 1897, Freud wrote to Fliess about his seduction: "… that in my case the 'prime originator' was an ugly elderly but clever woman".

Freud did not name his seducer but went on to disclose his memory of her:

> *(between two and a half years) my libido towards matrem [mother]* was awakened, namely on the occasion of a journey with her from Leipzig to Vienna, during which we must have spent the night together and *there must have been an opportunity of seeing her madam [nude]*
>
> (Masson, 1985, p. 268, Letter from Freud to Fliess – October 3, 1897, italics added)

Freud's description in this Letter to Fliess has the feel of his describing his mother and his "other mother", his nursemaid, Resi Wittick. This may have indicated Freud's emotional reaction to having "two mothers" to take care of him. These were also moments and memories which clearly indicated that his "other mother" was his sexual seducer:

> Today's dream has, under strangest disguise, produced the following: *she was my teacher in sexual matters and complained because I was clumsy and unable to do anything... Moreover, she washed me in reddish water in which she had previously washed herself. [The interpretation is difficult; I find nothing like this in the chain of my memories; so I regard it as a genuine ancient discovery.*]
>
> (Masson, 1985, p. 219, Letter from Freud to Wilhelm Fliess – October 4, 1897, italics added)

We can interpret the reddish water as being Resi Wittick's menstrual flow, bathing young Sigmund in it, as she enjoyed her own sexual fantasy.

Krüll (1986), who identified Resi Wittick as his nursemaid and "other mother", stated:

> *Freud's nursemaid, ... played a role of extraordinary importance during his early life in Freiberg... I have recently discovered an entry in the list of visitors for 5 June 1857: 108, Amalia Freud merchant's wife with child, Sigmund and maid Resi Wittick.*
>
> (Krüll, 1986, p. 119, italics added)

Freud's early childhood experience with Resi Wittick also produced an abandonment trauma. His mother told him that his nursemaid was taken away from him because she was a thief, having taken money and toys from the household:

> I wrote to you that she induced me to steal zehners and give them to her... [his mother said]: Your brother Philippe himself fetched the policeman; she then was given ten months in prison.
>
> (Masson, 1985, p. 271, Letter from Freud to Wilhelm Fliess, October 15, 1897)

The maintenance of his positive feelings toward his nursemaid are clear when he states:

> If I succeed in resolving my hysteria, I shall have to thank the memory of the old woman who provided me at such an early age with the means for loving and surviving.
>
> (Masson, 1985, pp. 268–269)

Freud neither disclosed any negative reaction to having been sexually abused nor expressed any emotional despair that his "other mother" disappeared from his life, forever. Partridge (2014) had a more meaningful emotional reaction to Freud's nursemaid's troubling behavior than Freud did:

> [It] chills me because it reveals a detached and reified reflection on what is in effect the consequence of Freud's abandonment by his mother and abuse by his nurse.
>
> (p. 142)

I join Partridge (2014) and Coles (2003) in believing that Freud was not dismayed that his self-analysis revealed two traumatic experiences from his childhood. He did not report in any of his writings that he continued to analyze the meaning of these traumas and developed insight into his neurotic issues. What is more, his lack of insight did not inform his theories about seduction and abandonment traumas.

Sándor Ferenczi's childhood sexual experiences with "servant girls"

Sándor Ferenczi reported in his Clinical Diary (Ferenczi, 1988) that he was the survivor of childhood sexual abuse. Before I present the actual citation of this experience, it would be meaningful to describe how Ferenczi retrieved his memory of childhood sexual abuse. There is an interesting contrast between Freud and Ferenczi's report of their childhood sexual abuse. Freud, as we have seen, retrieved his childhood sexual abuse through his self-analysis. He had a need to verify his retrieval of his childhood sexual abuse, since his self-analysis was a one-person experience, not a two-person experience. Clearly Freud needed a person, other than himself to be sure he was retrieving a real memory of his nursemaid:

> I asked my mother whether she still remembered the nurse. 'Of course,', she said, 'an elderly person, very clever'.
>
> (Masson, 1985, p. 271 – Letter from Freud to Fliess, October 15, 1897)

Sándor Ferenczi's retrieval of his childhood sexual experience was a result of a two-person experience. It occurred as a result of a mutual analysis between his analysand Elizabeth Severn and himself. What is additionally important about Ferenczi's retrieval of his childhood sexual abuse was that his analysand, Severn, suggested that Ferenczi allow her to analyze him, in order to work on and through his negative countertransference reaction toward her. Ferenczi struggled to enter into the mutual analysis with Severn for a year, realizing his role as analyst might be compromised. He also questioned whether he could trust Severn to empathetically analyze his emotional issues. Ferenczi's capacity to concede to Severn to help him with his countertransference reaction was a realization that Severn needed an emphatic response to Ferenczi's negative feelings toward her. As we shall see as we examine Ferenczi's disclosure of childhood sexual abuse, Severn helped him retrieve, analyze, and develop insight into a fundamental personality issue, which was "my hatred of females" (Ferenczi, 1988, p. 61).

Ferenczi's mutual analytic experience with Severn produced the following revelation of sexual seduction:

> I submerged myself deeply in the reproduction of infantile experiences; *the most evocative image was the vague appearance of female figures, probably servant girls from earliest childhood; then the image of a corpse; whose abdomen I was opening up, presumably in the dissecting room; linked to this mad fantasy that I was being pressed into this wound in the corpse.* Interpretation: the after-effect of passionate scenes, which presumably did take place, in the course of which *a housemaid probably allowed me to play with her breasts, but then pressed my head between her legs, so that I became frightened and felt I was suffocating.*
>
> (Ferenczi, 1988, p. 60–61, Clinical Entry: March 1932, italics added)

The recovery of childhood seduction in the mutual analysis between Ferenczi and Severn went beyond retrieving childhood seduction. Their interaction can be considered an analytic experience. Ferenczi was able to analyze the material in the recovered memory of childhood seduction with Severn's help:

> To use R.N.'s [Ferenczi's code for Severn in his writings] mode of expression: in R.N. I find my mother again, namely the real one, who was hard and energetic and of whom I am afraid. R.N. knows this and treats me with particular gentleness; the analysis even enables her to transform her own hardness into friendly softness, … one must be content with obtaining pieces of the analytic insight from the patients in scattered fragments, and not allow them to concern themselves with our person any more than is necessary for *their* analysis.
>
> (Ferenczi, 1988, p. 45, Clinical Entry – 24 February 1932, italics added)

Ferenczi acknowledged in the examination of the mutual analysis that his "mutual analytic partner", Severn (Rachman, 2023), was to be credited in helping him retrieve, analyze, and develop insight into the trauma of being sexually abused by a household servant (Ferenczi, 1988). The question of Ferenczi's success in this "analysis" is raised by his willingness to credit Severn with success. We know Ferenczi was very critical of his primary analyst, Sigmund Freud:

> My own analysis could not be pursued deeply enough because my analyst [Sigmund Freud] (by his own admission, of a narcissistic nature), with his strong determination to be healthy and his antipathy toward any weaknesses or abnormalities, could not follow me down into those depths, and introduced the 'educational' stage too soon.
>
> (Ferenczi, 1988, p. 62)

As Ferenczi became an international figure in psychoanalysis, making friendships among his colleagues, Georg Groddeck, one could say, became his "second analyst". Ferenczi pursued a more open friendship with Groddeck as if they were brothers. They exchanged letters about self-analysis, mutual analysis, analyst subjectivity, and countertransferences, which brought them into greater emotional contact and shared subjectivities that he had with Freud (Fortune, 2000).

Ferenczi's description of his mutual analysis with Severn indicated that she could be considered his "third analyst" and his most successful (Rachman, 2017). The mutual analysis with Severn was pursued deeply enough so that he could reach the emotional depth of his sexual seduction determined by revealing disturbing images of sexual and physical abuse and he developed insight into his emotional relationship with his mother. This success with his "third analyst" completely contradicts the negative assessment of Freud, Jones, and the orthodox followers who condemned Severn as an untrained, emotionally disturbed individual who was not fit to be a psychoanalyst (they came to think and say the same thing about Ferenczi years later). Ferenczi did not share this negative view of Severn. He felt this analysis was a training analysis. Furthermore, when she left Budapest and opened up a psychoanalytic practice in New York City, she became a successful psychoanalyst (Rachman, 2018).

Freud abandoned the concept of childhood sexual trauma while ferenczi embraced it

There is a marked contrast between Freud and Ferenczi's analysis of their childhood sexual seduction which demonstrates why Freud abandoned his Seduction Hypothesis and why Ferenczi embraced it. The more Ferenczi analyzed his own childhood sexual abuse the more he understood the importance and meaning of psychological trauma (Ferenczi, 1933). Freud never returned to his personal disclosures about seduction and abandonment trauma, never mentioning it again anywhere in his writings. Freud never turned to fully analyze his childhood seduction because he dissociated from his sexual seduction experience. In so doing, the meaning and importance of childhood sexual experience was not intellectually or emotionally available to him to use in formulating a mature theory of psychological disorder and its treatment. In later years, when Jung and Ferenczi offered to analyze Freud, he turned them down. If Freud had allowed Ferenczi to analyze him, there would have been a possibility of an exploration of the two traumas. Ferenczi would have engaged in an emotional encounter that he had wished he had in therapy with Freud.

Ferenczi, on the other hand, continued to work with difficult cases, which were beyond Freud's preoccupation with what he thought was neurosis. Ferenczi's clinical experiences during his mature years were of individuals who suffered from borderline personality, somatic, and psychological trauma disorders. Freud obsessively/compulsively clung to his Oedipal Complex theory, actually seeing individuals who were not neurotic. Freud published his Case Study of Dora as evidence of the Oedipal Complex theory. Dora was actually an adolescent who was sexually harassed by a 40-year-old male friend of her family and who was a survivor of sexual abuse trauma (Rachman & Mattick, 2023). Masson (1984) reported that Muriel Gardner had told him that the Wolf Man's second analyst, Ruth Mack Brunswick, had written an unpublished paper that the Wolf Man was anally raped by a family member as a child. I investigated Masson's report and I found Ruth Mack Brunswick's paper verifying that the Wolf Man was anally raped. Freud did not know this, and Mack Brunswick never revealed this to Freud. The material was stored in the Library of Congress, U.S.A. (Rachman, 2018). I have the Ruth Mack Brunswick unpublished paper on the Wolf Man as well as unpublished notes from the Brunswick analysis. I plan to publish this historically important material.

Ferenczi's Confusion of Tongues theory (Ferenczi, 1933) made it clear that his analysis of difficult cases was not Oedipal Complex neurotic cases. His case of R.N., described in his Clinical Diary (Ferenczi, 1988), exemplified a non-Oedipal case. Masson (1984) identified R.N. as Elizabeth Severn, realizing she was more likely to be a borderline personality or trauma survivor.

The very important difference between Freud and Ferenczi's sexual seduction self-reports was that Ferenczi was able to analyze his sexual seduction, in mutual analytic sessions with his analysand, Elizabeth Severn (Rachman, 2018). Once again, Freud had no idea that child sexual abuse was an important psychodynamic in the Wolf Man case. Freud thought this case was a classical Oedipal experience. The availability of Severn, who was a psychotherapist when she entered into the mutual analytic sessions with Ferenczi, made an important therapeutic difference. Ferenczi, with Severn's help, was able to develop the insight that his childhood sexual seduction was emotionally connected to his negative emotional experience with his mother during childhood. Ferenczi's mutual analytic experience with Severn allowed him to analyze the meaning that the childhood sexual seduction had on his personal and professional functioning. Rather than dissociating from the sexual seduction, he was able to integrate it into his adult personality. When Severn revealed her childhood sexual abuse by her father, he was able to empathically respond to the abuse, helping Severn to work through the emotionally devastating psychopathology that haunted her as an adult. It was Ferenczi's capacity to accept and understand his seduction that allowed him to analyze Severn's childhood sexual trauma. Freud, Jones, and the orthodox analytic community did not understand the essential importance of empathy in the analysis of a trauma disorder (Rachman, 2018, 2022; Rachman & Mucci, 2024).

Sexual abuse of children in the United States in the year 2023: Fulfilling Ferenczi's prophecy

There is no better way to demonstrate that Jeffrey Moussaieff Masson's attempt to revive Sándor Ferenczi's iconic contribution about the incidence of the sexual abuse of children than to outline data from the present, over 90 years after the Confusion of Tongues paper, was given. A list of the statistics for child sexual abuse in the U.S.A. for the present year, 2023, clearly illustrates how prophetic Ferenczi was when he introduced the Confusion of Tongues concept to establish the incidence of sexual abuse of children as an important psychodynamic in the development of psychopathology and personality. Here is some important data about the incidence of child sexual abuse in the U.S.A gathered by The United States National Center For Victims of Crime (https://victimsofcrime.org):

1. In 2010, the U.S. Department of Health and Human Services Children's Bureau reported that 9.2% of victimized children were sexually assaulted.
2. Studies by David Finkelhor, Ph.D., Director of the Crimes Against Children Research Center indicated:
   a) One in 5 girls and one in 20 boys are a victim of child sexual abuse.
   b) Self-report studies show that 20% of adult females and 5–10% of adult males recall a childhood sexual assault or sexual abuse incident.
   c) Sixty-three percent of women who had suffered sexual abuse by a family member also reported a rape or attempted rape after the age of 14.
   d) A child who is the victim of prolonged sexual abuse usually develops low self-esteem, a feeling of worthlessness, and an abnormal or distorted view of sex. The child may become withdrawn and mistrustful of adults and can become suicidal.
   e) Child sexual abuse is not solely restricted to physical contact; such abuse could include non-contact, such as exposure, voyeurism, and child pornography (Brown & Finkelhor, 1986; Finkelhor, 1990).
   f) Children are most vulnerable to sexual abuse between the ages 7 and 13 (Brown & Finkelhor, 1986; Finkelhor, 1990).
   g) Three out of four adolescents who have been assaulted were victimized by someone they knew well (Brown & Finkelhor, 1986; Finkelhor, 1990).

Freud's neglect of the importance of childhood sexual abuse in the development of psychological disorder and personality development set a template for psychoanalysis and society to use the same mechanisms as analysands employ, dissociation and denial, to wash away the pain of real trauma. But dissociation has not erased the incidence or pain of sexual abuse in our lives. Rachman (2022) has recently outlined the world-wide epidemic of sexual abuse in present-day society, and the continued neglect of psychoanalysis to use its significant resources to treat the epidemic.

There are signs that we may be on the cusp of a Zeitgeist change as society has begun to confront sexual abuse. The activities of investigative reporters, social activists, and abuse survivors have highlighted the sexual abuse activities within the Catholic Church, the Harvey Weinstein scandal in the entertainment industry, the sexual abuse of female gymnasts by Dr. Nassar, and the development of the #MeToo movement (Rachman, 2022). Psychoanalysis can contribute to the Zeitgeist change by integrating Sándor Ferenczi's *Confusion of Tongues* paper, Jeffrey Moussaieff Masson's book *The Assault on Truth* (Masson, 1984), and now, Warwick Middleton and Martin Dorahy's (Eds.), *Contemporary Perspectives of Freud's Seduction Theory and Psychoanalysis: Revisiting Masson's, "The Assault on Truth"* (Middleton & Dorahy, this volume). Clara Mucci and I have recently contributed our attempt to encourage psychoanalysis to realize that Ferenczi's

Confusion of Tongues paper was as relevant in 1932 as it is today by accepting childhood sexual abuse as a significant psychodynamic in the development of psychological distress (Rachman & Mucci, 2024).

References

Berger, L. (2009). *A dream of undying fame: How Freud betrayed his mentor and invented psychoanalysis*. Basic Books.

Brothers, D. (1995). *Falling backwards: An exploration of trust and self experience*. Norton.

Brown, A., & Finkelhor, D. (1986). Impact of child sexual abuse: A review of the research. *Psychological Bulletin, 99* (1), 66–77.

Coles, P. (2003). *The importance of sibling relationships in psychoanalysis*. Karnac.

Coles, P. (2011). *The uninvited guest from the unremembered past: An exploration of the unconscious transmissions of trauma across the generations*. Karnac.

Ferenczi, S. (1933). The Confusion of Tongues between adults and children: The language of tenderness and passion. In M. Balint (Ed.), *Final contributions to the problems and methods of psychoanalysis*, Vol. 3 (pp.156–167). Brunner/Mazel, 1980.

Ferenczi, S. (1988). *The clinical diary of Sándor Ferenczi*. J. Dupont (Ed.) (trans. M. Balint and N.Z. Jackson). Harvard University Press.

Finkelhor, D. (1990). Early and long-term effects of child sexual abuse: An update. *Professional Psychology: Research and Practice, 21*(5), 325–330. https://doi.org/10.1037/0735-7028.21.5.325

Fortune, C. (2000). *The Ferenczi-Groddeck Letters, 1921-1933*. Open Gate Press.

Freud, S. (1896). *The aetiology of hysteria*. J. Strachey (Ed.), The Standard Edition (Vol. 30, pp. 187–221). Vintage Arrow.

Freud, S. (1939). *Moses and monotheism*. Hogarth Press.

Goldwert, M. (1986). Childhood seduction and the spiritualization of psychology: The Case of Jung and Rank. *Child Abuse & Neglect, 10*(4), 555–557. https://doi.org/10.1016/0145-2134(86)90062-1

Herman, J. (1981). *Father/daughter incest*. Harvard University Press.

Izenberg, G. N. (1991). Seduced and abandoned: The rise and fall of Freud's seduction theory. In J. Nue (ed.) *The Cambridge Companion to Freud* (pp. 25–43). Cambridge University Press.

Krüll, M. (1986). *Freud and his father*. Norton.

Marcel, M. (2005). *Freud's traumatic memory: Reclaiming seduction theory and revisiting Oedipus.* Duquesne University Press.

Masson, J. M. (1984). *The assault on truth: Freud's suppression of The Seduction Theory*. Farrar, Strauss, & Giroux.

Masson, J. M. (Eds. & Trans.) (1985). *The complete letters of Sigmund Freud to Wilhelm Fliess, 1887–1904*. The Belknap Press.

Middleton, W. (2018). Robert Fliess, Wilhelm Fliess, Ernest Jones, Sándor Ferenczi and Sigmund Freud – ISSTD President's Editorial. In W. Middleton, A. Sachs, & M. J. Dorahy (Eds.), *The abused and the abuser: Victim – perpetrator dynamics* (pp. 234–250). Routledge.

Miller, A. (1981). *Thou shall not be aware: Society's betrayal of the child.* Giroux.

Partridge, S. (2014). The hidden neglect and sexual abuse of infant Sigmund Freud. In K. White, & O. B. Epstein (Eds.), *Attachment: New direction in psychotherapy and relational psychoanalysis, 8*, 139–150.

Rachman, A. W. (1997a). *Sándor Ferenczi: The psychotherapist of tenderness and passion*. Aronson.

Rachman, A. W. (1997b). The suppression and censorship of Ferenczi's Confusion of Tongues Paper. *Psychoanalytic Inquiry*, 17(4), 459–485. https://doi.org/10.1080/07351699709534142

Rachman, A. W. (1999). Death by silence. (Totschweigen): The traditional method of dealing with dissidents in psychoanalysis. In. R. Prince (Ed.) *The death of psychoanalysis: Suicide murder, or rumor greatly exaggerated* (pp. 154–164). Aronson.

Rachman, A. W. (2016). *The Budapest school of psychoanalysis*. Routledge.

Rachman, A. W. (2017). The three analyses of Dr. F. Unpublished manuscript.

Rachman, A. W. (2018). *Elizabeth Severn: The "evil genius" of psychoanalysis*. Routledge. https://doi.org/10.1080/00207578.2022.2067043

Rachman, A. W. (2022). *Psychoanalysis and society's neglect of the sexual abuse of children, youth, and adults.* Routledge. https://doi.org/10.4324/9780429298431

Rachman, A. W. (2023). *Elizabeth Severn: Sándor Ferenczi's "mutual analytic partner"*. Presentation. 150th Anniversary Sándor Ferenczi Conference. Budapest, Hungary, June 9.

Rachman, A. W., & Mattick, P. (2023). *Freud and Dora: A confusion of tongues*. Routledge.

Rachman, A. W., & Mucci, C. (2024) *Sandor Ferenczi's confusion of tongues theory of trauma: Neurobiological and relational perspectives*. Routledge.

Roazen, P. (1975). *Freud and his followers*. Alfred A. Knopf.

Roazen, P. (2002). *The trauma of Freud: Controversies in psychoanalysis*. Transaction Publishers.

Rush, F. (1980). *The best kept secret: The sexual abuse of children.* Prentice Hall. The United States National Center For Victims of Crime (2023). https://victimsofcrime.org.

Vitz, P. (1993). *Sigmund Freud's Christian unconscious*. Gracewing.

Wolff, L. (1995). *Child abuse in Freud's Vienna. Postcards from the end of the world.* New York University.

4 The Perpetuation of Deliberate and Inadvertent Insensitivities within Psychoanalysis

Origins, Rhymes, and Reasons

Richard P. Kluft

Jeffrey Moussaieff Masson's scholarship confronted mainstream psychoanalysis with its failure to address the plight of sexually exploited women. Masson's contributions generated a powerful backlash, destroying his promising analytic career (Masson, 2017). It is difficult to overlook the many parallels between the ways psychoanalysis failed these women and the ways psychoanalysis failed Jeffrey Moussaieff Masson. Unwarranted misunderstandings and mistreatments of "disturbers of the psychoanalytic peace" have occurred since the earliest years of psychoanalysis. Contemporary scholars often single out the circumstances of women for special study. However important and overdue, privileging these concerns overlooks a more general problem. Misunderstandings and mistreatments of both patients raising unwelcome issues and dissident or innovative colleagues seem to stem from similar sources.

Sigmund Freud's influence upon subsequent generations of psychoanalysts remains profound. Whenever one person in a field is so dominating and idealized, difficulties in that person's contributions may pass unnoticed.

Sigmund Freud's unique impact upon the direction and values of his remarkable body of work was marked by his profound defensiveness, intolerance of dissent (e.g., Ratner, 2019), narcissism (Breger, 2009; Makari, 2008), and willingness to make inaccurate statements to advance his arguments (Kluft, 2018 b, c; Ratner, 2019). Freud took offense quickly, insisted upon loyalty, and found disagreement and criticism intolerable. He worked to develop a paradigm in which he would always be the ultimate authority (Freud, 1914). He could react angrily when reviews of his efforts were not completely favorable (Ratner, 2019). Letters to Fleiss document Freud's struggles to contain his rage. Rationalized patterns of defending associates and overlooking the pain of the victimized were apparent in Freud's defense of Fleiss' egregious malpractice.

Freud's personal issues and zealous efforts to promote psychoanalysis remain potent influences, still largely unaddressed.

DOI: 10.4324/9781003431466-5

Contextualizing Masson

In the 1970s, the incidence of father–daughter incest was stated to occur in one in a million North American families (Henderson, 1975), an inaccuracy congruent with both societal denial and psychoanalytic beliefs that allegations of incest likely represented Oedipal fantasies (see Simon, 1992).

The 1980s witnessed explosive increases in both awareness of trauma and powerful reactive pressures countering that awareness. Acknowledging the importance of exogenous trauma and the relevance of external realities in the etiology of psychological difficulties challenged established psychoanalytic thinking. In the main, however, psychoanalysis continued along its way, confident in the basic correctness of its premises, paradigms, and practices.

Jeffrey Moussaieff Masson, Ph.D., had seemed destined to become a star of the first magnitude in the analytic firmament. His fervor for the study of Freud and Freud's work made him welcome among prestigious senior colleagues. After becoming Director of the Freud Archives, Masson found previously unpublished correspondence between Freud and Fleiss related to abuse and to the fate of the seduction theory.

While others deemed these materials irrelevant or detrimental, Masson believed they had scientific and historical importance. Anna Freud sanctioned their publication. Permission notwithstanding, many considered his actions no less than a betrayal of Sigmund Freud, Anna Freud, and psychoanalysis itself.

Masson's work, pre-eminently his 1984 *The Assault on Truth: Freud's Suppression of the Seduction Theory*, questioned the legitimacy of Freud's repudiation of this theory and his covering up Wilhelm Fleiss's horrific malpractice in the treatment of Emma Ekstein. It was not welcomed within the analytic mainstream. His swift and brutal repudiation, expulsion, and exile from the analytic community followed the model of Sigmund Freud's ruthlessly severing connections with those who disagreed with him and his theories (e.g., Sándor Ferenczi).

A calmer, circumspect consideration of Masson's work might have reawakened analytic interest in trauma and encouraged greater toleration of differences of opinion (see Eisold, 1994). Instead, psychoanalysis continued its privileged veneration of Freud and a theoretical model that marginalized the importance of trauma and the lived experience of patients. However rationalized and congruent with analytic paradigms, such stances constitute *a priori* dignity violations (see Hicks, 2012; Kluft, 2016). Models of therapy that minimize or marginalize respectful consideration of patients' experiences bring ongoing elements of invalidation, narcissistic injury, humiliation, derealization, and disrespect into the heart of what should be a safe therapeutic process (Kluft, 2016).

Not only sexual traumatizations were discounted. Discussing Israeli analyst Ilany Kogan's (2003) treatment of a second-generation Holocaust victim, C. Brenner (2003) insisted that her patient's improvement was due to analysis of Oedipal themes, not those Kogan raised. Ferro (2003) opined that Kogan's work, tied to trauma, lacked creativity and imagination. To them, the Holocaust lacked standing as a matter of analytic interest, distracting from a preferable focus on psychological reality.

Masson's repudiation mirrored Ferenczi's. He was attacked and rejected by former friends and colleagues, as well as by many who did not know him, but reacted to what they perceived as his attack on a heroic and revered figure, his body of work, and, by virtue of their identification with Freud and his work, as an attack upon themselves and their professional identities.

Considering concepts advanced by Volkan (1986, 1997, 2009), perhaps those who identified with an admired individual being shamed experienced that perceived insult as a "chosen trauma," an indignity visited upon not Freud alone, but upon them individually and collectively, and became righteously vengeful, determined to redress the injustice they felt Masson had perpetrated. Reactions to Masson by many traditional psychoanalysts took the form of an "attack other" shame script (i.e., shame those whom you believe shame you [Nathanson, 1991]).

Masson's repudiation cannot be explained by his dissemination and discussion of newly published materials alone. Psychoanalysts learn to listen, think, empathize, and intervene guided by understandings, both explicit and implicit. Their models influence their perceptions. They are responsive to suggestions and concerns remote from the immediate clinical encounter. Role models, paradigms, and personal backgrounds and histories influence how their thinking proceeds.

Masson urged a reexamination of not only the specific matters he raised but of the entire manner of analytic understanding. One shorthand for such requests is an "ask." Such asks may offer unwanted confrontations, which commonly evoke knee-jerk aversions.

A matter of long-standing concern

American Psychoanalytic Association (APSAA) Past-President Robert Glover (2023) noted predecessors' concerns that the "splendid isolation" which protected and nurtured the emergence and development of psychoanalysis also held the potential to diminish Freud's creation.

"Psychoanalysis is my creation," said Freud (1914, p. 7). "For ten years I was the only person who concerned himself with it… even today no one can know better than I what psychoanalysis is… ." Idealizing often protects personal attitudes and positions from close scrutiny. Freud's bold assertion bypasses Emma Ekstein, Freud's patient and a victim of Fleiss' malpractice, who became the second analyst and first female analyst in 1897.

Many APSAA presidents expressed concern over psychoanalysis' resistance to change and its reluctance to join the academic and scientific mainstreams (Glover, 2023). Such concerns notwithstanding, the idealization of Freud's heroic individualism and uncritical acceptance of his defensiveness have discouraged explorations of psychoanalysis from perspectives other than his own. These influences have rationalized and supported the isolation of psychoanalysis from other academic and clinical disciplines and what they have to offer. Glover described this form of dissociation as "excessive social closure."

We must ask, "How has a profession ostensibly so dedicated to freeing minds from oppressive ensnarement accepted and assiduously guarded its own largely self-imposed intellectual and attitudinal 'house arrest?'"

Considerations

Waelder (1962) identified six levels or parts of "psychoanalysis or Freudian doctrine." First are data of observation (i.e., that which is evident and what can be inferred as derivatives of the unconscious [sic!]). The second, clinical interpretation, appreciates the interconnection of one set of clinical observations with other behavior or conscious content. From groups of observations and interpretations comes a third level, clinical generalizations. Clinical theory is the fourth level: "… clinical interpretations permit the formulation of certain theoretical concepts which are either implicit in the interpretations or to which the interpretations may lead, such as repression, defense, return of the repressed, regression, etc." (p. 620).

Beyond lies a fifth level of more abstract concepts, metapsychology, often not clearly demarcated from those in level four. Examples include cathexis, psychic energy, Eros, and the death instinct. The sixth level concerns Freud's philosophy, his way of looking at the world. Waelder (1962) described Freud's philosophy as "in the main, the philosophy of positivism, and a faith in the possibility of human betterment through reason – a faith which in his later life, in consequence of his psychoanalytic experience, became greatly qualified though not altogether abandoned" (p. 620).

For Waelder's audience, mostly philosophers, this sufficed. However, personal philosophies generally consist of a person's amalgamation of values and attitudes, not an approximation to a major school of philosophical thought. Taken together, Freud's writings, Freud's attitudes and actions, and relevant historical information suggest different perspectives on Freud's "philosophy."

Waelder considers the data of observation and clinical interpretation indispensable. Clinical generalizations and clinical theory are important, but less so. Freud observed that metapsychology is composed of hypotheses, "not the bottom but the top of the whole structure [of science], and they can be replaced and discarded without damaging it" (1914, p. 77). They are neither essential nor fixed. Waelder added that "Freud's philosophy is largely a matter of his time and has little bearing on psychoanalysis" (1962, p. 621).

That notwithstanding, historically, psychoanalysts as a group have defended Freud's unproven abstract concepts tenaciously and protected much of what they understand to be Freud's attitudes and philosophy. If Freud's attitudes and personal perspectives permeate psychoanalytic thinking, it is possible that at times "dispensable" elements may become privileged and empowered to warp or drive the "indispensable." When the indispensable becomes vulnerable to contamination by the dispensable, it may be treated as dispensable. Should we not wonder whether this has been the fate of trauma, dissociation, and external reality?

A patient reports incestuous material. If the analyst's frame of understanding privileges the likelihood it expresses a fantasy, the material *per se* may not be accorded meaningful respect. Accounts challenging privileged abstractions risk receiving dismissive treatment.

This concern is not hypothetical. Waelder included derivatives of presumed unconscious fantasies among data of observation [sic!]. Clearly, the pressures of metapsychology, philosophy, personal attitudes, as well as social forces may influence, even contaminate, both the perception and clinical management of clinical observations. Treating a patient within a paradigm unable to accommodate or predisposed to invalidate the truths of that patient's experience risks contaminating an ostensibly caring and helping enterprise with dignity violations (Hicks, 2012, Kluft, 2016), inflicting narcissistic injuries (Kohut & Wolf, 1978).

Masson's work insists that psychoanalysis recovers what it left behind when Freud abandoned the seduction theory and accord due attention to external as well as psychological reality. This is an enormous "ask," the rethinking of positions held in psychoanalysis since the 1890s. Small wonder Masson's ideas were perceived as disruptive and unreasonable attacks on a system of thought and intervention that most of its practitioners held in high esteem and were not motivated to revise.

Biblical scholarship includes exegesis (i.e., applying rules of searching and understanding to a text to discover and understand its message). The goal of exegesis is to comprehend the truth and meaning of the text under study.

In another methodology, eisegesis, scholars bring their own ideas to the study of the text, making efforts to discover within or impose upon the text preconceived ideas of what should be found. The desired result is the discovery that the text's meaning is congruent with what the scholars want it to mean. While the word is unusual, the phenomenon is not. We encounter it every time a public figure comes to the same invariable and preferred understanding of matters, regardless of the circumstances and/or available information to the contrary.

Given Freud's profound influence, psychoanalytic efforts to understand his work often have proceeded within an unrecognized eisogetic frame of reference. Generations of analysts expected to find what they would find, found it, and taught it, perpetuating a self-reinforcing cycle. Masson implicitly challenged this gold standard of finding and re-finding classical Freudian constructs by taking into consideration matters beyond the realm of inner, or psychological, reality.

How did psychoanalysis evolve into a top-down eisogetic culture representing itself as a bottom-up culture, paradoxically preaching the importance of the freedom of the mind for the creative, productive, loving, and gratifying human lives of analysands while too often attempting to impose severe, doctrinaire limitations upon the thinking of those involved in its study and practice? Why do Masson's early experiences at his institute, dating from before he became controversial, so clearly bring to mind Freud's style of asserting authority and stifling dissent?

The narcissism, authoritarianism, favoritism, and challenges to personal honesty Masson witnessed and experienced during his training cannot be dismissed as disgruntled complaints. Although less frequent today, similar unfortunate incidents persist. That such abuses have been and remain part of the largely undocumented culture and oral history of a profession dedicated to compassionate healing seems jarring until we ask, "Were they not manifest in behaviors modeled by its idealized founder?"

Sequelae of Freud's defensiveness

In *The Psychoanalyst's Aversion to Proof*, Ratner (2019) describes Freud's defensiveness and reviews the assimilation of such patterns into the ongoing intellectual fabric and culture of psychoanalysis. He demonstrates the importance of personal matters in the development of psychoanalysis and in the often isolationist nature of its defensive stances.

Freud's letters demonstrate that he was both excited and anxiety-ridden over his findings concerning sexuality (Ratner, 2019). Sometimes he felt he had the courage to go forward, sometimes his efforts induced hysteria and exhaustion. He struggled with misgivings about his discoveries and ideas, which he claimed had led to a decade of social isolation after breaking with Breuer. Ratner further observed that Freud was uncomfortable and ashamed about going forward with forbidden knowledge and hypothesizes that Freud projected his own self-criticism over his shame and over his ambitious desire for recognition onto his critics, seeing many as more hostile than they were.

Freud avoided direct confrontation, choosing audiences carefully and occasionally enlisting surrogates. When challenged, Freud often criticized his critics and acted as if offering proof would be both a distraction and a submission to authorities unworthy of acknowledgment. Beneath the pleasant exterior he tried to cultivate, Freud harbored rage he feared he could neither express nor sublimate.

Freud could let potentially problematic matters go unaddressed, as if hoping they would pass (Kluft, 2018 b, c, 2022; Ratner, 2019). Freud shared the insight that the parental seductions reported by his hysterical patients were repressed fantasies, not accurate memories, in an oft-cited 1897 letter to Fleiss. This "realization" is often discussed as if it had been openly stated at that time, part of his effort to pacify strong reactions to his ideas about sexuality. However, Ratner notes that Freud wrote Fleiss about his fears of possible adverse consequences if he reversed himself at that time. He would not "go public" with his retraction for another eight years, in his 1905 *Three Essays on the Theory of Sexuality* (see Ratner, 2019). Likewise, he would attack hypnosis most trenchantly two years after Bernheim's death in 1919, 26 years after he abandoned its use.

Ratner makes it clear that Freud's narcissistic vulnerability, his inability to face and contend with disagreement and opposition while hungering for recognition, his unsublimated rage, plus his willingness to bend truth to his own needs, for his own safety, and for convenience, contributed to a set of unconstructive attitudes operative in overt and subtle ways throughout the history of psychoanalysis (Ratner, 2019; also Breger, 2009; Kluft, 2018a, , cb, d; 2022).

Sigmund Freud's "philosophy" as expressed by his choices – I

Freud's personal concerns and attitudes affected what might otherwise appear to be scientific decisions. Their persistent influences lead naturally to the depersonalization, dehumanization, and inappropriate treatment of those ideas, persons, groups, and data seen as threats to the core of psychoanalysis. Perhaps by studying what motivations were expressed in Freud's choices and behavior, they can speak for themselves.

In 1882, 26-year-old Sigmund Freud noted his use of Bernheim's self-suggestive methods. Foreshadowing his drive to make a name for himself, Freud's preface to his 1888 translation of Bernheim's *Suggestion* goes beyond thoughtful observations; he critiques Charcot and takes issue with Bernheim himself.

Freud co-authored a paper with Forel for the 1889 First International Congress of Hypnosis in Paris. Scholars there debated whether hypnosis could compel a person to do unwanted antisocial acts. Bernheim's Nancy School affirmed this possibility, which Charcot's Paris School disputed. Congress participants were unaware that an as-yet-undiscovered event had occurred that would position their disputes at the center of a world-wide sensation (Levingston, 2014).

Con man Michel Eyraud knew hypnosis. His accomplice, Gabrielle Bompard, was an experienced hypnotic subject. After murdering an affluent libertine and minor official, they became the subjects of a world-wide dragnet and media frenzy. Bompard claimed that anything she had done had been done at Eyraud's command while she was under the influence of hypnosis. Eyraud met his fate at the guillotine in early 1891. Young and attractive, Bompard received a lighter sentence, perhaps mitigated by infatuated public sentiment and lingering concerns about her allegations concerning hypnosis.

Their infamous crimes inspired George du Maurier's *Trilby*, serialized in 1894 and published as a novel in 1895. Through 1894–1895, the world was fascinated with *Trilby*, the first best-seller of the modern era. *Trilby* recounts the domination of the lovely young Trilby by Svengali, an evil Jewish hypnotist. Svengali, du Maurier's vehicle for expressing his fervid anti-Semitism, was not only an Eastern European Jew; he was from the homeland of Freud's parents. Dramatized, *Trilby* became a hit on the stages of Europe, North America, and elsewhere. While the first edition of Freud's *The Interpretation of Dreams* (1900) would sell less than 100 copies per year, *Trilby* sold 200,000 copies in one market in two months in 1895. Two years later, its sales would be surpassed by another novel about an evil hypnotist, Bram Stoker's *Dracula*.

Anti-Semitism was rife in Europe in the late 1800s. For example, the same year that *Trilby* first appeared (1894) saw the fraudulent trial and conviction for treason of Captain Albert Dreyfus, a Jewish officer in the France army with a spotless reputation, a heinous act of anti-Semitism. In Austria, Karl Luger, a rabid anti-Semite, was rising to power. He would become Vienna's mayor (1897–1911). Although Freud took no public stance in the matter of Dreyfus and left no mention of *Trilby*, he was painfully aware that he lived in an anti-Semitic time and place. It is arguable that anti-Semitism was a potent factor in his abandoning hypnosis (Kluft, 2022). Amidst these events, Freud and Breuer (1893–1895) wrote and published their *Studies on Hysteria.*

Freud had changed his birth name, Sigismund Schlomo, to Sigmund when he entered the army. He celebrated Christian holidays, not the Jewish ones. Freud feared that his contributions would be dismissed as "Jewish science." Hence, his later efforts to install the conspicuously Aryan Carl Jung as his successor in psychoanalysis.

Freud felt professionally isolated. He repeatedly bemoaned the state of his practice, complaining that his office was often empty. He wrote Fleiss that his mood seemed determined by how his practice was doing. Years later, in his address to B'Nai B'rith, Freud spoke of the warm acceptance accorded him in this Jewish fraternal organization during those years of isolation.

During the 1890s, he was both aggressively determined to make a mark for himself and apprehensive about his efforts (Breger, 2009). He entered the 1890s still burdened by his cocaine fiasco of the 1880s. He wrote the masterful neuropsychophysiological *Project*, a work so far ahead of its time that it would not be published in his lifetime. Freud reinvested himself in hypnosis and worked with Breuer until they parted ways. Thereafter, Freud distanced himself from hypnosis. As noted, his solo practice was often marginal, and he was fretful. He presented his seduction theory, which was controversial, and developed his ideas on sexuality further. In 1897 he "realized" that his seduction theory was incorrect but declined to make a prompt retraction. For a rejection- and criticism-sensitive man driven to achieve recognition, this decade represents the mortifying failure of one heroic effort after another.

Small wonder that after developing a paradigm based on unconscious fantasies that he would know better than anyone else (see Freud, 1914), Freud may have felt he had finally reached a relatively safe haven. His emerging model was based on internal, psychological reality. He had finally found a realm in which he could, in fact, reign supreme. His paradigm could withstand denial by an analysand, minimize the external as less meaningful than inner psychological reality, and was fortified by authoritative reasoning, the ultimate truths of which only he could decree.

Now, Freud's unconscious constructs defied the challenges of time and space. He "circled his wagons" and defended his "turf" as best he could.

Sigmund Freud's "philosophy" as expressed by his choices – II

Mainstream psychoanalysis understands Freud's abandonment of hypnosis as a moment of exciting progress. His few publications on hypnosis routinely referenced by psychoanalysts present hypnosis negatively. The best-known (1921) accords great power to the hypnotist, cautioning against the possible misuse of hypnosis. However, the Psychoanalytic Electronic Publishing attributes to Freud over 70 hypnosis-relevant contributions. Taken together, with some input from modern sources, they call his charges against hypnosis into question.

Freud's self-description in a 1900 letter to Fleiss remains eloquent and revealing:

> On the whole, I have noticed that you usually overestimate me greatly. The motivation for this error, though, disarms any reproach. For I am actually not at all a man of science, not an observer, not an experimenter, not a thinker. I am by temperament nothing but a conquistador – an adventurer, if you want it translated – with all the curiosity, daring, and tenacity characteristic of a man of this sort. Such people are customarily esteemed only if they have been successful, have really discovered something; otherwise, they are dropped by

> the wayside. And that is not altogether unjust. At the present time, however, luck has left me; I no longer discover anything worthwhile.
>
> (Freud, 1900a, p. 398)

Freud compares himself to men who are intrepid explorers, prepared to take what they want (however rationalized), and crush or destroy opposition. Although this analogy is jarring, Freud repeatedly demonstrated his willingness to attack those he saw as inimical to his "cause."

Freud did not discuss his 1895 decision to abandon hypnosis in detail for years. When he did so, he offered criticisms and misrepresentations of hypnosis left largely unchallenged by generations of analysts. I found no psychoanalytic sources in which Freud's arguments received close scrutiny or their accuracy was not taken for granted. A few of Freud's complaints are addressed briefly below. For detailed considerations, see Kluft (2018 a, b, c, d; 2022).

Elkins, Barabasz, Council, and Spiegel (2015) developed a modern definition of hypnosis: "A state of consciousness involving focused attention and reduced peripheral awareness characterized by an enhanced capacity for response to suggestion" (p. 6).

Hypnosis may be brought about by a ritual of induction performed by another (heterohypnosis), or by oneself (autohypnosis). "Spontaneous" hypnosis may occur in response to particular stimuli (internal or external) or circumstances (Kluft, 2015). Normal forms of dissociation are linked to many aspects of spontaneous trance (Butler, 2006).

Debate continues on whether hypnosis should be defined by antecedent interventions (preferable for some forms of research but failing to define the phenomenon per se) or by a particular state of consciousness (defining the phenomenon *per se* but more difficult to study directly). In Freud's era, hypnosis was often "defined" by the hypnotist's procedures. Ergo, when Freud discontinued using such procedures, he could claim that he had put hypnosis behind him. He tried to distance himself from all the negative implications that hypnosis had recently acquired in the minds of the public. However, his mentor, Bernheim, practiced both formal trancework using inductions and waking hypnosis involving focus, concentration, and suggestion alone. He had developed self-suggestive (autohypnotic) methods. Even subsequent to his "abandoning hypnosis," Freud noted the advantage of utilizing the spontaneous trances into which his patients fell on the couch to pursue additional associations in *The Interpretation of Dreams* (1900). Therefore, Freud knew of all three forms of hypnosis. His stating he had abandoned hypnosis was a selective, incomplete, and perhaps disingenuous assertion.

Freud complained that hypnosis, which involves suggestions, distorted the transference. Certainly, the demand characteristics of the hypnotic situation and the nature of suggestions made may do so, but Freud's complaints were oversimplified.

Suggestion is ubiquitous, not restricted to particular moments or procedures. Whether or not suggestions might induce detrimental distortions depends on what is suggested, how it is presented, and the relational field in which it occurs. Gabrielle Bompard was a hypnotic virtuoso. She followed suggestions to manifest many phenomena. But, following suggestions with which she disagreed was not among them (Levingston, 2014)!

The words Freud (1913) proposed for use in beginning an analysis instruct the patient what to do. They pass as unremarkable but are expressed in the language of a hypnotic suggestion. Freud speaks of this basic rule as the sole exception allowing the use of suggestion, instructing patients that this is the only rule they must follow.

> So say whatever goes through your mind. Act as though, for instance, you were a traveller sitting next to the window of a railway carriage and describing to someone inside the carriage the changing views which you see outside. Finally, never forget that you have promised to be absolutely honest, and never leave anything out because, for some reason or other, it is unpleasant to tell it.
>
> (Freud, 1913, p. 133–134)

Similar imageries, following inductions, are taught in contemporary hypnosis workshops. The basic rule determines the overall atmosphere, expectancy, and work ethic of the analysis. It is renewed, implicitly, with every analysis of resistance. The idea that suggestion is inevitably dangerous is absurd, remaining credible only if left unexamined. It is true that a carefully misled subject can become subject to mind control techniques (Sheflin & Opton, 1978), but such efforts are far from the realm of standard clinical hypnosis.

Freud's most trenchant criticisms of hypnosis were voiced in *Group Psychology and the Analysis of the Ego* (1921). Freud describes the hypnotist as tapping into uncanny and primitive powers of domination. Again, his portrait of the hypnotist is unsettlingly reminiscent of Svengali, not of Bernheim, Liébeault, Charcot, or Breuer.

Freud describes approaches attributing powerful dominance to the hypnotist, who can easily use them to pursue evil designs. He looks back to Mesmeric beliefs in "animal magnetism" discredited by the 1784 French Royal Commission. The implication of Freud's commentary is that the sort of person who uses hypnosis may be one who exercises inordinate dominance and control by the force of his uncanny powers.

However, thanks to the media and popular literature of the era, Freud's misrepresentations of the hypnotist struck a familiar note with the public and professionals alike. In presenting his readers with a description of the fictional Svengali as the hypnotist, his most famous attack against hypnosis and the hypnotist was a misleading deception, not a bold stance against coercive control. This shameful fictional mischaracterization continues to be referenced in mainstream analysis and persists in the minds of the public. Freud had a wider understanding of hypnosis than he drew upon in discussing his abandonment of hypnosis.

Another rationale Freud (1914) cited was his discovery that not all patients could be hypnotized adequately for therapeutic purposes. His presenting this as a realization is unsettling. Bernheim knew and taught that patients were not equally hypnotizable. In his preface to Bernheim's 1888 *Suggestion*, Freud cautions that not all patients are suitable for hypnotic treatment. Indeed, when Freud once brought a patient he could not hypnotize to see Bernheim in consultation, Bernheim failed as well. Long before Freud "discovered" that he could not hypnotize all patients, and pondered whether he was no more than a "mediocre" hypnotist, he was already fully aware that all patients were not equally hypnotizable, and that there were patients with whom the world's greatest experts could not succeed.

Toward the end of his career, Freud (1937) would level against psychoanalysis many of the same accusations he had made against hypnosis decades before, as if unaware of these ironic parallels. Freud was already mature and experienced when he made his most disparaging statements against hypnosis. It is reasonable to understand them as politicized polemics rather than objective scientific observations and reasoned conclusions.

Freud often lionized psychoanalysis irrationally. Discussing the possible blending of "the copper of suggestion" with "the gold of analysis," Freud (1919) asserted that should such a treatment prove helpful, the benefit would be due to the contribution from analysis, not "suggestion." In "Wild Analysis," Freud (1910) insisted that in any misadventure, psychoanalysis would suffer more injury than the patient. Freud enlisted hyperbole, exaggeration, twisted reasoning, and inaccurate or dishonest assertions in the service of his cause.

Together, Freud's personal concerns and the urgency with which he tried to advance his cause are quite consistent with his portrayal of himself as a conquistador. They express a set of attitudes in which his defensiveness and determination combine to rationalize and condone dismissiveness and mistreatment in dealing with problematic individuals and issues.

Discussion

Sigmund Freud's personal issues and the stressors of his era helped shape a defensive, risk-aversive personal philosophy and inculcated and rationalized a stance of isolation from and insulation against disagreements and demands for proofs of the merits of his ideas and approaches. At times he withheld information, at others, he made inaccurate statements and offered embarrassing mischaracterizations to better promote his "cause." Some instances suggest dishonesty and historical revisionism.

The power of Freud's influence and the attractions and strengths of his ideas was such that much he asserted was left unchallenged. Whatever or whoever proved unwelcome to or unsettling to Sigmund Freud became unwelcome, treated dismissively or with overt hostility, and/or received minimal attention subsequently. Conflicts and issues beyond Freud's model were not deemed fit subjects for analysis.

Many unexamined but problematic notions have been passed along, unquestioned, for over a century. Eisogetic distortions built into what was represented and promulgated as improved understanding became transgenerational identifications (i.e., aspects of a group culture paying homage to feelings and concerns remote from the present and protected by the institutionalized perpetuation of Freud's efforts to evade confrontations and demands for proof of his ideas). However rationalized, these archaic misadventures still may unduly influence otherwise dedicated and accomplished professionals, compromising both optimal patient care and the encouragement of thoughtful progress.

Hence Emma Ekstein, the first female analyst; Sándor Ferenczi, who sought to reinvigorate interest in the seduction theory; Heinz Kohut, a distinguished senior analyst who proposed a new understanding of narcissism; and the promising young scholar Jeffrey Masson, who declined to suppress unsettling information, were all perceived as threats and treated poorly. These mistreatments were rationalized to counter perceived threats to valued ideas and reputations, and to prevent opposition to those invested in preserving established ideas and practices.

Kohut (1970; Kohut & Wolf, 1978) described selfobject transferences, which are useful in studying aspects of Freud's behavior. His three major selfobject constellations described mirroring, the idealized object, and alter ego or twinship. Freud was very eager to be validated and confirmed; that is, he sought interactions with those who served a positive "mirror" function, returning acceptance, approval, and agreement with his ideas.

Freud became his own omnipotent object, his own grandiose citadel of strength. Disillusioned by his father, critical of subsequent mentors and colleagues, Freud was determined to be the one who knew the most about psychoanalysis (Freud, 1914), and he assumed the role of arbiter of what psychoanalysis would and would not accept. He identified himself with the conquistadors … plunderers, enslavers, and perpetuators of genocide.

With regard to his sense of twinship, or sameness with others, Freud did best with those who in many ways were his alter egos. Most of his close circle came from similar backgrounds. A man preoccupied with protecting and promulgating his own ideas would find unacceptable ideas, data, and individuals whom he saw as threats to his "cause."

Once trauma had been removed from the center of his concerns, Freud both remained aware of trauma and remained hostile to efforts to make trauma a central focus of analytic concern. His stances established an orthodoxy in which exogenous traumata became marginalized as non-analytic concerns, as distractions from core analytic concerns. He was not above marginalizing the dissociative pathologies and hypnosis despite, or perhaps because, he himself was hypnotizable, he suffered dissociative symptoms, and he feared that he might be endangered by deep trance experiences (Kluft, 2018 a, b, c).

Attempts made by several senior analysts to prevent Masson from making known unwelcome and embarrassing information were painfully reminiscent of Freud's delaying publication of his withdrawal of his original trauma theory in order to protect his reputation. Inappropriately aggressive attacks on Masson and unwarranted mischaracterizations of him and his work bore unwanted resemblances to Freud's putting forward a false Svengali-like hypnotist to disparage hypnosis.

Both public and professional attention to Jeffrey Masson's scholarly contributions (e.g., 1984, 2017) have focused on his forceful exposition of the consequences of Freud's withdrawal of the seduction theory; Freud's protection of his friend,

Wilhelm Fleiss, from the consequences of his malpractice in his treatment of their mutual patient, Emma Ekstein; and his abject betrayal of Emma Eckstein' best interests. Freud's dubious behavior opens him to charges of misogyny and more. By claiming that no one but he took an interest in psychoanalysis for a decade (1914), he "erased" Emma Ekstein from his preferred history of psychoanalysis.

The discussions above demonstrated how personal matters in the life of Sigmund Freud played a role in bringing unscientific elements into the heart of the psychoanalytic enterprise and contributed to their perpetuation. However, they do not indicate that Freud should be held accountable for their persistence into the present day. Psychoanalysis has had well over a century to make a thoughtful reassessment of what it long defended against objective scrutiny and scientific study. Many have been discouraged and harmed by the unfortunate tenacity of ideas and stances that are inaccurate and/or incomplete and, in their inaccuracy and incompleteness, potentially hurtful.

Contemporary psychoanalysis faces the burden of addressing matters that have received undue protection from overdue scrutiny for over a century. It is as unfair to blame today's psychoanalysts for their persistent problems as it is to blame Freud, but it does fall to today's psychoanalysts to address them forthrightly.

There is no excuse for any healing discipline to condone ignorant and insensitive approaches to the issues of women, mistreated/traumatized groups and individuals, and entire diagnostic categories (such as hypnosis-related symptomatology and the dissociative disorders). Likewise, there is no excuse for gratuitous attacks upon those who advance new/different/unwelcome ideas. Psychoanalysis began as a new modality, far from the mainstream. It grew to become legitimized, respected, and sufficiently established to resist accommodating many further understandings and innovations.

The work of psychoanalysts who have grappled with the importance of addressing external as well as psychological reality, and who have studied the transmission of trauma and issues of importance across generational lines, may have much to offer in identifying the dysfunctional persistence of ideas and stances that have long outlived their usefulness. I believe that their insights can teach psychoanalysts of today how to preserve what is strong and valid in psychoanalysis, carefully dissect out problematic influences, and restore to the psychoanalytic mainstream a circumspect and comprehensive appreciation of hypnosis and hypnotic phenomena, exogenous trauma, and the dissociative disorders, in addition to the dissociation linked to relational trauma.

Placing these responsibilities before the psychoanalytic community may be the most lasting, healing, and helpful impact of Masson's efforts. While irrational and inaccurate elements are commonly discovered within the origin stories, cultures, and operational procedures of most groups and enterprises, psychoanalysis has resisted allowing and participating in the objective examination and careful scrutiny of its foundations, despite clear indications that this has resulted in the persistence of attitudes and practices with harmful potential. Analytic education reinforces the retracing and rediscovery of Freud's findings. However, assuring that the discovery, exploration, and resolution of problematic concerns be granted appropriate recognition at the center of analytic attention – clinically, scientifically, educationally, and organizationally – must become an ongoing commitment by the entire profession.

References

Breger, L. (2009). *A dream of undying fame: How Freud betrayed his mentor and invented psychoanalysis.* New York, NY: Basic Books.

Brenner, C. (2003). Commentary on Ilany Kogan's "On being a dead, beloved child." *Psychoanalytic Quarterly, 72*, 769–776.

Butler, L. (2006). Normative dissociation. *The Psychiatric Clinics of North America, 29*(1),45–62. https://doi.org/10.1016/j.psc.2005.10.004

Eisold, K. (1994). The intolerance of diversity in psychoanalytic institutes. *The International Journal of Psychoanalysis, 75*(4), 785–800.

Elkins, G., Barabasz, A., Council, J., & Spiegel, D. (2015). Advancing research and practice: The revised APA Division 30 definition of hypnosis. *The International Journal of Clinical and Experimental Hypnosis, 63*(1), 1–9. https://doi.org/10.1080/00207144.2014.961870

Ferro, A. (2003). Commentary on Ilany Kogan's "On being a dead, beloved child. *The Psychoanalytic Quarterly, 72*(3), 777–783. https://doi.org/10.1002/j.2167-4086.2003.tb00652.x

Freud, S. (1888). Preface to the translation of Bernheim's *Suggestion.* In J. Strachey (Ed. & Trans.), *The standard edition of the complete psychological works of Sigmund Freud* (Vol. I, pp. 73–87). Hogarth.

Freud, S. (1900a). Letter from Freud to Fliess, February 1, 1900. In J. Masson (Ed. & Trans.), *The complete letters of Sigmund Freud to Wilhelm Fliess, 1887–1904* (pp. 397–398). Harvard University Press.

Freud, S. (1900b). The interpretation of dreams. In J. Strachey (Ed. & Trans.), *The standard edition of the complete psychological works of Sigmund Freud (Vol. IV)*. Hogarth.

Freud, S. (1905). Three essays on the theory of sexuality. In J. Strachey (Ed. & Trans.), *The standard edition of the complete psychological works of Sigmund Freud* (Vol. VII, pp. 123–246). Hogarth.

Freud, S. (1910). Wild analysis. J. Strachey (Ed. & Trans.), *The standard edition of the complete psychological works of Sigmund Freud* (Vol. XI, pp. 219–228). Hogarth.

Freud, S. (1913). On beginning the treatment. J. Strachey (Ed. & Trans.), *The Standard Edition of the Complete Psychological Works of Sigmund Freud* (Vol. XII, pp. 123–144). Hogarth.

Freud, S. (1914). On the history of the psycho-analytic movement. J. Strachey (Ed. & Trans.), *The Standard Edition of the Complete Psychological Works of Sigmund Freud* (Vol. XIV, pp. 1–66). Hogarth.

Freud, S. (1919). Lines of advance in psycho-analytic therapy. J. Strachey (Ed. & Trans.), *The Standard Edition of the Complete Psychological Works of Sigmund Freud* (Vol. XVII, pp. 157–168). Hogarth.

Freud, S. (1921). Group psychology and the analysis of the ego. In J. Strachey (Ed. & Trans.), *The standard edition of the complete psychological works of Sigmund Freud* (Vol. XVIII, pp. 65–144). Hogarth.

Freud, S. (1937). Analysis terminable and interminable. In J. Strachey (Ed. & Trans.), *The standard edition of the complete psychological works of Sigmund Freud* (Vol. XXIII, pp. 209–254). London, UK: Hogarth.

Glover, W. (2023). Psychoanalysis – More than a profession. Unpublished manuscript.

Henderson, J. (1975). Incest. In Sadock, B., Freeman, A., & Kaplan, H. *Comprehensive textbook of psychiatry – II (2 volumes)*. Williams & Wilkins.
Hicks, D. (2012). *Dignity: Its essential role in resolving conflict*. Yale University Press.
Kluft, R. P. (1995). The confirmation and discontinuation of memories of abuse in dissociative identity disorder patients: A naturalistic clinical study. *Dissociation, 8*, 253–258.
Kluft, R. P. (2015). The revised APA division 30 definition of hypnosis: An appreciation, a commentary, and a wish list. *The American Journal of Clinical Hypnosis, 57*(4), 431–438. https://doi.org/10.1080/00029157.2015.1011495
Kluft, R. P. (2016). You have to be carefully taught: Dignity considerations in clinical practice, scholarship, and trauma treatment. In S. Levine, (Ed.), *Dignity matters: Psychoanalytic and psychosocial perspectives* (pp. 141–158). London: Karnac Books.
Kluft, R. P. (2018a). Reconsidering hypnosis and psychoanalysis: Toward creating a context for understanding. *The American Journal of Clinical Hypnosis*, *60*(3), 201–215. https://doi.org/10.1080/00029157.2018.1400810
Kluft, R. P. (2018b). Freud's rejection of hypnosis: Part I: – The genesis of a rift. *The American Journal of Clinical Hypnosis, 60*(4), 307–323. https://doi.org/10.1080/00029157.2018.1426321
Kluft, R. P. (2018c). Freud's rejection of hypnosis: Part II: – The genesis of a rift. The *American Journal of Clinical Hypnosis*, *60*(4), 324–347. https://doi.org/10.1080/00029157.2018.1426326
Kluft, R. P. (2018d). Freud's rejection of hypnosis: Perspectives old and new: Part III of III—toward healing the rift. *The American Journal of Clinical Hypnosis*, *61*(3), 208–226. https://doi.org/10.1080/00029157.2018.1544432
Kluft, R. P. (2022). The mysterious case of the suspiciously silent psychoanalyst. *Journal of Controversial Ideas, 2*(2), 99–125.
Kogan, I. (2003). On being a dead, beloved child. *The Psychoanalytic Quarterly*, *72*(3), 727–804. https://doi.org/10.1002/j.2167-4086.2003.tb00650
Kohut, H. (1970). *The analysis of the self.* University of Chicago Press.
Kohut, H., & Wolf, E. (1978). The disorders of the self and their treatment: An outline. *International Journal of Psychoanalysis, 59*, 413–425.
Levingston, S. (2014). *Little demon in the city of light: A true story of murder and mesmerism in Belle Epoque Paris*. Doubleday.
Luborsky, L. (1996). *The symptom-context method: Symptoms as opportunities in psychotherapy*. American Psychological Association.
Luborsky, L., & Crits-Cristoph, P. (1998). *Understanding transference: The core conflictual relationship method (2nd ed.)*. American Psychological Association.
Makari, G. (2008). *Revolution in mind: The creation of psychoanalysis*. Harper.
Masson, J. (1984). *The assault on Truth: Freud's suppression of the seduction theory*. Farrar, Straus, & Giroux.
Masson, J. (2017). A personal perspective: The response to child abuse then and now. *Journal of Trauma and Dissociation, 18*, 476–482. https://doi.org/10.1080/15299732.2017.1295429
Nathanson, D. (1991). *Shame and pride*. Norton.
Ratner, A. (2019). *The psychoanalyst's aversion to proof.* International Psychoanalytic Books.
Scheflin, A., & Opton, E. (1978). *The mind manipulators: A non-fiction account*. Paddington Press.
Simon, B. (1992). "Incest—See Under Oedipus Complex": The history of an error in psychoanalysis. *Journal of the American Psychoanalytic Association, 40*, 955–988. https://doi.org/10.1177/000306519204000401

Volkan, V. (1986). The narcissism of minor differences in the psychological gap between opposing nations. *Psychoanalytic Inquiry*, *45*, 255–273.
Volkan, V. (1997). Chosen trauma-unresolved mourning in *Bloodlines – From Ethnic Pride to Ethnic Terrorism* (p. 36–49). Farrar, Straus, and Giroux.
Volkan, V. (2009). Large group identity, international relations and psychoanalysis. *International Forum for Psychoanalysis, 18*, 206–213. https://doi.org/10.1080/08037060902727795
Waelder, R. (1962). Psychoanalysis, scientific method, and philosophy. *Journal of the American Psychoanalytic Association*, *10*, 617–637. https://doi.org/10.1177/000306516201000310

5 Jeffrey Moussaieff Masson Revisited

The Seduction Controversies about Reality versus Fantasy

Henry Zvi Lothane

Four decades ago, Jeffrey Moussaieff Masson published his sensational book, *The Assault on Truth: Freud's Suppression of the Seduction Theory* (1984a). The current essay is a reappraisal of Masson's life drama and an appraisal of psychoanalysis as a method and theory. It is my purpose to parse the pith and pitch of Masson's predication about seduction, procured by his perusing a particular letter Freud sent Fliess in 1897.

Jeffrey and I are both octogenarians, Jewish, polyglots, and admirers of Freud, the German language, and its literature. I am an American psychiatrist and psychoanalyst, he is an American PhD and former Canadian psychoanalyst. We were disappointed by our training analyses, we did not learn anything new about ourselves, our books were not liked by orthodox Freudians, and we got involved[1] with Janet Malcolm (1981, 1984). In the 1980s we met at Malcolm's townhouse in New York. The atmosphere was friendly, and I was impressed by Jeffrey, but we did not communicate thereafter. There were also some differences: Jeffrey was a son of a Sephardic father and Ashkenazi mother; both my parents were Ashkenazi; Jeffrey's first wife Terri was born in Poland, as was I; my wife was a Sephardic born in Jerusalem and raised in Panama.

The provocative title of Masson's book calls for a preliminary disambiguation of seduction, assault, and suppression. Assault is either a violent bodily attack or an attack with words, and only the latter is relevant here. To suppress means to subdue bodily, prevent information from being known, or to block something from consciousness. Freud did not use the term seduction *theory*, other authors used this term, for example, Ernest Jones (1953, p. 356).

In my 1987 essay on Masson's book, I discussed the various meanings of seduction. Seduction, derived from the Latin root *se*, apart, and *ducere*, to lead, to guide, means an interaction of influence, persuasion, and participation between a person acting as seducer and another who yields to being seduced. In the 1984 book, Masson claimed (a) that there was a factual and precise truth about seduction, and (b) that "Freud's Renunciation of the Theory of Seduction" (p. 107 ff.) was an indisputable fact. These claims were based solely on Freud's letter to Fliess of September 21, 1897:

DOI: 10.4324/9781003431466-6

> I no longer believe in my *neurotica* … from the continual disappointment in my efforts to bring a single analysis to a real conclusion … the running away of people; … the absence of complete successes; … I was ready to give up two things: the complete resolution of a neurosis and the certain knowledge of its etiology in childhood.
>
> (Masson, 1985, pp. 264–265)

How did Freud differentiate genuine cases from faked or fantasized ones? How were childhood traumas related to the present illness? And Freud wondered: "Can it be that this doubt merely represents an episode in the advance toward further insight?" (Masson, 1985, pp. 264–265). Indeed, how could so much hinge on an episode?

Laplanche and Pontalis (1973) noted Freud's definition of sexual trauma (*Standard Edition*, 1, pp. 221–223):

> dropping the seduction theory in 1897 as a decisive step in the foundation of psycho-analytic theory … calls, however, for some qualification. Right up to the end of his life, Freud continued to assert the existence, prevalence, and pathogenic force of scenes of seduction actually experienced by children.
>
> (pp. 405–406)

Let us review Freud's qualifications. Freud discussed precocious childhood sexuality in (1) 1896a, (2) 1896b, (3) 1896c, and (4) 1905.

(1). In 1896a Freud wrote:

> hysterical symptoms are traced back to their origin … . Travelling backwards into the patient's past … I finally reached the starting point of the pathological process … . The event of which the subject has retained an unconscious memory is a *precocious experience of sexual relations with actual excitement of the genitals resulting from sexual abuse committed by another person* … up to the age of eight to ten before the child has reached sexual maturity.
>
> (pp. 151–152; italics in original)

But there were also conscious memories.

(2). In 1896b Freud stated:

> what I have to add here, [is] a uniform outcome of the analyses carried out by me on thirteen cases of hysteria … Furthermore, hysteria is far and away more frequent in the female sex; for even in childhood they are more liable to provoke sexual attacks.
>
> (p. 163)

In 1924 Freud added this footnote:

> This section is dominated by an error which I have since repeatedly acknowledged and corrected … Seduction retains a certain etiological importance, and even today I think some of these psychological comments are to the point.
>
> (p. 168)

Freud restated these remarks in 1925:

> I do not believe that I forced the seduction phantasies on my patients, that I 'suggested' them. I had in fact stumbled for the first time upon the *Oedipus complex* … in its disguise of phantasies … . Moreover, seduction during childhood retained a certain share, though a humbler one, in the etiology of neuroses but the seducers turned out as a rule to have been older children.
>
> (pp. 34–35; italics in original)

Freud first mentioned the Oedipus complex to Fliess on October 15, 1897 (Masson, 1985 p. 272) but did not discover it working with patients:

> (between the ages of two and two-and-a-half years) my libido was stirred up towards *matrem* [mother], namely on the occasion of a journey from Leipzig to Vienna, during which we must have spent the night together and I must have had the opportunity to see her *nudam* [nude].
>
> (Masson, 1985, p. 268)

(3). In 1896c, Freud mentioned "eighteen cases … *all* the cases on which I have been able to carry out the work of analysis" (p. 200, italics in original) and delineated three "groups" of experiences:

> (a) assaults … abuse on female children by adult strangers; (b) a nursery or governess or tutor, a close relative has initiated the child into sexual intercourse and has maintained a regular love relationship with it … which has often lasted for years; (c) child relationships proper—sexual relationships between two children of different sexes, mostly a brother and a sister.
>
> (p. 208)

Freud did not renounce this "important finding" (p. 203).

(4). Remarkably, Freud discussed the seduction theory in the 1905 *Three Essays*:

> The reappearance of sexual activity is determined by internal causes and external contingencies … . In the foreground we find the effects of seduction, which treats a child as a sexual object prematurely and teaches him, in highly emotional circumstances, how to obtain satisfaction from his genital zones … which he is then usually obliged to repeat again and again by masturbation. An influence of this kind may originate either from adults or from other children.

> I cannot admit that in my paper on "The Aetiology of Hysteria" (1896c) I exaggerated the frequency or importance of that influence, though I did not then know that persons who remained normal may have had the same experiences in their childhood … . Obviously, seduction is not required in order to arouse a child's sexual life; that can also come about spontaneously from internal causes.
>
> (pp. 190–191)

In 1914a Freud reminisced:

> At last came the reflection that, after all, one had no right to despair because one has been deceived in one's expectations … if hysterical subjects trace back their symptoms to the traumas that are fictitious … then … they create such scenes in *phantasy*, and this psychical reality requires to be taken into account alongside actual reality.
>
> (pp. 17–18; italics in original)

This overview shows that for Freud seduction was a search for an equilibrium between fact and fantasy, perception and imagination, the external environment and the internal environment, a question of emphasis, not a repudiation.

In 1916 Freud wrote in Lecture XXIII: "The phantasies possess *psychical* as contrasted with *material* reality, and we gradually learn to understand that *in the world of the neuroses it's the psychical reality which is the decisive kind*" (p. 368, italics in original[2]). However, if real means an *existent*, then seeing real things and persons with the bodily eye and "seeing" nonexistent things and persons, as Hamlet said, with the mind's eye, as in dreams and daydreams, then both are real *events* that can be remembered and narrated by both the neurotic and the normal. Thus, having fantasies cannot be used as evidence against the reality of true memories of trauma.

Trauma expert Bessel van der Kolk (2015), who cited Freud repeatedly, did not consider fantasy as a relevant factor in his studies of trauma and he emphasized memory. It is necessary to investigate whether a given memory is truth, lie, or error. Trauma can be overcome without causing disorder, but where there is stress disorder, there is always trauma. Whereas traumatic seduction in childhood may become a problem in the sexual life of an adult, it does not apply to nonsexual traumas. Moreover, fantasizing (i.e., imagining) is a basic, normal ability to visualize thoughts and feelings in mental *images* (Lothane, 1982, 2007a, b; Russell, 1921; Ryle, 1949). Therefore, I suggested defining psychical reality as *emotional reality* (Lothane, 2015): it creates a feeling of conviction and suggests a flexible boundary between neurotic and normal.

Since we live in the external world of events and actions, these make up a drama (derived from the Greek *dran*, to act). The Greeks invented *dramaturgy*, the art of composing and staging dramas, we show dramas in film and television. In 2009, I introduced *dramatology* as a method of studying real dramas, the events of a lifetime. An event is an unchangeable historical fact, but the stories told about it are as varied as the narrators (e.g., as shown in Kurosawa's film *Rashomon*). Dramatology and narratology go hand-in-hand. Lived drama is lived trauma in two forms: (1) dramatization in *images* of dreams and daydreams and (2) dramatization in spoken words and acts in the waking state. Anna O[3] enacted her thoughts and feelings: "since she lived through these things, she partially dramatized these through talking" (A.A. Brill's translation[4]), "so that the people around her became aware to a great extent of the content of these hallucinations" (Breuer & Freud, 1895, p. 27). Anna Freud (1966) observed that "the child's ego may maintain and dramatize his pleasurable fantasies" (p. 89). Scenes of seduction were dramas and traumas.

In the "Conclusion" of *The Assault on Truth,* Masson asserted that "Freud gave up the [seduction] theory not for theoretical or clinical reasons, but because of a personal failure of courage … when he shifted his attention from external trauma to internal fantasy as the causative factor in mental illness. But that does not mean it represents the truth" (p. 189). I argue this claim is not true or at least not the whole of the truth, nor did Freud lack courage. Freud himself spoke of his own fortitude:

> I am by temperament nothing but a conquistador—an adventurer, if you want it translated—with all the curiosity, daring, and tenacity characteristic of a man of this sort."
>
> (Masson, 1985, p. 304)

Masson's use of hyperbole resulted in the following report by Malcolm (1984):

> The abandonment of [seduction], far from being a triumph, was something of a disaster for psychoanalysis … . Speculating about the effect of "the new view of "the seduction theory" on psychotherapy, he [Masson] said, with inspired impudence, "They would have to recall every patient since 1901. It would be like the Pinto [motor car]" (p. 19). [Kurt Eissler and Anna Freud] sensed that I could single-handedly bring down the whole business—and, let's face it, there is a lot of money in that business. And they were right to be frightened because what I was discovering was dynamite."
>
> (p. 35)

The columns of the temple were not brought down, but "impudence" was Malcolm's disparaging editorializing. Ironically, the orthodox apostles and apostate Masson were saying the same, that Freud abandoned the seduction theory! Anna Freud put it pithily:

> Keeping up the seduction theory would mean to abandon the Oedipus complex, and with it the whole importance of fantasy life, conscious or unconscious fantasy. In fact, I think there would have been no psychoanalysis afterwards.
>
> (p. 63)

Masson was also attacked by analysts for seeking publicity in the *New York Times*. Here is how it happened. In 1979 Dr. Milton I. Klein, a New York analyst, and his coworker Dr. David Tribich, published "On Freud's 'Blindness,'" arguing that,

> in his five major cases Freud described destructive behavior on the part of his patients' parents, but he did not see it as destructive, showing how a "parent deceived, threatened, bullied, beat and tortured their children, remaining himself peculiarly blind to the effects of such mistreatments.
>
> (p. 52)

In the fall of 1981, I was introduced to Dr. Klein by Dr. Joseph Reppen, publisher of the journal *Psychoanalytic Books*, who knew of my interest in seduction. In 1981, Klein claimed that in giving up seduction "Freud made neither a *'discovery' nor an 'error' nor did he almost make a 'fatal mistake.' What he did was to reinterpret the theoretical significance of his clinical data while having little scientific reason to do so*" (pp. 186–187, italics in original).

Klein, who had heard about Masson's work from several sources, told Tribich about it, who then passed it to his brother-in-law, Ralph Blumenthal, staff reporter for the *New York Times*. In the early summer of 1981, Blumenthal got so excited by learning that Masson had discovered Freud's unpublished letters that he traveled to California to interview Masson, who then also handed him his "Yale lecture," the fateful paper he had just read in New Haven at the June meeting of the Western New England Psychoanalytic Society. Upon his return, Blumenthal published two articles in the science section of the *New York Times*, "Subtleties in Origin of Master's Theories Sought in Documents" (August 18, 1981) and "Did Freud's Isolation, Peer Rejection Prompt Key Theory Reversal" (August 25, 1981). When Janet Malcolm read these reports, she also traveled to San Francisco to interview Masson obtaining materials for her publications in 1983 and 1984. Masson did not rush to advertise himself, he was approached by interviewers and told them what happened.

Dr. Klein also corresponded with Anna Freud and received this letter from her:

20 Maresfield Gardens London, NW3 55X
13th January 1982

Milton I. Klein, Ph.D.,
145 East 27th Street
New York, N.Y. 10016 USA

Dear Dr. Klein,
Thank you for your letter of December 31st. I never thought that there was any doubt why my father gave up the seduction theory. Certainly, it was his clinical work and constant contact with patients. That it occurred in the patients' material so frequently could in the long run not be attributed to reality, but only to a fantasy of overwhelming generality. It seemed to me that that is the opinion that he himself expressed in his writings.

Yours sincerely,
Anna Freud [handwritten]

What finally brought Masson down was calling psychoanalysis sterile in the lecture to Yale analysts. In the brouhaha that ensued, childless benefactor Kurt

Eissler—for whom Masson was like an adopted son—yielding to pressure by many analysts, fired Masson as project director of the Freud Archives. Masson (1990) described his fall from grace as follows:

> And when, after I was fired at a meeting of the board of directors of the archives, Eissler said goodbye to me, he said we would probably not meet again. We are both close to tears. Something that had begun with such enthusiasm on both sides, with so much respect, so much love even, was now ending like this. Why? I felt as though I was leaving a deeply loved father who said that unless I lived life as he lived it, I could not stay in his house. I had no choice but to leave.
> (p. 47)

In my opinion, Eissler and Anna Freud could have kept Masson had they wanted to, but he was cut loose, not because Masson had challenged a "bastion of male supremacy" (Masson, 1990, p. 47), but because he dared to criticize Freud; for them Freud was infallible, thus above all criticism.

The alleged recantation by Freud was only an episode, and yet it lured Masson to overstate its importance and psychoanalysts en masse to resort to generalizations and formulaic interpretations such as the Oedipus complex and the sexual drive theory, instead of viewing seduction as a dyadic (i.e., interpersonal action analyzable with the method of free association; Lothane, 2018).

In the September 21, 1897 letter to Fliess, Freud relapsed to viewing hysteria as an etiologically, diagnostically, and prognostically monadic medical illness. Moreover, his reasoning was that

> future cases will work out like the past ones. It is the attribution of similar behavior to similar things. This familiar method of framing a general hypothesis, by generalizing from observed cases to all cases of the kind, is called *induction*.
> (Quine & Ullian, 1970, p. 55)

However, there is a difference between observing objects, persons, and actions and *theorizing* about objects, persons, and actions. A theory operates with the method of *subsumption*. One day an apple fell on Newton's head, so he discovered the theory of gravity, subsuming his apple under a law applying to all apples. But interactions with people can only be explained with the method of *individuation*, as unique real-life dramas (i.e., traumas) that give rise to a variety of narratives. The subsumption theory of seduction lured analysts to resort to generalizations and formulaic interpretations (e.g., the Oedipus complex or drive theory), also trumpeted by the prominent German historian of psychoanalysis Ilse Grubrich-Simitis in 1987 (Freud, 1987). Earlier that year (1987), she was the publisher and editor of Freud's phylogenetic fantasy that neuroses had evolved as a result of the Ice Age. In her second essay in 1987, she concluded that "Freud transformed the trauma model of etiology of the neuroses into the drive model" (p. 995). She argued that "the trauma model in his most poignant version is in keeping with the so-called seduction theory, but the drive model is the essential psychoanalytic etiological theory" (p. 997). Here she should have cited Jeffrey Masson, whose 1984 book she listed in her references. Goethe said this about theory: "Gray, worthy friend, is all theory and green the golden tree of life" (Faust, Part 1). Freud cited his mentor Charcot who said: "*la théorie, c'est bon, mais ça n'empêche pas d'exister*," (theory is good but it does not prevent things from existing; Freud, 1893, p. 13).

> There is a difference between speculative theory and a science erected on empirical interpretation … . For these ideas are not the foundation of science, upon which everything rests; that foundation is observation alone. They are not the bottom but the top of the whole structure, and they can be replaced and discarded without damaging it.
>
> (Freud, 1914b, p. 77)

In 1976, in a long footnote, Masson wrote, "It is worth remarking that Freud never retracted the [seduction] theory in *toto* as has too often been erroneously assumed" (p. 354).

Here again we see it was not Freud, but Masson who changed.

Freud as a love therapist

The patients treated by Freud around 1890–1892 and described in 1895, told Freud about their adult traumatic sexual experiences and conflicts. Emmy von N. (Fanny Moser), Cäcilie (Anna von Lieben Tedesco), Katharina, and Elisabeth von R. (Ilona Weiss) did not report any childhood traumas; and Freud was a theoretical minimalist, primarily interested in the psychological treatment of his patients.

In 1895, Freud drew an essential distinction between treating a patient with a medical illness and one with psychological problems and dysfunction, describing psychotherapy as follows:

> The procedure is laborious and time-consuming for the physician. It presupposes great interest in psychological happenings, but personal concern for the patient as well. I cannot imagine bringing myself to delve into … hysteria in anyone who … would not be capable of arousing human sympathy.
>
> (pp. 265–266)

Max Scheler (1954) elaborated "sympathy" as "fellow feeling," "love and hatred," and "empathy," as an ability to project oneself vicariously into the mind of another.

What's love got to do with it?

The first time Masson broached love as related to himself was in the December 1984 issue of *Mother Jones* magazine. It was a breath of fresh air to read Masson directly and not through the filter of Malcolm. The headline on the cover story was: "Seduced And Abandoned: How Jeffrey Moussaieff Masson Was Betrayed

By The Freudian Establishment" and Masson's story was entitled *The Persecution & Expulsion of Jeffrey Masson As Performed by Members Of The Freudian Establishment & Reported By Janet Malcolm Of The New Yorker* (Masson 1984b). It was introduced by Deidre English:

> Masson disputes the objectivity of Malcolm … and it is no wonder that he does. "Many of the statements attributed to me are, at best, distortions of my words and ideas, at worst, outright fabrications … . She presents a caricature of my views, in a language foreign to me and in a tone I do not recognize."
>
> (p. 6)

Malcolm's writing about Masson's "impudence" and personal attacks by analysts could fairly be seen as character assassination. In his dealings with Malcolm, Masson should have known that Sir William Osler had warned physicians to shun the

> temptation to toy with Delilah of the press … there may be times when she may be courted with satisfaction, but beware! Sooner or later she is sure to play the harlot, and has left many a man shorn of his strength, namely the confidence of his professional brethren.
>
> (Osler, Aphorism 91; Bean, 1950)

In the opening paragraph Masson harks back to seduction, noting his wait for Anna Freud to return to Freud's house in London one late October afternoon in 1980 (p. 34) to tell her about his latest discovery, an unpublished letter Freud wrote to Fliess on December 22, 1897 about a patient whose father had "brutally deflowered her" at age two "and infected her with his gonorrhea … and her life was endangered by the loss of blood and vaginitis" (Masson, 1985, p. 288; see also Masson, 1984a, p. 117). Again, this does not square with the idea that Freud absolutely abandoned seduction on September 21 of that year.

Another partial disclaimer by Freud of the absolute denial of the reality of parental sexual abuse was his letter to Fliess of December 12, 1897:

> my confidence in paternal etiology has risen greatly. Eckstein[5] deliberately treated her patient in such a manner as not to give her the slightest hint of what would emerge from the unconscious and in the process obtained from her among other things the identical [seduction] scenes with the father.
>
> (Masson, 1985, p. 286)

But this passage is also quoted by Masson in 1984a on page 114. Freud did not change, he wavered; it was Masson who changed.

Masson told how while teaching Sanskrit he realized

> that nothing interested [him] as much as this [psychoanalysis]: a humane response to mental suffering … Rather improbably … . I was accepted as a

> candidate at the Toronto Institute of psychoanalysis and thus began an eight-year training analysis program that was … to transform my life.
>
> (Masson 1984b, p. 37)

In the US only MDs were accepted for training. "Thoroughly disgusted with … the provinciality of psychoanalysis in Toronto," Masson settled in San Francisco, where "things were no different … only slightly less blatant." The solution was "to associate [himself] … with people like Kurt Eissler and Anna Freud" (p. 42).

The other breath of fresh air was Masson's 1990 book, "Final Analysis," with the subtitle, *The Making and Unmaking of a Psychoanalyst.* This book is both a moving story about his therapy and of his training analysis as well as a fiery critique of organized psychoanalysis (a "guild" and "fraternity") and its training system in Canada. Here is what led up to it. After my 1987 essay, I invited Masson in 1989 to present his 1988 *Against Therapy* in a meet-the-author event at the spring meeting of the American Academy of Psychoanalysis in San Francisco. In that book Masson overstated his condemnation of all psychotherapy as a form of abuse. Already in 1999, I wrote: "his therapy-bashing book and his [1990] autobiography … confirm the suspicion I had all along: Masson saw himself as the seduced-abused, traumatized step child of the psychoanalytic establishment" (p. 158).

In 1962, the twenty years old Masson saw an analyst recommended by Erik Erikson: "My problem is that I am not able to fall in love, although I sleep with many women," to which the analyst responded with a joke: "*I* should have such a problem." Masson felt this to be "in bad taste and unhelpful"; he "was looking for a strong father figure to help" (Masson 1990, p. 9). Therapy was once a week and it lasted one year.

In 1970 Masson moved to Toronto and found a psychiatrist, "a man of broad interests" who was "a lot of fun. Too much fun … . Soon I was invited to his house and eventually became friendly with his whole family. That was the end of our therapy" (p. 10). At that time he was dating Terri, his future wife, who introduced him to a professor of humanities who was in psychoanalytic training and suggested to him to apply for psychoanalytic training. After a screening Masson was approved for starting a "trial analysis" during the first year, and if successful, he would be admitted to start a training analysis (p. 13). On September 12, 1971, for the first time, Masson saw his training analyst Irvine Schiffer, who he described as "the best." After being instructed "to say *everything* that came to [his] mind" (p. 13), Masson told Schiffer that the furniture in his office was "tacky and ugly" and got the repartee: "Listen—this is my office. I furnish it any way I please. You don't like it? Leave. As for the 'tacky furniture—fuck you, my mother died recently, and those were her things. I am proud to have them here" (p. 25). Schiffer repeatedly used the sexual expletive, an odd and unorthodox behavior for a Freudian psychoanalyst. No training analyst in New York would have spoken like Schiffer.

Masson wrote, "When the analysis ended in 1976 … I did not actually feel "healthier" than when I had come in. I still had, basically, the same problems" (p. 81).

During that period Masson had lunch with Schiffer and told him he was leaving for Berkeley and planning to apply for membership in the San Francisco

Psychoanalytic Society, where he would read an inaugural paper written with his wife Terri, entitled "The Navel of Neurosis: Trauma, Memory, and Denial." Schiffer's reaction stunned Masson: "You are a thief, Masson, that is my paper [desist] … or I will tell the membership committee that you have not finished your analysis … you have a choice" (pp. 82–84).

In Chapter Seven, "Illusions," of *Final Analysis,* Masson told how in 1978 he read *The Navel of Neurosis: Trauma, Memory and Denial* at his inauguration as a member of the San Francisco Psychoanalytic Society, emphasizing "the central position that trauma must occupy in any theory of therapy" and "the reality of sexual abuse of young children" (p. 136); and Terri was there, too. Masson was criticized by the very people who had invited him to join: Victor Calef was "disappointed" and "angry … women do actually fantasize sexual seductions"; Edward Weinshel: "Jeff, Freud abandoned the seduction theory" (p. 137). Norman Reider complained: "Terri, why have you included your own personal experiences in the Warsaw Ghetto? This is bad form and irrelevant to the theoretical issues. Such remarks have no place in a scientific paper" (p. 138). Masson felt "snubbed," "embarrassed," and "isolated" (pp. 137–138). "I just didn't belong" (p. 144). Masson consulted a senior analyst about a woman he was treating and was told: "Well, Jeff, you are incompletely analyzed. You have never overcome this problem [feelings toward women]. Well, maybe you shouldn't analyze anybody then" (p. 148). And Masson concluded: "True, maybe I just wasn't analytic material, either as a patient or as an analyst, but I was beginning to wonder if that was such a bad thing after all" (p. 148). Masson's career as a psychoanalyst was over and done with.

In Chapter Eight of *Final Analysis*, "Anna Freud and I," the themes of trauma and the Holocaust were captured, and the chapter focused on 1980, two years before she died. Anna Freud had been questioned by the Gestapo but thanks to Princess Bonaparte she and her father were able to escape to London; Freud's elderly sisters were murdered in a death camp. Anna Freud declared: "psychoanalysts [don't] have any … reason to be interested in the holocaust … . How, for example, has it affected psychoanalytic theory?" (p. 155)[6]

One day that year Masson was invited to a conference at the Freud House and he

> talked about the new material relating to the sexual abuse of children in the letters of Freud. "The American Professor started the discussion by saying, 'This is a very provocative talk, and I feel provoked.' Leonard Shengold came to my assistance but from a certain distance … . 'Jeff, I have to tell you that I agree with what you say, but I deplore your way of saying it'."
>
> (p. 165)

Muriel Gardiner also tried to be helpful:

> I see that you are having a tough time here, where there are a few researchers and many clinicians. Maybe you should think of doing pure historical research and give up the idea of practicing analysis.
>
> (p. 166)

It looked like killing the messenger. This time Masson drew Anna Freud, whom he described as "remarkably trusting and open" (p. 171), into a discussion of "this whole 'episode' as she insisted calling it" (p. 178): "He (S. Freud) told me (A. Freud) that he changed his mind based on his clinical work with patients" (p. 179); Masson riposte was:

> But there was no proof that that is true. There are no case histories. There is no evidence for it in his own clinical notes. In fact … [there is] proof that he was seeing the reality of sexual abuse in his own private practice, *after* he supposedly abandoned the theory.
>
> (p. 179, italics in original)

Supposedly abandoned, isn't that another self-contradiction? Masson feared: "I knew I was taking a risk. She could revoke her permission to publish the letters at any time" (p. 180). It paid off: publishing the unexpurgated Freud letters, that replaced the expurgated version in the *Standard Edition*, was Masson's greatest contribution to Freud's historiography and scholarship.

Chapter Nine, "Disillusion" is the last. Again, Masson revisited his Yale lecture that met with "a deathly silence" (p. 190) and he declared, "Yes, I do think Freud committed a giant mistake. Every patient whose memory of abuse was treated as nothing but wishful thinking would have to be recalled … it reminds me of the Pinto" (p. 191). Back in Berkeley he was interviewed by Ralph Blumenthal. After his articles were published, Masson described that "Eissler's rage knew no bounds" (p. 194) but he "could not … explain to me what precisely I had done to bring the entire psychoanalytic world upon my head" (p. 196). On November 14, 1981, Masson faced the thirteen members of the board of directors of the Freud Archives. The members voiced a variety of objections:

> the articles in the *New York Times* made analysis look bad; my supposed hunger for publicity; an analyst should not allow his picture to appear in the paper, this could disturb patients; I abandoned all the major tenets of psychoanalysis.
>
> (p. 199)

But the real zinger was that Masson "had accused analysis of being sterile," and here something unexpected took place: Eissler could stand it no longer: "Stop it. Of course, Masson is right about the aridity of psychoanalysis today … . But the point is, who is to blame for this? Masson would blame Freud. That is outrageous" (p. 200). "You called Freud a coward" (p. 201). Masson was unable to appreciate that Eissler was a Freud fanatic, that for him Freud could do no wrong. All the bridges were burned: he was fired from the Freud archives, lost his membership in the International Psychoanalytical Association and the Canadian Psychoanalytic Society, "was stripped of all rank, like a disgraced soldier," like Alfred Dreyfus. But his last words were: "I ought to have felt terrible. Instead, I felt free" (p. 204).

Masson's critique of psychotherapy

In the first sentence of his 1988 book, *Against Therapy,* Masson says: "This is a book about why I believe psychotherapy, of any kind, is wrong" (p. ix). The conclusion is stated in the book's subtitle: "Emotional Tyranny and the Myth of Psychological Healing." Once more the title is both provocative and riveting, which immediately suggests Thomas Szasz's 1961 *The Myth of Mental Illness*, about whom Masson noted: "Perhaps the best-known critic of psychiatry is Thomas Szasz. But he has not widened his criticism to psychotherapy" (p. 186). But Szasz did that in his 1978 book *The Myth of Psychotherapy, Mental Healing as Religion, Rhetoric and Repression.* While both these books are fascinating, the incontestable fact remains that therapy is basically a conversation, and conversation is no myth, as expounded in two books by Pedro Lain Entralgo (1969, 1970) in which he discussed Freud as well.

As before, Masson's historical research is interesting and valuable, and I am particularly interested in what he said regarding Sabina Spielrein. It was for me a great satisfaction to read Masson on Sabina Spielrein and her "affair" with her analyst Carl Jung. Masson made several factual mistakes. Referring to Magnus Ljunggren, the renowned Swedish expert on Slavic literature, Masson labeled him as a journalist. He stated that Spielrein suffered from "psychotic hysteria" (p. 170), contrary to a certificate by hospital director Eugen Bleuler that she never was. Masson noted in "1908 Sabina was still being treated by Jung"—she was not, he had treated her only as an inpatient. Nonetheless, Masson concluded correctly: the affair "does not seem to have led to actual intercourse, only kissing. Spielrein refers to 'poetry' sessions, but she never makes clear what they consisted of" (p. 171). I fully confirmed Masson's hunch, and I showed what Spielrein really meant by poetry (i.e., sensual exchanges such as touching, holding, kissing, looking into each other's eyes, and swooning romantically), in my 2023 book based on her unpublished Russian diary and correspondence.

Conclusion

My analysis and reappraisal of Masson's work show that Freud never completely abandoned the realness of seduction. The significance of the September 21, 1897, episode was misread both by Masson and orthodox Freudians. The latter also erred in claiming that the sex drive theory superseded the realness of seduction as trauma.

Freud was a careful clinician, but he conflated two kinds of history, the universal and the particular, and two kinds of theory, subsumption and individuation. Moreover, infantile sexuality is normal, but as important as infantile sexuality is, it cannot fully explain either adult sexuality or nonsexual trauma and its consequences. The proper study of lives both personal and public is offered by dramatology, which captures the reality of one's experience and the internal resonance in its various forms which plays out.

As expressed in W. H. Auden's elegy to Freud, "to us he is no more a person now but a whole climate of opinion." Rather, thanks to his neurosis and activity as a psychoanalyst, Freud bequeathed to us the profession of psychotherapy.

Notes

1 Janet Malcolm interviewed me in 1983 and I gave her my paper in press (Lothane, 1983). She explained why I was not mentioned in her 1984 book: it would reveal the identity of my Aaron Green, the hero of her 1981 book. But his identity was an open secret: he was the late Leon Balter, a classmate at the New York Psychoanalytic Institute. See Balter et al. (1980).
2 Freud's two other papers that shed light on psychical reality are the 1908 "Creative Writers and Day-dreaming, *Standard Edition* Volume 9 and the "Two Principles of Mental Functioning" Volume 12.
3 Pseudonym for Bertha Pappenheim, about whom Freud wrote to his bride Martha on October 10, 1882: "Yesterday I was with Breuer until 12 o'clock; among other things he told me the interesting story of the illness of Miss Pappenheim" (pp. 377–378) (Freud, 2011). In 1885 Freud would tell this story to Charcot, but he showed no interest.
4 Published in 1936 in the Nervous and Mental Disease monograph series by the Nervous and Mental Disease Publishing Company.
5 Emma Eckstein, the first analyst, see the 1984 Chapter 3 "Freud, Fliess and Emma Eckstein."
6 There was a great deal of interest in the Holocaust among analysts, e.g., Bergmann and Jucovy (1982), Lothane (2020).

References

Balter, L., Lothane, Z., & Spencer, Jr., J. (1980). On the analyzing instrument. *Psychoanalytic Quarterly*, 49, 474–504.
Bean, B. B. (1950). *Sir William Osler, Aphorisms from his bedside teachings and writings*. Henry Schuman, Inc.
Bergmann, M. S., & Jucovy, M. E. (1982). *Generations of the Holocaust*. Basic Books, Inc.
Breuer, J., & Freud, S. (1895). Studies on hysteria. *Standard Edition*, 2.
Entralgo, P. L. (1969). *Doctor and patient*. McGraw-Hill Book Company.
Entralgo, P. L. (1970). *The therapy of the word in classical antiquity*. Yale University Press.
Freud, A. (1966). *The ego and the mechanisms of defense*. International Universities Press, Inc.
Freud, S. (1893). Charcot. *Standard Edition*, 3.
Freud, S. (1896a). Heredity and the aetiology of neuroses. *Standard Edition*, 3, 148–156.
Freud, S. (1896b). Further remarks on the neuro-psychoses of defence. *Standard Edition*, 3, 162–185.
Freud, S. (1896c). The aetiology of hysteria. *Standard Edition*, 3, 191–221.
Freud, S. (1905). Three essays on the theory of sexuality. *Standard Edition*, 7, 135–243.
Freud, S. (1914a). On the history of the psycho-analytic movement. *Standard Edition*, 7, 7–66.
Freud, S. (1914b). On narcissism: An introduction. *Standard Edition*, 14, 73–102.
Freud, S. (1916). Introductory lectures on psycho-analysis. *Standard Edition*, 16.
Freud, S. (1925). An autobiographical study. *Standard Edition*, 20, 7–73.

Freud, S. (1987/1915). *A phylogenetic fantasy Overview of the transference neuroses*. Edited and with an essay by Ilse Grubrich-Simitis, 1987.
Freud, S., & Bernays, M. (2011). Die Brautbriefe Band I (the engagement letters volume 1). Fischer.
Grubrich-Simitis Königstein, I. (1987). Trauma oder Trieb—Trieb oder Trauma (trauma or drive-drive or trauma). Lektionen aus (lessons from) Freuds phylogenetischen Phantasie von 1915. *Psyche*, *41*(11), 992–1023.
Jones, E. (1953). *The life and work of Sigmund Freud*, Volume 1. Basic Books, Inc.
Klein, M., & Tribich, D. (1979–1980). On Freud's 'blindness'. *Colloquium*, 2(2) & 3(1), 52–59.
Klein, M. I. (1981), Freud's seduction theory: Its implications for fantasy and memory in psychoanalytic theory. *Bulletin of the Menninger Clinic*, 45, 185–208.
Laplanche, J., & Pontalis, J. B. (1973). *The language of psychoanalysis*. Norton.
Lothane, H. Z. (2009). Dramatology in life, disorder, and psychoanalytic therapy: A further contribution to interpersonal psychoanalysis. *International Forum of Psychoanalysis*, 18, 135–148.
Lothane, H. Z. (2015). Emotional reality: A further contribution to dramatology. *International Forum of Psychoanalysis*, *24*(4), 191–203.
Lothane, H. Z. (2018). Free association as the foundation of the psychoanalytic method and psychoanalysis as a historical science. *Psychoanalytic Inquiry*, 38(6), 416–434.
Lothane, H. Z. (2020). Lessons learned. In I. Brenner (Ed.), *The handbook of psychoanalytic Holocaust Studies International Perspectives* (pp. 3–17). Routledge.
Lothane, H. Z. (2023). *The untold story of Sabina Spielrein: Healed and haunted by love/ Unpublished Russian diary and letters*/Translated by Henry Zvi Lothane with the collaboration of Vladimir Shpilrain. The Unconscious in Translation.
Lothane, Z. (1982). The psychopathology of hallucinations – a methodological analysis. *British Journal of Medical Psychology*, 55, 335–348.
Lothane, Z. (1983). Reality, dream, and trauma. *Contemporary psychoanalysis*, 19(3), 432–443.
Lothane, Z. (1987). Love, seduction, and trauma. *Psychoanalytic Review*, 76, 83–124.
Lothane, Z. (1999). The perennial Freud: Method versus myth and the mischief of Freud-bashers. *International Forum of Psychoanalysis*, 8(3–4), 151–171.
Lothane, Z. (2007a). Imagination as reciprocal process and its role in the psychoanalytic situation. *International Forum of Psychoanalysis*, 16, 152–163.
Lothane, Z. (2007b). Ethical flaws in training analysis. *Psychoanalytic Psychology*, 24(4), 688–696.
Malcolm, J. (1981). *Psychoanalysis: The impossible profession*. Alfred A. Knopf.
Malcolm, J. (1984/1983). *In the Freud archives*. Alfred A. Knopf.
Masson, J. M. (1976). Perversions, some observations. *Israel Annals of Psychiatry & Related Disciplines*, 14, 134–361.
Masson, J. M. (1984a). *The assault on truth: Freud's suppression of the seduction theory*. Farrar, Strauss and Giroux.
Masson, J. M. (1984b). The persecution & expulsion of Jeffrey Masson as performed by members of the Freudian establishment & reported by Janet Malcolm of The New Yorker" *Mother Jones* (December 1984), 34–37, 42–47.
Masson, J. M. (1985). *The complete letters of Sigmund Freud to Wilhelm Fliess 1887–1904*. The Belknap Press of Harvard University Press.
Masson, J. M. (1988). *Against therapy: Emotional tyranny and the myth of psychological healing*. Atheneum Publishers.

Masson, J. M. (1990). *Final analysis: The making and unmaking of a psychoanalyst.* Addison-Wesley Publishing Company.
Quine, W.V., & Ullian, J.S. (1970). *The web of belief.* Random House.
Russell, B. (1921). *The analysis of mind.* Unwin Brothers, LTD.
Ryle, G. (1949). *The concept of mind.* Evanston, Barnes and Noble Books.
Scheler, M. (1954). *The nature of sympathy.* Yale University Press.
Szasz, T. S. (1961). *The myth of mental illness. Foundations of a theory of personal conduct.* A Hoeber-Harper Book.
Szasz, T. (1978). *The myth of psychotherapy Mental healing as religion, rhetoric, and repression.* Anchor Press/Doubleday.
Van der Kolk, B. (2015). *The body keeps the score/Brain, mind, and body in the healing of trauma.* Penguin Books.

6 Power, Courage, Trauma, Betrayal, and Memory

An Interview with Professor Jennifer Freyd

Jennifer J. Freyd and Warwick Middleton

Warwick Middleton (WM):	When did you first meet Jeffrey Masson?
Jennifer Freyd (JF):	That was when I went on sabbatical the first time to New Zealand in early 2002, and I was officially a guest of the University of Auckland. He found out I was there, so somebody must have connected us. He invited me over to his house. One time he also came over to the house we were living in. The only times I met him in person were those two visits.
WM:	What was your first reaction to reading "*The Assault on Truth*"?
JF:	I was not a clinical psychologist by training, so I was learning a lot quickly. I had very superficial knowledge, and still do really, of psychoanalysis and psychodynamic theory. I had heard about the Oedipus complex, but I knew nothing about the history of Freud's life or anything like that until I read the book. It was incredibly eye opening, and it all made sense, because at the same time I was learning about the actual prevalence of child sexual abuse including in families, so what Jeff exposed was consistent with the empirical evidence that was emerging already in the 1990s.
WM:	How important do you think "*The Assault on Truth*" (Masson, 1984) has been?
JF:	That's hard for me to answer. I think it's probably been very important but the problem in social movements and intellectual movements is that peoples' work builds on other peoples' work, so it wasn't like he was all alone out there changing people's understanding. You had activists and survivors, other theoreticians, and researchers, all pointing to similar truths. I think what *The Assault on Truth* gave us was a historical understanding of why Freud's initial insights were suppressed, and how he changed his mind. I don't know – maybe some other people knew that before

DOI: 10.4324/9781003431466-7

Jeff's book, but I think Jeff's book brought that to people's awareness and that was probably very radical. But, if it was just that, if he had written the book but there wasn't also the emerging information about the prevalence rates and so on, I don't know that the book on its own could have done that. I think it was synergy, right? Different forces coming together.

WM: Given what happened when Freud first offered a "seduction" theory for hysteria, and given the fate of those prior to Masson who followed a broadly similar theoretical path, what is your take on why the modern trauma field, despite at times very vocal opposition, gained the traction to become substantial and enduring over a period now of decades?

JF: These are really hard questions and they're kind of outside of my expertise in the sense that I'm not a historian or cultural critic. I also don't totally understand how people's consciousness about things changes over time. If you look at Bessel van der Kolk's earliest work and Judy Herman's writings, they describe these periods of 'amnesia' and of knowing, of this cyclical awareness of trauma, and how it would get buried, between moments of awareness. My experience, since I first delved into this field in the early 90's, has been that it [i.e., appreciation of the extent and impact of trauma] has not gone away. Sure, there's always ups and downs, but I have not seen awareness of trauma completely suppressed the way it clearly had been, at different times in history.

It's 40 years since 1984. Maybe that's too short a period, maybe in 20 years it'll all be suppressed again. I hope not, and I don't think it will because there's the other thing, which is the Internet. Something may have shifted in the current acknowledgement of the impact of trauma, and it may be just that it was like a critical mass thing, like enough force pushing awareness, that it could not be pushed back down this time. And it could be a combination of factors, like *The Assault on Truth* showing us how it came to be that Freud flip-flopped, at the same time as data from researchers were saying "No, really large numbers of people are being sexually abused in this way – including by fathers", and at the same time as what we called the "women's movement" found traction. It all happened somewhat in parallel, but it's interesting because all through the 90's, where there was this bitter fight about false memories, it seemed like a period of suppression was going to happen again.

I think it's really interesting that around the year 2002, the Boston Globe had their big Spotlight series where they devoted enormous resources, and then newspaper coverage to the sexual abuse of children in the Catholic Church. I think that was a watershed too. Some people think it all started with "#MeToo". No way! This was all building up over decades until #MeToo emerged. #MeToo pushed general awareness that sexual violence happens into yet another level of awareness, but even #MeToo is still more about adults in the workplace than about children. There's still a long way to go. There's still insufficient attention to the plight of children I would say, but there's been ongoing progress … There's Dr Nassar and his abuse of US gymnasts and all these things, and I feel like it's out. I think it would be really hard to put it back under the covers now. Then there's the Internet... That information is much more retrievable and permanent than it used to be. I do think about Freud's letters being so important in understanding what really happened. If those had been on the Internet it would be really different, right?

WM: That's one of the things that Jeffrey did: he had access to original Freud material that no one else had ever published before and he made that public, which is different to everyone else that commented on these issues.

JF: Yes, his approach was very empirical too. It was just that the tools of his discipline were different from those used in psychological science.

WM: What parallels do you see between the "Oedipal fantasy" explanation of reported memories of childhood sexual abuse and the later "False Memory Syndrome" explanation of reported memories of childhood sexual abuse?

JF: That's a good question. Not surprisingly, I see this a little bit in terms of this concept I have developed of DARVO (Deny, Attack, and Reverse Victim and Offender) where you kind of flip things around. So, in both these cases the credibility of the person saying "this bad thing happened to me" is attacked and the abuse is denied. But then it makes the false memory people sort of complicit through Freud's Oedipus theory – that the wronged party is the father who is being accused: he is the true victim. And then by default the perpetrator is the person saying they were abused. So, it just flips victim and offender very effectively and serves the purpose of suppressing the information about the abuse. It's very effective.

WM: What is your take on the thesis that Jeffrey Masson put forward in the *The Assault on Truth* – that Freud suppressed his own theory on the aetiology of hysteria? He would have known from first-hand contact during his time at the Paris morgue of deadly abuse perpetrated on children which included significant sexual components. Then, without providing any hard evidence by way of proven fantasy, he found it professionally expedient to adopt a "fantasy" explanation for the accounts that his patients provided regarding childhood sexual abuse? In other words, Freud seemed to pivot on a dime and then, without any hard evidence, introduced a new theory which he defended endlessly and with very little reference from then on to actual childhood sexual abuse?

JF: Yes, I feel like a lot of people know more about this than me.

WM: I'm interested in your take on it because you've absorbed this sort of controversy, I guess, in multiple ways, for a long time.

JF Yes, I find it very understandable. Another concept that we're developing is called the "betrayal blindness", which is an ability to not know about the betrayals in one's midst because in not knowing you get to retain your relationships with people when those relationships are dependent upon the suppression of information. Clearly for Freud, it was extremely costly for him to know about the sexual abuse. It was costly financially and socially, so if he could sort of unknow it, then he regains a much more comfortable position in society. I know he could be accused of selling out, but I think that's a judgement that we must be cautious about, because we don't know what it would've been like to be alive then and maybe it was just too much to know. It was like knowing had become too dangerous and it was a survival thing to unknow it. So, I feel some compassion for him. I wish he could have been, in some sense, stronger and stood up against the denial, but people are human and there was really no space in society for his point of view, it was so threatening to the patriarchy.

WM: What do you think of psychoanalyst Bennett Simon's (1992) conclusion after an extensive review of the psychoanalytic literature that *"[n]either Freud, nor, to my knowledge, any other analyst, published a case wherein a woman, not psychotic, told of an incestuous relationship with the father and then in the course of the treatment it turned out to be a fantasy!"*? So, he could not find anywhere, within the entire publications of psychoanalysis, a single study that supported Freud's Oedipal Fantasy being the focus of analysis whereby the victim of the Oedipal Fantasy recovered from the fantasy?

JF: That doesn't surprise me because the whole hypothesis is so absurd. The world is very big and there are billions of people, so anything you can imagine a person can do, probably somebody has done it. Therefore, probably somebody has had this fantasy and made it all up. Probably such a thing has happened, but it is so implausible that it would happen very often and therefore be the foundation of most psychiatric distress, so it's not surprising that it is not documented because it's probably so rare.

WM: Yes, but Bennett Simon did something that no other analysts did. He was enraged, like most psychoanalysts seemed to be at the time, by Masson's theory, but instead of just leaping into print castigating him publicly – like putting him in stocks in the village square and throwing things, he at least resolved to test his hypothesis. And then he did an exhaustive review of the psychoanalytic literature and ended up effectively saying, "Well, actually Jeffrey is right".

JF: Yes. So, he gets credit for that. I love it when data overrides people's biases. It's great.

WM: And Bennett Simon went on to be co-author of a book on the first psychoanalytic case after Freud's Dora for which the case notes survive (written by Louville Eugene Emerson). It was in America and dates to 1912. The case was of a victim of severe ongoing incest into adulthood. Fantasy in that case wasn't pushed at all. Bennett Simon was a co-author of that book (Lunbeck & Simon, 2003). I appreciate your point about data overriding dogma. Jeffrey has made the point that when he was training as a psychoanalyst, the issues of Oedipal fantasy and hysterical mendacity were endlessly emphasized, not to mention penis envy, and all the rest that goes with it… which probably haven't stood the test of time very well outside certain closed, entrenched analytic groups.

JF: Now it sounds like a spoof! It sounds like if you were going to make up a silly satire of the patriarchy you would come up with something like "penis envy", right? You'd invent these as satirical extensions?

WM: Yes. Have you ever come across the writings of Florence Rush?

JF: No.

WM: She occupied the same sort of area that Masson did. They did not meet prior to the publication of *The Assault on Truth*, and yet, she's a great writer from back in the 70s, about these issues.

You had for over two decades been the editor of *The Journal of Trauma and Dissociation.* (And by the way, congratulations on what an amazing achievement that is!) How significant was it in terms of the recognition of child sexual abuse that Freud himself did not embrace the construct of dissociation?

JF: Well, I don't know, but it was inevitable that the concept would come to light again because of the data. It is so fundamental to the survival of many child sexual abuse victims, that it was inevitable. It's interesting, back maybe 10 or 15 years ago I did a project with librarians at the University of Oregon to put together an archive of the work on dissociation over time and while different words were used for it on some occasions, nevertheless, people kept observing it. So, whatever kept Freud from embracing it, it didn't stop it from becoming understood.

WM: Yes. Joseph Breuer wrote about "hypnoid states", which were pretty much dissociation. Janet beat Freud into print on some of these areas, but Freud seemed to massively need to distance himself from Janet.

JF: Yes. Have you ever looked at the archives we have?

WM: Yes, I have. You have made available all the old editions of the journal, *Dissociation*?

JF: There are two archives. One is with the old books, and then one is with all the old issues of *Dissociation.* It was hard to find them all. That was part of the challenge – getting those hard copies because there was no electronic record at all.

WM: Yes, when you look back on it, *Dissociation* as a journal, was quite a monumental feat. Richard Kluft carried that.

JF: Yes, he was doing it all. He was trying to be editor and publisher. That's crazy. It's really hard.

WM: You would know that more than anyone. You can see how hard it is just being an editor, let alone doing the rest! Without in any way seeking such a role, you found yourself a reference point for public polarizations regarding childhood sexual abuse and "recovered memories" of trauma. In navigating such challenges, were there guiding principles that you employed?

JF: Probably not. I'm pretty intellectual, so I tend towards wanting to understand and so I tried to read things and do research and understand at an intellectual level, and I really value honesty and truth, so those things were there but it was a really strange time. It was very weird. I didn't really have anything. Nothing prepared me for it, and I didn't have a sense of other people or situations I could sort of draw from. It was this weird thing of being in a situation that was very unfamiliar to me and so I was just trying to understand it. People were behaving in ways that I could not entirely understand, like my own colleagues joining the False Memory Syndrome Foundation – it just did not make sense to me and so I was really trying very hard to make sense of it.

WM: Looking back now, because you actually have in an exemplary way navigated your way through it, it seemed like you were very careful about not being baited into conflict and it can be tempting to sort of charge into battle, but it's much smarter to take a mindful, careful, considered approach and not be drawn into grandstanding activities. This, I guess, is what a lot of those associated with the false memory syndrome perspective wanted to do. Some colleagues were being picketed.

JF: Totally. I got picketed but I think one of the benefits I had was that I'm really shy in a lot of ways and really a pretty private person and so part of what was so horrifying for me was my privacy being so violated and people talking about me all the time, with my name in the newspapers, those things... I didn't want to do anything to increase that. I was really trying to protect my privacy, but at the same time, I want to say I didn't entirely avoid conflict because a lot of what I ended up writing was pretty much questioning all that stuff. I just think I had a more academic approach.

WM: A word that comes to my mind is that you exhibited dignity.

JF: Thank you. I think it helped too that I had my husband, JQ (John Quincy), who you met. He was incredibly supportive. I had this wonderful nuclear family with JQ and our children and I had friends. So, I had a really secure situation. I think if I was all by myself and wasn't educated, there's lots of circumstantial things that would have made it much harder to hold on to my dignity.

WM: Did you have a reaction to the folding of the False Memory Syndrome Foundation in December 2019?

JF: One of my reactions to this whole thing has been embarrassment. I just find the whole thing embarrassing and the fact that I share a pretty rare last name with my parents makes it sort of cringey. I think it was primarily relief.

WM: Were you surprised at all that it folded when it did?

JF: I didn't know about it directly. I think I read about it from somewhere and so there was a little bit of surprise at new information, but it wasn't shocking. Back in the early 90's they definitely had the upper hand culturally, but by the time they folded they really didn't. There's still really a problem with the influence of the false memory syndrome movement on textbooks, and on the court system, at least in the US. But compared to the way it was in the early-to-mid 90s when all the media believed it, they really lost that hold and I think it was just because the research that had come forward through those many years did not support the position of the False Memory Syndrome Foundation (FMSF). So again, given the data it wasn't shocking to me that they would fold.

WM: One of the things that I've done over the years is kept a tab on where their website was going. Back when they founded the FMSF in 1992, with great fanfare, there was the formation of a Scientific and Professional Advisory Board. The thing that struck me was that it virtually never changed from the early 90s, and over the years as members of this group progressively died, they maintained their membership on the board! So, by the time the FMSF formally folded, virtually half the members of the Scientific and Professional Advisory Board were actually dead!

What is your take on why psychoanalysis became so fixated on "Oedipal Fantasy" and historically placed so little emphasis on actual childhood sexual abuse despite it being Freud's initial focus?

JF: I think it's in the same category of answers in terms of people's comfort level and the status quo. It's very threatening to the social order to accept that reality, so although the whole fantasy explanation is implausible really, it is much less threatening to the power structure.

WM: What do you think of the fact that a movement, or an organisation, that's supposedly so focused on understanding psychology and human behaviour and motivation should have been so aligned with a theory for which there was so little evidence, as Bennett Simon pointed out, and yet people were steeped in this belief system?

JF: You know it's not just that theory, the histories of mental health fields have been complicit with the forces of oppression. That's pretty bad: there were theories in diagnostic manuals about the mental state of slaves that essentially justified slavery, where it was a disorder for slaves to want to run away. And at various times there have been diagnoses for women who are being abused or want freedom or whatever. Mental health fields do not have a clean record on social justice, just the opposite. So, I see this as one more example of that. Even more recently, the American Psychological Association (APA) have been complicit in work on psychological torture – it's just a repeated problem, but fortunately it's not the whole story.

There's also been wonderfully important liberatory forces as well from the mental health fields. But one of the things I think should be corrected is how people are trained in the mental health fields, all of them. They should learn these histories, because what they currently get is so whitewashed. They get exposure, whether its psychiatry or psychology or social work or whatever it is, to a narrative that their field only does good. They don't learn about these terrible collusions with oppressive forces and therefore they are more prone to fall prey to that same dynamic. It's the old adage, "You're going to repeat history if you don't learn about it". We need to avoid repeating all this.

WM: What do you think the mental health field in the broader sense needs to do to safeguard against perpetuating these sorts of mistakes?

JF: This is probably time for this concept I have of "institutional courage" because I think that there are certain steps organisations can take to be less prone to these betrayals and in this case, education has got to be a big piece of it. For a couple of years before I retired, I was teaching a course that historically had been called "History and Systems" and it was required for clinical psychology students and required by the APA. The textbooks tend to be an example of whitewashing, focussing on all the glory moments, like 'psychology did this, it's so wonderful' and when I taught it I tried to balance that with all the times psychology went the wrong way and did harm so that the students would learn both things. But without that education I think students are just going to go out there and think that by virtue of their degree they are immune from doing anything harmful. That's a very dangerous thing. You need to learn all these dangers so that you don't act them out.

WM: As you know, Jeffrey wrote, among other books, one called *Against Therapy* (1988) and another one called *Final Analysis* (Masson, 1990) which represented his critique of mental health and also psychoanalysis.

JF: I assigned *Against Therapy* in the graduate seminar I taught and it's very threatening to students in clinical psychology. And I argued with Jeffrey about that book because I felt he had gone a bit further than I could accept, and then I gave him this example of a psychologist therapist I know who believes in kindness and in her power to be truly respectful of her clients and honestly helpful. She is a counterexample to the sort of sweeping claim by Jeffrey that there's no possible way that therapy is not going to be corrupt. We were arguing about this, and he said, "Are you saying your whole argument is that you know one person?" And he kind of got me there because I was sort of arguing from one example. But I think he makes an extremely important point, and whether his most radical position is correct or not, it's a really important point or position for people to grapple with because if he's not correct that it's inevitably bad, it's often bad. So many people get mistreated in the context of therapy and it's a power abuse as he points out.

WM: One of the people he mentions is Masud Khan who was one of those baying for his expulsion from the Freud Archives. But Khan, of course, was an appalling abuser, with the full extent of his abuse only coming out in later years. Unfortunately, we see this happening repeatedly with very prominent people in this psychoanalytic saga, individuals who have very questionable backgrounds in terms of their own abuse tendencies. Another one that comes to mind is Ernest Jones, who was to Freud what Saint Paul was to Jesus. He was the propagator of psychoanalysis and yet very credible evidence would indicate that he had very poor sexual boundaries and that he sexually abused children.

JF: Well, I think it is really a problem for all of us that there are abusers in our midst and some of those abusers have a lot of power, not just in their relationships with others, but in their ability to define knowledge through their professional positions and it's dangerous of course to go around accusing people you don't agree with of being personally motivated. That's a risky position to take. On the other hand, sometimes it's true. Sometimes people are personally motivated to hold certain viewpoints. Maybe we all are to some extent. There are some people who I have interacted with who I know from other sources are abusive people in particular contexts and then when I'm dealing with them in some other context, they are espousing a viewpoint that conveniently in some sense justifies their abusiveness, or denies it, or whatever.

Do I keep the argument entirely intellectual? Do I just take them at face value? What do I do with this knowledge of their behaviour in this other context? I find that very challenging. If someone tells me about somebody, I try to keep an open mind about it because sometimes it's just not true and you can do reputational damage to somebody with just a rumour. But, if I have directly seen this person behave in an abusive way in the workplace, it's often an abuse of power but not a crime per se, and then they are in this other context in which they are speaking with the authority of an intellectual, but the particular thing they're saying is in some way relevant to excusing or denying their other behaviour, I find that a challenging situation. I ask myself; how do I hold those bits of information? Do I just focus on the pure intellectual context or content? I don't really have the answer to that, but when it's occurred, I have found that very hard.

WM: It's slightly amusing that when Jeffrey first mentioned to me about doing this book, he had a sense of wry humour about asking, of all people on earth, a psychiatrist to edit it.

JF: But you know, one of the things that I remember so distinctly about you … you said something to me that changed things for me, and part of it was that you were a psychiatrist who said this to me, because I didn't necessarily have the most flattering view of psychiatrists…

WM: And Jeffrey certainly didn't either.

JF: But you picked me up, I think it was like our first car ride soon after I met you, and you were driving me somewhere, and you said to me something like, you've "never encountered a case of a person who was really suffering, their mental health was really suffering, who did not have some experience of mistreatment". That mental health problems and distress are related to the mistreatment that people have experienced. It was a radical thing to hear from you because I had not put it myself that clearly. And as soon as you said it, I knew it was absolutely true. But I also was really shocked you would say it because it's the opposite of the pathologizing viewpoint that dominates, and maybe dominates a little bit less now than it did, but it's still been the dominant paradigm – that people who are suffering from emotional distress or other mental health issues have something wrong with them. And the way you put it shifted that. What was wrong was the mistreatment and people have now said this in a million different ways, but you said it to me a long time ago and it was striking to me that here you were, this white male psychiatrist, clearly with professional success, saying this to me. So, thank you.

WM: Thank you. You make a focus in your writings on "betrayal trauma" (Freyd & Birrell, 2013) and the role played by institutions. Indeed, you have established the Centre for Institutional Courage, which applauds the role of whistleblowers within institutions. What has been the role of institutions in facilitating or covering up the sexual abuse of children? Do you conceptualize Jeffrey Masson as a whistle-blower?

JF: I don't know if before your question I would have come up with the term but as soon as you asked, I thought it is appropriate. Jeffrey was being a whistle-blower – at least at the time he was doing *The Assault on Truth*, and the response he got was typical of what happens to whistle-blowers. He was retaliated against. He was ostracised. He was turned into the perpetrator to dare to say these things. So yes, it's the right term.

WM: In the broader sense, what do you see is the fate of whistle-blowers? You've probably seen quite a few.

JF: Yes. Well, they get DARVO'd. What they say gets denied and they get their credibility attacked and they are put into the perpetrator role. But I think also they get ostracised, people stop talking to them, even people who don't disagree with the facts that they're putting forward. Even people who are not DARVOing them are afraid of them – like whistle-blowers are really scary and are threatening all sorts of relationships. If you are seen with a whistle-blower or affiliated with a whistle-blower, then you're going to pick up some of that stigma. So, it can be really costly to you to befriend a whistle-blower even if you are not saying anything about anything: just being their friend is costly. So, I think whistle-blowers are often very lonely and they get painted as if there's something weird about them. It's tragic because the people that blow the whistle usually are some of the most caring, loyal people who do it because they want things to be better and they care for and often love the organisation or whatever it is. They're identifying what is happening as a problem. So, it's really poignant, because they are the people who really should be revered and it's why one of the steps in institutional courage is to cherish the whistle-blower.

WM: Jeffrey's then-career was destroyed by his role as a whistle-blower, if we call it that, and he was dismissed from the International Psychoanalytic Association and from his local psychoanalytic association. He was pilloried and ostracised and attacked and people wrote incredibly harsh reviews about his book, and he ended up moving to the other side of the planet and writing about the emotional life of animals. It's an unusual trajectory, but in your experience do you see many whistle-blowers who have a reasonable outcome, or do they suffer the effects of their whistleblowing indefinitely?

JF: I've seen it all. I've certainly seen people be destroyed by it. I have seen people just crumble, the consequences of the retaliation and ostracism are just too much, and their life becomes small, and they often die prematurely whether it's through suicide or chronic illness. But I have seen people, I think Jeffrey is one of them, who emerge, get through it, and find their way. So, I think there's the whole range and where somebody is going to land probably has a lot to do with the social supports, they have around them, both at the time, but also earlier in life, like the things that support people developing their strengths. I really think we often try explaining variations in people's outcomes in terms of something intrinsic about them when probably so much of it's just about luck – like who was around you: like if you're an abused kid, was there another adult around who was giving you enough nurturing and support to counter that abuse? That's not a kid's choice, that's luck.

WM: What lessons can the modern trauma field take from the saga involving Jeffrey Masson, psychoanalysis, and the press?

JF: I think we have seen a few cautionary tales around the press. We can't assume the press is going to cover these issues very well. Doing more to educate the press is probably important for the field. One of the things I found the hardest in the 90's concerning the FMSF was the fact that the press seemed so gullible about it. They would just publish repeatedly the same sort of fluff pieces about these poor innocent accused fathers and these deranged daughters and therapists. That was very disillusioning to me. I had thought such organisations had more of an educated sceptical mind and they seemed to just fall prey to the forces of protecting the status quo. It's probably important to figure out ways to educate the press and to some extent the field has done that. There are awards that get given to good press coverage. The Dart Center for Journalism and Trauma is famous for fostering better journalism around trauma. So, I think there's been some efforts but probably we could keep doing more of that.

WM: Is there anything in respect to what happened to Jeffrey Masson regarding his treatment by the press that you'd comment on because he's not been without controversy. He obviously had the saga not only of the *Assault on Truth* but of suing Janet Malcolm.

JF: You know he's feisty, like where I'm shy, he's not shy. So, he'll go out there and do battle. So, part of it is somewhat – that's him.

WM Yes, I don't think there's an introverted bone in his body really. Now there is a question that you have touched on and will no doubt say more about. What are the implications for the modern trauma field of advances in communication technology and online interconnectivity that have become available in the years since the publication of "*The Assault on Truth*"?

JF: Yes, I think that the main thing is that it makes it harder for information to disappear because you can search for a word and get all these documents, so in that sense I think it's been very beneficial. But we know from all the pitfalls with social media in particular, that there are also dangers out there and now we've got this explosion in AI sophistication too. I think that this part of the human experience is becoming so dominant, it's so much more of our reality than I think, especially people our age, can really comprehend. But the trauma field totally needs to stay on top of this. What happens around these topics is really important now and there are scary things that happen out there in social media. Echo chambers, rather than helping people heal, can increase people's suffering through the electronic media so I would say that the field just really needs to take advantage of and celebrate the ways that information technology can help preserve information and help maintain awareness. But the field should also be wary of the ways it can be used to harm people.

WM: How strong are the forces in the world that seek to discredit, disbelieve or nullify the testimony of victims of trauma, including victims of child sexual abuse?

JF: Very, very strong. The forces of denial are very, very strong.

WM: Do you see any changes?

JF: I think those forces still are there and it's not so much that the forces have changed, the counterforce has changed. I think there's more counterforce. The nature of social liberation movements is that as soon as you start to make real headway towards liberation, the backlash strengthens. We saw it around Q Anon, where people (it's sort of very insidious) use the claim that they are against paedophiles to discredit anyone they don't like. So that's a really dangerous thing for our field and we must really be on guard against that. The awareness that child sexual abuse is real can be weaponised in these bad ways because that label, 'paedophile', can be attached to your enemy whether they are, or not, a paedophile.

WM: Do you think it would have been possible for Jeffrey Masson to have got his message outlined in The *Assault on Truth* in a way in which it provoked less polarisation or controversy? Or was the dynamic always going to be there no matter who was the speaker or how it was said?

JF: Well, probably the answer is that it was always going to be there to some extent, but my guess is that if he were to write that book now the opposition would have way less power and there would be more acceptance of what he had to say, because it fits in better with what we know. But this is so counter factual because the very fact that we've gotten to the point of awareness that we have now, is probably dependent in part on that book – like somebody must be first, somebody must be out there trailblazing, and that's what he was doing. But then of course, he had the reception of a person who was viewed as really, really threatening.

WM: Jennifer, is there anything that, in a more broad global sense that you would like to comment on?

JF: I'm not sure how well formed this is but I do think there's something that we could have more of in this world which is what I refer to in institutional courage writings as a sort of acknowledgement and apology, and which some people might call truth and reconciliation. So, whatever happened with the initial reception of Jeffrey's book or with the false memory reception in the 90's, there's still room for some repair involving those people: like not everybody is dead, and there's also the institutions. I know for me it would be extremely beneficial if the people or institutions who had joined my parents and ostracised me, were to actually apologise to me. That would be an amazing gift. Nobody has done that. Nobody. And I mean I would imagine this has probably been Jeffrey's experience too, that probably some of the people that were so up in arms about his book have come round to some extent, but have they really taken ownership for the way they treated him at the time? Maybe, but probably not. So, I think if we could figure out how to encourage more of that, it would go a long way to healing. That is a kind of accountability and apology.

WM: I know that Jeffrey's closest friend back around the time he was writing the book was Charles Hanly, who subsequently went on to become president of the International Psychoanalytic Association. He severed his friendship with Jeffrey, completely severed it, wouldn't speak to him, and published a derogatory review of Jeffrey's book.

JF: I know, I want it, but no, I don't rationally think it's coming. Maybe it is a project for future generations – to figure out how to make it more likely that there's repair because I do really think it would be valuable. I think people are surprisingly defensive, like we are just very defensive creatures, and that defensiveness gets in the way of acknowledgement and apology, and it doesn't serve anyone's interests in the long run.

References

Freyd, J. J., & Birrell, P. J. (2013). *Blind to betrayal: Why we fool ourselves we aren't being fooled.* Wiley.

Lunbeck, E., & Simon, B. (2003). *Family romance, family secrets: Case notes from an American psychoanalysis, 1912.* Yale University Press.

Masson, J. M. (1984). *The assault on truth: Freud's suppression of the seduction theory.* Faber and Faber.

Masson, J. M. (1988). *Against therapy: Emotional tyranny and the myth of psychological healing.* Atheneum.

Masson, J. M. (1990. *Final analysis: The making and unmaking of a psychoanalyst.* Fontana.

Simon, B. (1992). Incest – see under Oedipus complex: The history of an error in psychoanalysis. *Journal of the American Psychoanalytic Association*, 40, 955–988. https://doi.org/10.1177/000306519204000401

7 The Memories of Millions

Lynn Crook

In the 1980s acceptance of the reality and impact of child sexual abuse in the press and in society was high. Yet as more people started to accuse their alleged perpetrators, often family members, of sexual abuse during their childhood, a narrative began to develop in the early 1990s that memories of early sexual abuse could be false. This allowed the alleged perpetrator to become the victim and the person who was accusing them to be seen as acting on false and created memories of events that never occurred. This false memory narrative was fostered by the False Memory Syndrome Foundation and its $7.75M PR campaign along with the "lost in a mall" study (Loftus & Pickrell, 1995). The media ran with it, which changed societal perceptions about the reality and impact of childhood sexual abuse. Survivors were generally silenced with the idea that therapists were creating wholesale memories of clients being sexual abused in childhood by family members and others. This narrative meant that millions of adults molested as children could be told their accusations were and are false memories.

Over the past century, our beliefs that children are molested have vacillated from denial to shocked acceptance and then back to denial. We listen as victims describe the shocking experiences that shamed and embarrassed them as children. When their accounts become too much to bear, we turn to others who tell us the abuse did not happen. They assure us the accusations are fantasies, or false memories, or impossible. Such false memory narratives become louder and more pervasive when our acceptance of child sex abuse claims has already taken hold.

Sigmund Freud listened to his patients as they reported molestation by family members. His patients expressed feelings of anger, disgust, helplessness, and betrayal. Freud believed them. He concluded that early sexual trauma results in neurosis for victims. He reported his findings in 1896 to colleagues at the Society for Psychiatry and Neurology in Vienna. In doing so Freud had violated a taboo—he had discussed incest openly. His colleagues shunned him (Masson, 1984).

Freud replaced his "seduction theory" with a compromise. While his clients believed they were molested, their memories were not true. Instead, they were a result of fantasizing sexually about the opposite-sex parent. He called this the Oedipal complex, a normal part of child psychosexual development. These fantasies are then repressed and years later may be remembered as actual incidents.

DOI: 10.4324/9781003431466-8

Patients' expressions of anger and disgust at what was done to them were not the result of childhood trauma, Freud proposed. They were the internal experiences of emotional hysterics, borne out of fantasizing rather than reflecting actual memories of child sex abuse by a parent. Freud was welcomed back into the society. Secrecy and disbelief reigned once more.

Freud's seduction and fantasy theories were the subject of attention in the 1980s. Jeffrey Masson, PhD, had access to Freud's unpublished letters as the Projects Director of the Sigmund Freud Archives. Masson's *The Assault on Truth* (1984) supported Freud's earlier conclusion. Children are molested and this impacts their psychological development. Masson was subsequently dismissed from his position at the Freud Archives. Like Freud's early claims, Masson's claims were rejected. He was professionally isolated.

Breaking the silence of sexual abuse

Forty years ago, the press told us that child molesters are a reality. There was growing acceptance in the 1980s of the reality of child abuse and it impacted on adult life. Public silence gave way. Mandated reporting laws in the United States caused reports of child sexual abuse to soar. The media listened. An unspeakable topic—incest—became speakable. *ABC Theater*'s "Something About Amelia" in 1984 with Ted Danson and Glenn Close addressed the topic directly. The "something" was paternal incest. The film received three Emmys and two Golden Globes. The Associated Press followed with a five-part series, "America's Dirty Little Secret." Our secret? We tolerate child molesters. A *Los Angeles Times* survey in 1985 found that 22% of adults were molested as children. Predators had gained access to over 40 million children. And then came 1991.

The U-turn

Support for victims was growing by 1991 when states allowed adults to sue for damages based upon always- or recently remembered childhood molestation. *People Magazine* cover stories featured celebrities—Sandra Dee, Roseanne Barr, and former Miss America, Marilyn van Derbur. The women shared their experiences of childhood molestation by their fathers. Incest was recognized as a reality. Yet there were already signs of a return to denial.

Parents accused of molesting their children were working on a plan by 1991 to address the allegations and file potential lawsuits. With nearly half the states allowing accusers to sue for damages, the parents needed to silence their accusers. They needed an approach the media would adopt and disseminate to the public.

Pamela Freyd, PhD, the future leader of a non-profit organization for accused parents, tried gaslighting. When her daughter, Jennifer Freyd, PhD, recalled childhood sexual abuse by her father, Pamela, writing as "Jane Doe," claimed the role of victim. She published, *How Could This Happen? Coping with a False Accusation of Rape* (P. Freyd, 1991). She described "Susan" (the pseudonym she used for Jennifer) as "cruel and dramatic," "Gestapo-like," "insulting and degrading," and "temporarily deranged." Pamela sent copies of her article, with identifying details, to Jennifer's colleagues at the University of Oregon. The gaslighting approach was not successful. The media did not cover Pamela's story.

Jennifer went on to coin the term DARVO, which described the systematic oppression of alleged victims by accused sex offenders and their supporters: "Deny, Attack, and Reverse Victim and Offender." Pamela had DARVO'd Jennifer. Jennifer later published *Betrayal Trauma: The Logic of Forgetting Childhood Abuse* (J. J. Freyd, 1996). The book describes how memories of early abuse by a trusted individual can be forgotten, then remembered later when one reaches adulthood.

Professor Elizabeth Loftus at the University of Washington proposed some ideas to the media for silencing abuse accusations. She needed an explanation the media would accept so she tried out a few ideas: "The memories are suspicious … . They're driven by hatred and revenge … . They're 'unreliable …'" (Crook, 2022, p. 67–68). When Loftus suggested "implanted by therapists" to the *Washington Post*, the *Post* elevated Loftus's "implanted" theory to headline status in August 1991 as, "Alleged Victims Basing Actions on Memories Critics Say May Be Implanted in Therapy." The parents now had a defense the media would support. They initiated a PR campaign to promote "implanted memories" as a means to dismiss abuse accusations as false memories. Loftus's PhD credentials granted her expert status with the media. Her false memory claims were not challenged or fact checked. She assured the press that memories of long-ago incidents are malleable, unreliable, and faulty. She suggested that therapists might be implanting the memories. As evidence she explained that her student had convinced his younger brother he was present when the younger brother became lost at age 5 at the University City mall in Spokane. Next, she would need evidence suggesting that a memory of child sexual abuse could be implanted.

Promoting false memories

By 1992 the stage was set for accused parents to go public as falsely accused. They established a 501(c)(3), a non-profit they called the False Memory Syndrome (FMS) Foundation, with an office in Philadelphia and with Pamela Freyd as the Executive Director. Based on their IRS reports, the Foundation members invested $7.75M to silence their accusers and promote their false memory theory. Yet, at the very start, the media had little interest in and need for research on the validity of memories of child sex abuse. There was a scandalous, dramatic, human-interest story to cover. There were newspapers to sell.

However, "abuse accusations are false memories" became quite quickly a story the media wanted to hear. Dan Goleman, with his own PhD in psychology, was the first to disseminate the message with the July 1992 headline in the *New York Times* asking "Childhood Trauma: Memory or Invention?" Next was Bill Dietrich's (August, 1992) story for the *Seattle Times* and the Associated Press. He summarized the false memory story in his lead sentence, "Repressed memories of sexual abuse may be false and can be inadvertently suggested by therapists, University of Washington psychologist Elizabeth Loftus will tell the American

Psychological Association (APA) tomorrow." The Foundation recruited 34 media representatives for its first conference in 1993. By 1995, 300 stories in the popular press assured the public that abuse accusations are false memories. Disclosures of childhood sexual abuse were no longer met with compassion. Instead, victims were told, "I read about false memories like yours."

The FMS Foundation's October 1993 newsletter commended the media. "Reporters are the primary vehicle for the dissemination of information. The reporters who contact us have been extremely responsible about consulting with the Foundation's experts and getting their facts straight" (p. 2). The Foundation became a sponsor of continuing education credits for American Psychological Association members. The FMS Foundation and Johns Hopkins University co-sponsored meetings offering CEUs in San Diego, Boston, and Chicago. As the false memory story went viral, alleged victims were no longer believed and therapists were harassed.

Psychologist Ken Pope questioned in an open letter on his website how the APA could support an organization that harasses therapists. He explained, "Ridicule has escalated to explicit statements telling ex-patients to imagine engaging in violence against their therapists, claiming that the impulse is sane and natural and that violent cognitions about murdering ex-therapists can be pleasurable" (Pope, 1996). Professor Ross Cheit's Recovered Memory Project, dating from 1996, lists corroborated cases of recovered memories of childhood sexual abuse (see Kendall, 2021).

Crook v. Murphy

I was feeling the impact of the parent's campaign by early 1994 when the *Crook v. Murphy* trial began. I had sued my parents in September 1991 for damages related to childhood sexual abuse. The local newspaper covered the story and I received more than 70 letters supporting my decision to hold my parents accountable. False memory experts Richard Ofshe, PhD, and Elizabeth Loftus, PhD, testified for my parents during the trial. After a month-long trial, the judge declared in my favor, awarding me $140K in March 1994. Yes, I was aware of what the media was telling the public about memories like mine. But my case was corroborated. So I was surprised by the community response. Whenever I told someone about the trial, they assumed my memories were false. They had been reading about false memories like mine, they said. I stopped talking about my lawsuit. Still, I wondered why the media would believe a campaign run by accused sex offenders without fact-checking their claims. I decided to do some fact-checking myself.

Silencing tactics

FMS Foundation members have silenced their critics by gaslighting them. Martha Dean, PhD, and I experienced this tactic when we co-authored a review of the "Mall study" for *Ethics & Behavior* in 1999 (Dean & Crook, 1999). In the "Mall study" each participant was given four stories. Three were true. Loftus reported 2 participants (8–9%) of the 24 in her final report to the University of Washington Records Office developed false memories of being lost in a mall as children (Crook, 2022). For publication in *The Formation of False Memories* (Loftus & Pickrell, 1995), the result was inflated to 6 who thought the false memories of getting lost were true (p. 723). Loftus was given the opportunity to read our work before she responded. She called our article, "a misrepresentation … a misstatement … a distortion … partisan … disturbing … unscientific … incompetent … bizarre" (Loftus, 1999, pp. 51–60). Martha and I were shocked. We thought Loftus might be trying to embarrass us or bully us into silence. Our paper was meticulously referenced and footnoted. We decided to go ahead and submit our paper to *Ethics & Behavior*.

We hadn't realized the threat our article posed to Loftus back then. My co-author insisted I request a report on the final "Mall study" findings. On page 64 of our *Logical Fallacies and Ethical Breaches* reply to Loftus's response (Crook & Dean, 1999), we had quoted the final result—8%—that Loftus submitted to the UW Public Records Office. We still can't figure out how 8% in the UW documentation could go to 25% in the published paper. We have a hunch though. Loftus's student, Jim Coan, who induced a lost in the mall belief in his younger brother, initially oversaw the "Mall study." He took the first six subjects through the study and reported, "All [the first six] subjects were able to correctly identify the false story" (Coan, 1993, p. 16). Thus, the study designed to support parents' false memory claims had not elicited any false memories in the first six participants.

We had determined from the final university report (June 1, 1994) that 2 of the 24 participants (8%) thought they were lost. A copy of that report is included in Crook (2022, p. 205). The study had failed to produce meaningful indications to back up the false memory claims. Yet the parents had already invested over $2M in their PR campaign. In addition, the media believed in false memories. Rather than announcing the "Mall study's" failure, Loftus and Pickrell (1995) inflated their result to six subjects (25%) for publication in *Psychiatric Annals.* Interestingly, Murphy et al. (2023) published a study entitled "Lost in the mall again: A preregistered replication and extension of Loftus & Pickrell (1995)" and largely replicated the earlier published findings. Just over a quarter of the 123 participants came to believe they had been lost in a mall as a child. As with the original study, the participants were told their relative was present at the time of them being lost in the mall and provided the researcher with the "memory" that the participant had been lost in the mall. Yet even those claims (of someone "witnessing" their experience and providing the "memory") did not cause most participants to believe in the false memory that they were lost.

We wondered if Loftus had gaslighted others who challenged her work like she had done with us. We found she had used the occasion of receiving the William James Fellow Award from the American Psychological Society in 2001 to address those investigating the ethics complaint Nicole Taus had filed against her. "I am gagged at the moment, and may not give you any details," Loftus said. "But to me, that itself is the problem. Who after all benefits from my silence? Who benefits from keeping such investigations in the dark? My inquisitors. The only people who operate in the dark are thieves, assassins, and cowards" (Loftus, 2001, pp. 14–15).

Attorneys gathered at the Westin Hotel in Seattle in 1995 for a workshop on suing therapists. Joan Golston, MSW, covered the story for *Treating Abuse Today* (Golston, 1995). Dallas attorney Skip Simpson addressed the group,

> It doesn't matter what kind of law you practice, you can win in every case … I'm telling you, a blow-up doll can handle these cases … It's like shooting fish in a barrel. We sue the therapists, and the juries are eager to fill [our] dump truck with money.

Simpson added, "We have the studs on our side, the McHughs [i.e., Johns Hopkins Psychiatrist, Paul McHugh], and the Loftuses … In retractor cases, it's usually going to be a six figure plus settlement" (p. 25).

FMS Foundation advocate and accused parent Chuck Noah took to the streets, picketing therapists in his RV with large signs attacking their work. For three days he picketed psychology professor Jennifer Freyd's workplace at the University of Oregon. The students and staff who worked in her research laboratory were rattled by his activities in the street below. Freyd decided it was best to ignore him. Psychologist Wendy Maltz, another Eugene resident, wrote an early article in 1990 to help doctors identify symptoms of sexual abuse. A complaint was filed, claiming her article helped to implant false memories. The claim was quickly dismissed, and Noah showed up to picket Maltz's office. Noah and others picketed therapists David Calof and Laura Brown, PhD, in Seattle. Calof says that groups as long as two blocks demonstrated in front of his office (D. Calof, personal communication, October 23, 2023). Noah picketed the 1999 International Society for the Study of Dissociation (now the International Society for the Study of Trauma and Dissociation, ISSTD) conference in downtown Seattle. Security guards forcibly prevented Noah from entering the conference area.

The *Columbia Journalism Review* published Mike Stanton's story of how the FMS Foundation halted publication of an article. *Newsweek* had asked Katy Butler to write a story examining the uncritical acceptance of FMS Foundation claims, and to provide documented cases of recovered memory and traumatic amnesia, Stanton explained. FMS Foundation board members Richard Ofshe, Frederick Crews, and the Freyds wrote letters to *Newsweek* claiming that Butler was "a zealot masquerading as a journalist" and was "well known not only as a journalist in this area but also as a strong advocate" for recovered memory. In response, John Capouya, *Newsweek*'s senior editor, concluded, "We weren't too sanguine about getting into a huge pissing match with these people." Butler's article on documented cases was canceled (Stanton, 1997).

Arguably the FMS Foundation's greatest success was getting their claims into psychology textbooks where they remain today. Psychology 101 students molested as children learn their memories are malleable and unreliable. Those who were not abused learn that the allegations and disclosures of friends and family members are the result of suggestibility, rather than an experience with an alleged child molester.

Inflating the membership numbers

As Loftus was inflating the "Mall study" results for publication in 1995, the Foundation inflated its membership (see Dallam, 1997). There were 2,149 members for the fiscal year ending February 18, 1994 (IRS Form 990, p. 2) and this number peaked the following year at 2573.

Yet the January 1994 FMS Foundation newsletter announced, "We start the new year with almost 10,000 families" (p. 1). They had inflated their membership size as well as the size of the false memory problem. *Smiling Through Tears* by Pamela Freyd and Eleanor Goldstein in 1998 played down the impact of being raped as a child by a family member by offering dozens of political cartoons satirizing therapists and survivors.

Loftus asked a question at a false memory conference in 2000 that I attended. "How do we create a situation where people feel embarrassed about having these particular [false] beliefs [i.e., about being sexually abused as a child]?" She suggested public television, perhaps not realizing that survivors are typically more embarrassed by what the predator forced them to do as a child, than by false memory claims from accused parents and their supporters. The Foundation announced its success after four years:

> The success of the Foundation in helping to clarify the issues [i.e., of false memories of sexual abuse] can be seen in the gradual institutionalization of false memory claims in psychology textbooks, in reference works, in novels [sic], in television dramas, and in hundreds of scholarly papers. Indeed, the Foundation has been a corrective to a run-away belief system.
>
> (FMS Foundation Newsletter, 1996, p. 2)

Going after therapists

FMS Foundation members were encouraged to sue their accuser's therapist. The following accounts were not reported by the media. They are examples of the Foundation's early harassment efforts. They suggest the Foundation set out to (1) silence investigative reporting, (2) generate hefty financial settlements, and (3) criminalize therapy.

The November/December 1994 issue of Seattle therapist David Calof's bimonthly journal, *Treating Abuse Today* (TAT), included investigative reports of false memory activities (pp. 14–20). To prepare, investigative reporter Eva Doehr (1994) attended FMS Foundation chapter meetings in Seattle. She described members' efforts to promote lawsuits and ethics complaints against therapists. The picketing of Calof's office began in early 1995, causing Calof to move his office twice.

The stalking and harassment by accused parents and others impacted Calof's clients, his family members, his attorney, and his attorney's family members. He estimates their activities cost him over $1.5M in legal fees, lost speaker fees and moving expenses. Calof says in *Notes from a Practice Under Siege* (1998),

> [f]or over 3 years, members, officials, and supporters of the False Memory Syndrome Foundation, Inc., have waged a multimodal campaign of harassment and defamation directed against me, my clinical clients, my staff, my family, my attorney and others connected to me. I have neither treated these harassers or their families nor had any professional or personal dealings with any of them.
>
> (p. 161)

Calof's attorney, A. Stephen Anderson of Seattle, was awarded the Washington State Bar Association Courageous Award in 1998 for displaying "exceptional courage in the face of adversity."

Dozens of therapists were targeted for legal action including Mark Stephenson, PhD, in Idaho and Renee Fredrickson, PhD, in Minnesota. Gary Ramona was one of the first parents to sue his accuser's therapists. The jury awarded him $475K in 1994, enough to cover half of his legal expenses. Another lawsuit in 1996 showed how claims of implanted memories could generate millions of dollars for the plaintiffs' team. Pat Burgus and her two sons sued Bennett Braun, MD; Elva Poznanski, MD; and Rush Presbyterian Hospital in Chicago. The defendants were covered by separate insurance carriers. Deposed on January 17, 1997, Burgus testified that Braun did not implant any memories. Braun was not informed of Burgus's testimony. The "Mall study" raw data were subpoenaed. The "Mall study" researchers insisted on a gag order. Braun had paid a fee to ensure lawsuits could not be settled without his permission. The lawsuit settled for $10.6M without Braun's permission. The "Mall study" data were returned. Pat's share of the settlement was $3M minus her attorney's $1M fee and her share of the fees billed by six experts.

Therapists faced criminal charges in Houston. Defendants Judith Peterson, PhD; Richard Seward, MD; George Jerry Mueck; Gloria Keraga, MD; and Sylvia Davis, MSW at Spring Shadows Glen in Houston were indicted on 60 counts of mail and insurance fraud for diagnosing patients with dissociative identity disorder (DID) and billing through the mail. Some believed those charges were an attempt to criminalize therapy with DID patients. If found guilty, the defendants could spend the rest of their lives in prison. Each defendant hired their own attorney at a cost of approximately $500K. The government had presented its case for five months when the first false memory expert testified. False memory claims did not hold up well under cross-examination the court found. Elizabeth Loftus, who had not yet testified, resigned from the case. The government dropped all charges in March 1999.

Following the Houston trial, insurance carriers tried a new approach. A lawsuit in 1998 against two therapists in North Carolina went to trial rather than settling. Three trauma experts testified for the defense. Their testimony held up under cross-examination. *The Charlotte Observer* announced on August 20, 1998, "Jurors Believe Therapists."

With support waning and success applying the "false memory" rhetoric failing, the FMS Foundation limped along until December 2019, before closing its doors. The Foundation's message continues to strike a chord when efforts to deny childhood sexual abuse are mobilized, but it has lost some of its bite under the weight of scientific data that do not support its claims.

Celebrities and false memories

Celebrities charged with rape or murder often hire psychologist Elizabeth Loftus, PhD, as part of their defense team. She sets out to convince juries that the memories of alleged victims' and witnesses are unreliable. However, Loftus conceded under cross-examination by prosecutor Joan Illuzzi on February 7, 2020, in the Harvey Weinstein trial that our memory of the core details, what's important to us, is typically accurate. To date, many of Loftus's celebrity clients have been found guilty. Examples include the following:

2008—Loftus testified in the defense of record producer Phil Spector who was found guilty of the murder of Lana Clarkson.

2016—Loftus reviewed the cases of 13 women set to testify against media personality Bill Cosby. Their memories were all tainted she reported. She was not called to testify. She testified for Cosby in a civil suit filed by Judy Huth. A jury awarded Huth $500,000.

2018—She supported Judge Brett Kavanaugh in six media interviews regarding Christine Blasey Ford's sexual assault accusations against him. Loftus did not testify for Kavanaugh.

2019—Loftus was invited to testify in football coach Jerry Sandusky's appeal. Judge John Fedora dismissed Loftus's opinion as "having been rendered after an uncritical review of an absurdly incomplete record carefully dissected to included only pieces of information tending to support [Sandusky]."

2020—A judge ruled Loftus's testimony was unnecessary in the case of Kathie Klages, the first official informed by young athletes of Nassar's crimes. Klages was found guilty, but this verdict was overturned on appeal.

2020—Film producer Harvey Weinstein relied on the expert testimony of Loftus. He was convicted of sex crimes and sentenced to 23 years.

2021—Loftus testified for real estate heir Robert Durst who was found guilty of the murder of Susan Berman.

2021—Loftus testified for socialite Ghislaine Maxwell who was convicted of conspiracy and sex trafficking. For the first time in 30 years, the media used sneer quotes when describing Loftus as a "false memory" expert. *The Guardian* described Loftus as a professor of BugsBunnyology (Sweeny, 2021).

Our children's future

I attended a presentation by John Briere, PhD, some 30 years ago. He passed along a quote by Desmond Tutu, "We can keep rescuing people and pulling them out downstream, but eventually we need to go upstream and find out who is tossing them in." Briere's surveys in 1989 and 1996 found that 20% of males "upstream" are sexually attracted to young children. They would molest if they thought they could get away with it (Briere & Runtz, 1989; Smiljanich, & Briere, 1996). The

Australian Child Maltreatment Study in 2023 found that not much has changed. The world is not a safer place for children—28.5% are molested and go on to experience early and persistent harm. Yet 11 FMS Foundation leaders assured us that sexual contact with an adult does not harm a child (Crook, 2022).

Judith Herman (1992) tells us in *Trauma and Recovery*, "The perpetrator does everything in his power to promote forgetting. If secrecy fails, the perpetrator attacks the credibility of his victim. If he cannot silence her absolutely, he tries to make sure no one listens" (p. 8). The FMS Foundation successfully attacked the credibility of victims with false memory claims. They tried to make sure that no one listens to their alleged victims. They were successful for many years.

Are we prepared to deal with victims? Mia Fontaine wrote in 2013 for *The Atlantic* that we are not prepared to deal with the scope of child molesters and victims. Imagine what would happen if every kid currently being abused (60,000)—and every adult who was abused but stayed silent (40,000,000)—came out of the woodwork, insisted on justice, and saw that justice was meted out. The very fabric of society would be torn.

I am one of the 40 million. For me, surviving years of sexual abuse, then recalling, and then holding my parents accountable in court for their crimes was the biggest challenge I've ever faced. Is there another way for us to stop perpetrators and then hold them accountable for the crimes they commit against children? The justice system in the United States and in most other countries has not done well in listening to, or in believing and protecting, the children who experience sexual abuse.

References

Briere, J., & Runtz, M. (1989). University males' sexual interest in children: Predicting potential indices of pedophilia in a nonforensic sample. *Child Abuse & Neglect, 13*(1), 65–75.

Calof, D. L. (1998). Notes from a practice under siege: Harassment, defamation, and intimidation in the name of science. *Ethics & Behavior, 8*(2), 161–187.

Charlotte Observer (1998). *Jurors believe therapists*. Charlotte, NC.

Coan, J. (1993, August 18). Creating false memories. Senior Paper, Psychology Honors Program, University of Washington, p. 16.

Crook, L. (2022). *The deception that silenced millions*. Amazon.

Crook, L. S., & Dean, M. C. (1999). Logical fallacies and ethical breaches. *Ethics & Behavior, 9*(1), 61–68. https://doi.org/10.1207/s15327019eb0901_5

Dallam, S. J. (1997). Is there a false memory epidemic? *Treating Abuse Today, 7*(3), 29–37.

Dean, M., & Crook, L. L. (1999). "Lost in a shopping mall": A breach of professional ethics. *Ethics & Behavior*, *9*(1), 39–50.

Dietrich, B. (1992, August 13). UW expert challenges repressed memories—Says some sexual abuse may not be real. *Seattle Times.*

Doehr, E. (1994). The false memory movements political agenda. *Treating Abuse Today, 4*(6), 14–20.

False Memory Syndrome Foundation Newsletter (October 1993, volume 2, number 9).

False Memory Syndrome Foundation Newsletter (January 1994, volume 3, number 1).

False Memory Syndrome Foundation Newsletter (March 1996, volume 5, number 3).

Fontaine, M. (2013, January 24). America has an incest problem. *The Atlantic*.

Freyd, J. J. (1996). *Betrayal trauma: The logic of forgetting child abuse.* Harvard University Press.

Freyd, P. (1991). How could this happen? Coping with a false accusation of rape. *Institute for Psychological Therapies,* www.ipt-forensics.com/journal/volume3/j3_3_3.htm

Freyd, P., & Goldstein, E. (1998, January 3). Smiling through tears. *Social Issues Resources Series.*

Goleman, D. (1992). Childhood trauma: Memory or invention? *New York Times, July 21st.*

Golston, J. C. (1995). Current topics in law and mental health: False memory syndrome, multiple personality and ritual sexual abuse: The growing controversy. *Treating Abuse Today*, *5*, 24–30.

Herman, J. (1992). *Trauma and recovery.* Basic Books.

Kendall, J. (February 7, 2021) The false memory syndrome at 30: How flawed science turned into conventional wisdom. *Mad in America* www.madinamerica.com/2021/02/false-memory-syndrome/ https://doi.org/10.1080/09658211.2023.2198263.

Loftus, E. (1999). Lost in the Mall: Loftus, Loftus, E F. (1999) Misrepresentations and misunderstandings. *Ethics & Behavior, 9*(1), 51–60.

Loftus, E. (2001). When scientific evidence is the enemy. *The Skeptical Inquirer, 25*(6), 14–15.

Loftus, E. F., & Pickrell, J. E. (1995) The formation of false memories. *Psychiatric Annals, 25*, 720–725.

Masson, J. M. (1984). *The assault on truth: Freud's suppression of the seduction theory.* Farrar, Straus and Giroux.

Murphy, G., Dawson, C. A., Huston, C., Ballantyne, L., Barrett, E., Cowman, C. S., Fitzsimons, C., Maher, J., Ryan, K. M., & Greene, C. M. (2023). Lost in the mall again: A preregistered replication and extension of Loftus & Pickrell (1995). *Memory*. Advance online publication. https://doi.org/10.1080/09658211.2023.2198263

Pope, K. (1996) Open letter to the APA, p. 2/10. Online at https://astraeasweb.net/politics/fmsapa.html

Smiljanich, K., & Briere, J. (1996). Self-reported sexual interest in children: Sex differences and psychosocial correlates in a university sample. *Violence and Victims, 11*, 39–50.

Stanton, M. (1997). U-turn on memory lane. *Columbia Journalism Review*. Jul/Aug, 36(2).

Sweeny, J. (2021, December 18). Miss Sweden and Bugs Bunny add up to a bad day in court for Ghislaine Maxwell. *The Guardian*. https://tinyurl.com/5n6are8e

8 Another Suppression of Incest and Its Victims?

Christine A. Courtois

Overview

The rediscovery of incest by second wave feminists and social science researchers in the 1960s and 1970s ended the "Age of Denial" that resulted from Freud's reversal of his original seduction theory in favor of the Oedipal theory. Jeffrey Masson's book *The Assault on Truth* documented this reversal, its consequences, and the reasons for it using Freud's letters and other historical records. The book's publication – and Masson himself – were attacked by his peers for being disloyal to Freud and psychoanalytic orthodoxy as they were simultaneously heralded by feminists for challenging the orthodoxy and supporting the rediscovery of incest and its prevalence. This commentary presents some of the social/historical developments over the past 50 years that continue the dialectic between acknowledgment and denial.

Throughout human history and with few exceptions, incest has been prohibited across most cultures and ethnicities. Therefore, its actual occurrence was typically hidden in secrecy and silence, due to its taboo status. When witnessed, discovered, or disclosed, it was met with shock and horror, treated as scandalous, and its perpetrators and victims treated with contempt or shunned. The contemporary history of incest can be organized into three epochs: discovery (late 1800s/early 1900s), denial (early to mid-1900s), and rediscovery (1960s to the present). Although numerous forms of interpersonal and sexual violence have now been recognized, it is unclear whether incest is once again being singled out for suppression in response to a variety of social forces.

The original discovery of the prevalence of incest and other child sexual abuses, along with their high potential for negative impact over the lifespan, was made by Sigmund Freud and some of his contemporaries, constituting the "Age of Discovery". Based on reports of childhood sexual victimization by his patients, Freud developed the *seduction theory* postulating that incest and other childhood trauma were etiological to the development of psychological symptoms (notably hysteria and Briquet's syndrome, the disorders that mostly affected females and were of great interest to clinicians of the day).

As Jeffrey Masson documented in his book, Freud's courageous presentation of his provocative theory to his Victorian era contemporaries was not well-received

DOI: 10.4324/9781003431466-9

to say the least. In response to collegial scorn and disavowal and the likelihood they would impugn his reputation and derail his career, Freud reversed course. He replaced his original theory with the *Oedipal theory*, which emphasized fantasy or wish on the part of the child for sex with a parent rather than its reality. Despite this reversal, some of his contemporaries, notably Sándor Ferenczi, continued his belief in the reality of early childhood sexual victimization and its traumagenic and deleterious effects on children and over the entire life course. Their views made them outliers and outcasts as Freud's psychoanalytic method – with the *Oedipal theory* and repression at its core – prevailed and became the dominant form of psychotherapy until mid-20th century, constituting the "Age of Denial". The tragic consequence of this theoretical reversal was to virtually ensure that any individual who made a report of incest or other childhood sexual abuse during their treatment would be disbelieved or blamed for its occurrence by their analyst. And anyone who questioned or did not comply with the orthodoxy of the Freudian position was subjected to professional repudiation and exclusion as described so vividly by Dr. Masson in his introductory chapter of this text.

The 1960s and 1970s: Feminists and the "age of rediscovery"

The 1960s and 1970s were decades of great social turmoil. The rediscovery of incest prevalence was made in this context by feminists undertaking the study of gender-based discrimination and sexual violence as part of the women's liberation movement and who documented the prevalence of rape and sexual assault in both community and family settings. They wrote about how many families operated on principles of patriarchy/misogyny and sexual stereotyping that created "breeding grounds" for the roles of males and females. They made the provocative suggestion that incest was actually a form of conditioning of females to their submissive sexual status and roles vis-à-vis men who were simultaneously conditioned to be dominant and entitled.

Feminists also documented the range of appalling consequences of all forms of domestic violence at the time of its occurrence and over the life course. They roundly criticized psychoanalysis for its gender biases and stereotypes and its predisposition to disbelieve/blame, pathologize, and stigmatize women patients for their symptoms based on the Oedipal theory. Dr. Masson's *The Assault on Truth* buttressed their preliminary findings about both the prevalence and the suppression of incest by providing a psycho-social–historical account of Freud's theoretical reversal. In turn, feminist findings offered contemporary social–historical support for Masson's writings regarding Freud and for the calamitous consequences of his theoretical reversal for many women seeking assistance for their onerous symptoms.

This commentary traces the social–psychological history of incest since this rediscovery period. A bit about my interest and involvement with this topic: my first exposure came in the early 1970s due to phone calls to our newly developed university rape crisis center from girls desperate to escape repeated and ongoing sexual abuse at home by a parent or other close relative. Back then, the word "incest" was not one that I had heard or knew much about.

Yet, I was impacted by the plight of these trapped girls and set out to study their experience as my dissertation topic. This was the time when incest was "coming out of the Freudian closet" to paraphrase one writer and books by feminist researchers and memoirs by victims were being published. These were essential to my study, but I also discovered a body of qualitative research published earlier in the century. During that early period, father–daughter incest was studied by some social workers, psychiatrists, and criminologists who had worked with intrafamilial cases of physical and sexual abuse and who published their findings in case studies and case series. They documented common family dynamics and other sociological data in addition to long-lasting psycho-social, familial, and medical–physiological aftereffects suffered by victims. As these studies almost exclusively investigated socially and racially marginalized individuals from the lower socio-economic strata – those who would be most likely to be involved in the social services and criminal justice systems – this research contained a significant built-in bias. Unfortunately, it served to provide and reinforce misinformation that incest only occurred in chaotic, lower-class, underprivileged families, predominantly among African Americans. Moreover, some of these writings blamed mothers for colluding with their husbands in the abuse of daughters who were described as compliant, pleasing, and seductive in line with the Freudian Oedipal theory.

Faulty as it was, this work was the precursor and foundation for the more scientifically based contemporary study of all forms of violence and abuse in the family. Researchers documented that incest (and other forms of sexual abuse[1]) occurred regularly and prevalently in the lives of many children, the majority of whom were female, leading one feminist to remark that *the taboo is not on its occurrence but rather on its acknowledgment.* Acceptance and belief are most difficult issues when any type of sexual assault is disclosed or reported. When it occurs within the family and involves sexual transgressions by parents and other relatives (especially those in good standing – "pillars of the community", as well as any adults in roles of responsibility such as clergy, therapists, teachers, coaches, and military superiors), it is even more difficult to believe as it flies in the face of social norms and beliefs. Incest horror and personal revulsion are the most acute when the sexual contact is between a parent and a child. How much easier it was to exonerate a father and blame a daughter instead to keep the social order!

In the late 1970s and into the 1980s, several influential professional and lay books and articles were published on the topic of incest. Clinician/researcher and psychiatrist Judith Herman published her ground-breaking book *Father-Daughter Incest* (Herman, 1981) in which she outlined the typical dynamics and wide-ranging aftereffects at the time the abuse occurred and in later life. Sociologists Diana Russell (1983, 1986) published her community-based study of 930 individuals and David Finkelhor (1979) introduced findings about prevalence and consequences. Their aggregated findings about the prevalence of incest were alarmingly consistent as were their discussions of the effects on the child victim and later the adult survivor.

I added to this work with my dissertation research (Courtois, 1979), a qualitative study of women who volunteered to be interviewed about their incestuous abuse, using a detailed questionnaire derived from the available literature. My findings were very in line with those of the authors and researchers noted above.

The 1980s: The decade of trauma, dissociation, and treatment

Many different types of trauma were recognized and studied during this decade. Of singular significance to the mental health field was the inclusion of a new diagnosis of posttraumatic stress disorder (PTSD) in the *Diagnostic and Statistical Manual of Mental Disorders-III* (American Psychiatric Association, 1980). Derived primarily from the study of male combatants, PTSD legitimized the fact that an individual's distress and symptoms could result from exposure to overwhelming events and experiences outside of themselves rather than being purely intrapsychic (then the predominant perspective based on psychoanalysis). Mental health researchers and practitioners took note and began to apply this diagnosis to many trauma types, such as rape, incest/sexual abuse, other forms of child abuse, and domestic and community violence.

This decade also saw a resurgence of study of dissociation and the dissociative disorders alongside the study of psychological trauma. Pierre Janet (a French psychiatrist) along with Freud and some of their contemporaries had identified and studied dissociation at the turn of the century. Janet noted the connection between a history of child sexual abuse and the development of dissociative defenses in some of his patients. Unfortunately, his work was eclipsed by the ascendency of Freud's Oedipal theory as the basis of the analytic method and his emphasis on repression rather than dissociation.

The new research identified a continuum of dissociative processes, from those on the normative end that most individuals experience in daily life to those that are non-normative. The latter are the result of defensive reactions mobilized in response to high-intensity and repeated traumatic events, especially over the course of childhood. Researchers identified a cross-over between highly dissociative (formerly known as hysterical) individuals who frequently reported a history of severe sexual abuse (usually incest) and other types of family dysfunction and maltreatment in their backgrounds. From an early age, they somehow learned to "go away" or "space out" to defend themselves and to cope with repeated violations in an entrapping situation they could not easily escape. What began as "an escape when there was no escape" (Putnam, 1997) used in response to ongoing abuse and other adversities in childhood, continued into adulthood and, for some, it became automatic, out of their control, pathological, and disabling. Much like PTSD, dissociative disorders (which were included in the *DSM-III*) were given more attention among mental health practitioners than ever before.

The influence of the media

The media – including the talk shows of the day (i.e., Oprah, Donahue, Sally Jesse Raphael) – picked up the story of child sexual abuse and began extensive coverage that at the time was sensitive and sympathetic to victim/survivors and their stories.

The result: incest was *publicized and spoken about as never before in history*, prompting many heretofore "secret survivors" (mostly women but men as well) to come forward both to finally disclose their histories and to seek help. Therapists were unprepared for the influx of traumatized sexually abused clients and did not have an organized treatment model to use. Clinical training at that time (and to the present) did not include attention to psychological trauma and posttraumatic conditions, much less incest. This resulted in therapists doing their best with what they knew with clients who had complex and challenging needs and high acuity, not an optimal circumstance.

Before long, an issue came to the fore that further complicated the treatment: clients' memories of their trauma. Some reported having never forgotten and always having had full access, while others reported memories that were discontinuous. Still others did not remember anything about past abuse until they were flooded with memories ("recovered memories") often in the aftermath of exposure to some reminder, such as the media coverage. At the time, some therapists began overemphasizing the retrieval and processing of memory above all other concerns. Some utilized hypnosis and other procedures in attempts to unearth absent memories and did not question the accuracy of these memories, as they relied on the maxims of the day "always believe the client/clients never lie", developed as counterpoints to the Freudian position. In some cases, this approach led to plausible disclosures (some buttressed by witnesses and other evidence) and, in others, to increasingly bizarre recollections that defied belief.

It should be noted however that what many would consider bizarre reports of abuse have proven to be real, such as the infamous case of Josef Fritzl who held his daughter captive in the basement of the family home and impregnated her numerous times and other rigorously documented cases of incest that continued well into adulthood or never ended (Middleton, 2023). More recently, cases of parental trafficking of their children for money have been identified. The ongoing vulnerability of child victims to revictimization across the lifespan can occur to such a degree as to defy credibility leading to questions about the victim's complicity. Research supporting betrayal trauma theory has documented "betrayal blindness" in victims who are unable to recognize danger or to engage in self-protection, making them vulnerable to additional predation (Freyd, 1996).

Meanwhile, victimology studies documented psychological means of coercing victims used by abusers involving misrepresentation (i.e., grooming and gaslighting) that challenges the victim's reality and sense of self, sometimes supported by threats of or actual violence. There is now greater social awareness of how repeated misinformation can easily mislead and undermine child victims and adults alike. It also helps to explain the often ambivalent and confusing attachment patterns incest victims have to their abusers (trauma bonding), whom they report loving and hating. It must be remembered that incest occurs within established relationships and in a familial/relational context that involves confusing and crossed roles. Therapists must hold an appreciation of this ambivalence and not scapegoat the abuser as much as hold them accountable for their actions. While most incestuous abusers are male, there are significant numbers of female sex abusers and many who know of the incest without protecting their child. This is particularly the case where incest is ongoing into adulthood and in cases of intrafamilial sex traffic rings.

Early treatment development

Clinicians/researchers began to apply their findings to therapeutic practice, publishing articles and books and organizing professional training. Contrary to the psychoanalytic viewpoint, they believed that treatment required supporting the survivor/client to directly acknowledge and face the reality of the incest and additionally treating the long-term impact of the untreated original effects. However, it soon became clear that facing incest (or other complex trauma) too soon was emotionally overwhelming for many clients, some of whom decompensated. The highly disruptive symptoms of PTSD and the dissociative disorders and additional symptoms of anxiety, depression, and addictions, as well as life dysfunction and lack of personal safety, complicate the treatment and need to be addressed early in the process and the trauma processed once the individual is stabilized.

I wrote *Healing the Incest Wound: Adult Survivors in Therapy* (Courtois, 1988), the first book on treatment. I argued that incest was multifactorial and *potentially* if not usually traumatic for the victimized child and constituted a compounded form of interpersonal/relational victimization with aftereffects that themselves were complex and highly variable. The fact that the perpetrator was related or known to the victim created a betrayal trauma that compounded the victim's responses and made her vulnerable to additional victimization. A wide range of transdiagnostic aftereffects were to be expected and the most severe needed treatment attention either sequentially or concurrently. Soon thereafter, other treatment books from different therapeutic orientations were published.

Legal changes began to take place in response to these developments. Statutes of limitations for tort cases were lifted in some states and survivors began to file civil lawsuits against family members for the emotional and life damages caused by the incest. These cases were difficult for all involved and the credibility of the victim/plaintiff and her memories routinely came under intense scrutiny and challenge. Parents and other defendants protested that nothing like what was alleged had ever happened in their families and challenged the plaintiffs' memories as false and their motivation as vindictiveness and greed. Due to their novelty, the breaking of the silence imposed by the incest taboo, and the family conflict involved, these lawsuits also received extensive media coverage.

Along with others, I began to worry about a possible backlash especially from the accused but also from pedophiles (some in organized groups) who extolled sex with children and who were pro-incest. Herman had been prescient on this matter, having noted that backlash always accompanies social change and that the history of the study of trauma was replete with such disavowals and pushbacks. Concerning incest, these arrived in full force in the following decade.

The 1990s: Progress and backlash

Nineteen ninety-two (1992) was a hallmark year with two quite opposite major occurrences. Herman (1992) published *Trauma and Recovery* in which she described entrapping, repetitive, progressive, interpersonal/intrafamilial victimization in childhood as *complex trauma* and noted its potential for developmental impact above and beyond the posttraumatic. Based on factor analysis of available research on incest/child sexual abuse, she categorized seven criteria in addition to those of classic PTSD. She proposed the inclusion of an expanded diagnosis of complex posttraumatic stress disorder (CPTSD) in the next edition of the *Diagnostic and Statistical Manual* as a parallel or more compounded form of PTSD.

Herman also laid out a three-stage model of treatment. The first addressed personal and life safety as well as stabilization, education about trauma and posttraumatic responses, skill-building, emotional regulation, psychoeducation, cognitive description of the trauma, and the development of the treatment alliance. The second stage moved on to emotionally processing the trauma to some degree of resolution and the associated diminishment/remission of symptoms. This stage involved grief responses and, in some cases, confrontation of the perpetrator and other family members/bystanders or other courses of action. The third stage addressed life re-integration after trauma processing, including establishing healthy boundaries in relationships and increased assertion based on improved self-esteem and sense of self.

Field trials were successful in supporting the proposed criteria, importantly, the range of symptoms *in addition to* the standard criteria of PTSD. When the *DSM-IV* was published in 1994, CPTSD was not included as a freestanding diagnosis – even though it had received committee approval – but rather as an associated feature of PTSD (American Psychiatric Association, 1994). The reasoning for this exclusion was unclear and led to questioning of whether child abuse trauma was viewed as less important than combat trauma.

Nineteen ninety-two (1992) also marked the emergence of the "false memory" movement organized by a newly founded False Memory Syndrome Foundation (FMSF) whose advisory board consisted of prominent cognitive psychologists who researched memory. They challenged the prevailing views of clinicians about patterns of amnesia and the return of memories of past trauma in delayed form years later and suggested that memories of emotional or traumatic events would be *more memorable and therefore more remembered* rather than repressed, otherwise forgotten or disavowed memories that were later recovered. And, they noted, memories would not be recalled with great clarity and detail, as suggested by some therapists and trauma researchers.

Advisory board members published damaging critiques blaming naïve therapists for using suggestive techniques (referred to as "recovered memory therapy", not a term generally used by therapists) to encourage their clients to recall false memories of abuse that never happened. It was never made clear how the foundation determined that alleged abuse had not occurred and was therefore false, except to believe the denials of their accused members who had joined their foundation and their own tendency to disbelieve reports of abuse that had not always been remembered.[2] They further accused therapists of causing clients to decompensate through use of problematic techniques and of fostering overdependence on the therapist and alienation from their families. The FMSF claimed that thousands and even millions of families were saved from destructive therapists, a seemingly inflated claim with no research back-up. "Falsely accused" parents were encouraged to sue their adult child's therapists for malpractice and negligence and damages (for which advisory board members would serve as expert witnesses) and several such lawsuits were undertaken and won, some involving prominent clinicians and leaders in the field (especially those who treated dissociation).

The media quickly picked up on and sensationalized the FMSF position without a great deal of investigation or critique (Stanton, 1997), even though problematic terms such as "false memory syndrome" were not then and have never been substantiated nor was the prevalence of the problem ever scientifically determined. Media attention caused a pendulum swing in public perception from understanding and empathy for child victims and adult survivors to suspicion about their reliability and motivation. They questioned the credibility of both children and adults and warned of their suggestibility and instability.

The debate between mental health professionals (who had little working knowledge of memory) and memory specialists (cognitive psychologists who had little working knowledge of trauma – or of psychotherapy for that matter) was so ferocious as to be called the "Memory Wars", lasting for much of the decade. As mentioned above, there was concern about backlash, but it was not expected to be so organized or personalized in *ad hominem* attacks, innuendo, and lawsuits against therapists, nor was it expected to come from psychologists and the public. Many therapists were so frightened by the atmosphere (e.g., some prominent trauma therapists were threatened with lawsuits and violence, and some had their offices picketed by FMFS supporters) that they refused to treat incest survivors or other traumatized clients. Some left the field altogether.

I can personally attest to the vehemence as one of the six appointed members of the American Psychological Association Task Force on the Investigation of Memories of Childhood Abuse and an invited faculty member of a NATO-sponsored Advanced Scientific Institute on trauma and memory. Both were organized to study the issues and provide guidance and recommendations for therapists, researchers, and the public. The task force included three clinical psychologists specializing in the treatment of adult survivors of child abuse and three cognitive psychologists specializing in memory. This produced a composition of staunch advocates of their respective positions without other less polarized experts to temper the discussion, virtually guaranteeing a stalemate. Positions were so divergent to result in two separate reports and a critique and rebuttal of each other's positions before arriving at a set of guidelines for working on delayed/recovered memory issues in clinical practice, research, and policy (Alpert et al., 1996).

The NATO Institute included 100+ attendees from both the cognitive sciences and the traumatic stress/child abuse/psychotherapy fields who attended and intensely discussed faculty presentations. Conference participants were divided and strident at the start of the 11-day conference but over its course, a dialogue began that led to a tempering of the extreme positions. Some memory researchers began to understand more about trauma and its treatment and trauma clinicians and researchers learned more about memory and its malleability. Joint research projects were planned and developed. Among the major consensus items (that were also endorsed by numerous international and professional work groups empaneled during this same period): child abuse/incest is a highly prevalent societal problem; memory *could return* in delayed fashion in about a quarter (25%) to a third (33%) of cases; recollections are not pristine; false memories are possible; and suggestive techniques are to be avoided in psychotherapy (Lindsay & Read, 1997).

I came away from these experiences outraged by what I believed to be a highly organized and overgeneralized attack on all therapists, but especially those treating incest. Like Dr. Masson's account of his experience as the "truth teller", the hostility and derision directed towards the believer/therapist were palpable and frightening. I tried to hold a middle ground between the two polarities because I also knew that there were therapists who had gotten caught up in the challenges, treatment traps, and relational dilemmas that routinely emerge in this treatment and who, in their lack of training or knowledge, had made some major and costly mistakes. I was particularly worried that the advances in the relatively nascent field would be totally lost, and that incest would go back in the closet, resulting in children and adults again being disbelieved, silenced, and isolated. In my view, the whole field was set back by the "false memory" controversy (the critics of course hold the opposite view), and incalculable damage was done to real victims.

To provide clinicians, memory researchers, and lay readers with "middle ground" information, I published *Recollections of Sexual Abuse: Treatment Principles and Guidelines* (Courtois, 1999) that consolidated the recommendations of numerous aforementioned national and international professional task forces with guidelines I had developed for the NATO Institute. I suggested a consensus model of treatment for incest and other forms of complex trauma that established a neutrally supportive position from which to treat clients that neither suggested nor suppressed reports of abuse. I also endorsed the tri-phasic model of treatment geared to client stabilization before trauma processing.

The new millennium: Where we are now

At the close of the millennium, the atmosphere concerning recovered/false memory calmed. The field of traumatic stress studies became more established and accelerated in the aftermath of major societal traumata (i.e., the 9/11 attacks, transportation accidents, climate disasters, interpersonal assaults). The study of war trauma continued due to the ongoing wars in the Middle East and more localized conflicts and the impact on warriors, civilians, and displaced refugees alike. In 2000, the National Child Traumatic Stress Network was funded by Congress to systematically study traumatized children and their treatment in parallel to the VA's National Center for PTSD, the premier scientific organization investigating trauma and its treatment in adults. In 2002, the clergy abuse scandal in the Catholic Church erupted after a *Boston Globe* investigation identified the scope of the problem and its cover-up. Male survivors began to come forward in greater numbers making it obvious that the sexual abuse of males was more widespread than previously known. Some were incestuously abused by family members and some by others in fiduciary roles such as clergy, coaches, choirmasters, and scout leaders, among others.

Herman's complex trauma formulation opened the way for a continued emphasis on how a child victim's maturation is impacted when trauma begins early in life. The findings of developmental and attachment studies and the developmental/affective neurosciences supported a more sophisticated and nuanced understanding of both initial and long-term responses. A diagnostic formulation, developmental trauma disorder (DTD) (Van der Kolk, 2005), the child counterpart to complex PTSD in adults, was introduced and field tested, again with the hope of inclusion in the *DSM*. To date, neither CPTSD nor DTD has been accepted in the latest edition; CPTSD remains an associated feature of PTSD.

Complex PTSD was finally formalized as a diagnosis in the *International Classification of Diseases-11* (World Health Organization, 2018), the result of factor analyses that differentiated complex PTSD and classic form PTSD. In the *ICD*, CPTSD is a "sibling diagnosis" to PTSD that requires the endorsement of two symptoms from each of the original three criteria for PTSD and the additional three criteria of CPTSD (identity disturbance, emotional dysregulation, and relationship disturbance, organized under the heading of Disturbances of Self-Organization).

Treatment guidelines

Treatment guidelines became increasingly important in providing recommendations to clinicians and researchers about the effectiveness of treatment methods for a variety of psychological conditions. The first published trauma treatment guidelines were consensus-based, derived from a survey of identified authorities in traumatic stress and its treatment. Since then, as research methodology has developed and become more sophisticated, research findings have supplanted clinical consensus. Treatment guidelines are now based on systematic reviews and quality assessments of treatment efficacy studies to provide evidence-based treatment recommendations. Approximately 11 such guidelines for PTSD are now available, all finding primary support for the efficacy of exposure-based treatments, known as Trauma-Focused Treatments (TFTs), for the remission of *symptoms of PTSD*. Considerable debate exists about whether these treatment recommendations are applicable to the *additional symptoms of CPTSD* and whether sequencing of treatment is necessary. Based on their research findings, developers and proponents of TFTs argue for their immediate application at the start of treatment, while proponents of CPTSD counterargue for more gradual application within the sequenced model.

No similar evidence-based treatment guidelines are currently available for complex trauma as a research base is lacking, although currently developing. Several consensus-based guidelines for CPTSD have been published and several texts on the treatment of complex trauma are now available. Interestingly, none of the additional books are specific to the treatment of incest, and until more research emerges, an empirically based understanding of best practices for the treatment of all forms of complex trauma including incest is not possible.

What happened to incest?

In *Healing the Incest Wound*, I quoted the audacious phrase "Incest: If you think the word is ugly, take a look at its effects". I was not arguing for the eradication of the word, but instead that it be recognized as a word with ugly connotations, and whose even worst effects must be addressed (Courtois, 1988, 2010). Despite being 40+ years into the "Age of Discovery", it appears that the word incest is again being quashed. When revising *Healing* in 2010, a search of the literature using the keyword "incest" did not result in many hits.[3] The word had been subsumed under the more generic "child maltreatment" or "child sexual abuse". *This, despite the aggregate of research findings on child sexual abuse that perpetrators are most often parents or are otherwise related to or known to the child, making incest the correct term for this form of sexual violation and relational betrayal, and significant to the understanding and treatment of the victim's symptoms.* This suggests that professionals as well as society at large remain unwilling or unable to face the sexual exploitation and abuse of vulnerable children by family members and intimates using accurate terminology, so it gets "dumbed down" in a process of "language muting". Instead, society remains fixated on "stranger danger" rather than "intimate danger". In so doing, we look away from both the reality of this type of sexual abuse and the relational and betrayal conundrums its victims face at the time of its occurrence and in later life. We also embolden abusers by denial. The effect of this mislabeling is to reinforce secrecy and silence, re-establish the taboo, and again imply the word and experience are unspeakable or the experience is not real and is, rather, a fantasy.

The recent incredibly widespread response to the *#MeTooInceste* hashtag posted on social media in France is a testament to incest prevalence and to the fact that victims/survivors will disclose when there is a forum to do so and where they can anticipate being believed, protected, and supported. Mondragon et al. (2022) analyzed the content of the response tweets and concluded "[t]his wave of testimonies represents a turning point as it has broken the law of silence and allowed the victims to exist in the media space without being questioned" (p. 1). So, we can conclude that making openings for disclosure and ensuring that these are met with support and understanding, and not denial and degradation, will allow exposure of what has continued to be hidden and out of sight. In doing this, we remove part of what was so traumatizing, the secrecy and inability to seek help without additional shame and angst.

Meanwhile, the deniers and those involved in the previous backlashes have not gone away. Their efforts to aggressively challenge incest disclosures using the now outdated "false memory syndrome" persist. It can be expected that they will continue their efforts, and it can be argued that their efforts have metastasized to yet another domain, abortion rights.

Another retraction: Denied an abortion in the case of forced pregnancy

Obviously, rape and incest involving intercourse can result in pregnancy, another topic often shrouded in secrecy and shame. It is not an uncommon occurrence as now being documented by DNA testing (Zhang, 2024), and children born in such circumstances can suffer a variety of adverse consequences. They are often born in a condition of stigma to mothers whose reproductive options might have been curtailed and who may have difficulty attaching to or nurturing them due to cues associated with the circumstances of their conception. I have worked with several mothers filled with guilt and shame for their ambivalence and even hatred toward their child, whom they simultaneously love and who they know is not to blame for their birth circumstance. This is another conundrum of the violation that is incest – and still another has developed concerning abortion rights.

Abortion has been severely restricted in the US since 2021, the result of the Supreme Court's Dobbs decision. Since then, many states have nullified long-standing reproductive rights and banned the common exceptions for rape and incest. To date, little has been written about the plight, stigma, and welfare (including medical status and risk) of the girl or woman who become pregnant because of rape or incest, much less the stigma and welfare of a child born of such a conception.[4] In fact, in some states and jurisdictions, alleged and even convicted rapists are being given custody rights! Imagine raising a child in such a circumstance and what it would be like for both mother and the child. Once again, the mother/victim's circumstance is being dismissed or minimized, their choice eradicated, and many will be forced to have continued contact with their assailant if these decisions stand. Victims are not being seen or understood and are being made to carry additional lifelong consequences of what was imposed on them in non-consensual and illegal assaults. This is yet another travesty and punishment by those who put their ideology ahead of a living child or woman whose life will be put at risk and whose welfare and safety compromised by these restrictions. Is this yet another suppression of incest (and rape) being imposed in a draconian way by those who cannot or will not see the havoc that it has already caused and will continue to cause in the future? Reproductive rights groups are currently fighting these changes, citing the major consequences on privacy and other rights of victims. This can include causing those with forced pregnancies to avoid seeking needed medical care and again being silenced into keeping the secret. Yet another travesty is the punishment being meted out to those who seek out-of-state abortions and those who assist them, along with abortion providers themselves.

Conclusion

Major changes have occurred over the course of the past half century in the identification and the documentation of incest, its high degree of prevalence, and its often dire posttraumatic, developmental, and dissociative consequences for victims as well as its negative social impact. There is now an extensive and ever-expanding body of research on these issues that offers irrefutable evidence of their occurrence. This exposure, although initially accepted and responded to, was thereafter met with denial, pushback, and backlash, some of it vicious and even life-threatening. Victims again had their credibility and the accuracy of their memories challenged and their stories dismissed. Those who supported them were reviled.

Language muting in both professional and lay literature resulted in replacing the word "incest" with less direct and accurate terminology, itself a censoring of reality. Adding a further burden on its victims, long-established legal reproductive rights were severed and exclusions for rape and incest removed in many states. Incest victims deserve much better: to be seen, heard, protected, and saved from current and future indignities and loss of rights. They must also have avenues for justice and repair.

Proponents must continue to organize and fight back against the backlash and any similar organized censorship efforts that might arise in the future, even if they pay the price of being vilified or ostracized for doing so, as Masson was in the mid-1980s. It's time to reclaim the word and to not be afraid to call this form of interfamilial sexual abuse what it is: incest! And then to use the term to help those who have been most affected to understand its significance and impact and to recover sufficiently to have a less encumbered life and one worth living. It is also imperative that mental health and associated professions whose work involves responding to incestuous abuse continue to develop more effective intervention, and ultimately, to find ways to bring about prevention.

Notes

1 In the 2010 revision of my book, *Healing the Incest Wound*, I suggested that many forms of abuse involving non-relatives but within the context of a significant or fiduciary relationship with role and power differentials have incestuous connotations. Having a pre-existing relationship, or having the relationship used as a means of entrapping and sexually exploiting an individual or group, makes it very different from stranger assault and abuse as it involves intention and pre-meditation and is often repeated and blamed on the victim, thus compounding its dynamics and making them more like incest.

2 This stance was challenged directly by Dr. Jennifer Freyd (quite ironically, a heralded memory researcher) whose parents established the foundation after she recalled incestuous abuse by her father and subsequently asked her parents to cut short a holiday visit to shield her children from them. In a presentation she gave at a conference in Ann Arbor in 1993, she pointedly asked why her word (as both a well-functioning, mature adult and a well-recognized professional) was less credible than her father's and described some of the family dysfunction in her upbringing including his alcoholism.

3 I again searched this literature for this chapter and found some but not a great number of articles that particularly mentioned incest.

4 Here I am not discussing the genealogical problems that are possible resulting from inbreeding, but I have seen no mention of those either, although they are quite relevant to this issue.

References

Alpert, J. L., Brown, L., Ceci, S., Courtois, C. A., Loftus, E., & Ornstein, P. (1996). *Final report: Working group on the investigation of memories of childhood abuse*. American Psychological Association.

American Psychiatric Association (1980). *Diagnostic and statistical manual of mental disorders* (3rd Ed.). Author.

American Psychiatric Association (1994). *Diagnostic and statistical manual of mental disorders* (4th Ed.). Author.

Courtois, C. A. (1979). Characteristics of a volunteer sample of adult women who experienced incest in childhood and adolescence. *Dissertation Abstracts International*, 40A, Nov.-Dec. 1979, 3194-A.

Courtois, C. A. (1988). *Healing the incest wound: Adult survivors in therapy*. W. W. Norton.

Courtois, C. A. (1999). *Recollections of sexual abuse: Treatment principles and guidelines*. W. W. Norton.

Courtois, C. A. (2010). *Healing the incest wound: Adult survivors in therapy* (2nd ed.). W. W. Norton.

Finkelhor, D. (1979). *Sexually victimized children*. Free Press.

Freyd, J. J. (1996). *Betrayal trauma: The logic of forgetting childhood abuse*. Harvard University Press.

Herman, J. L. (1992). *Trauma and recovery: The aftermath of violence-from domestic to political terror*. Basic Books.

Herman, J. L., & Hirschman, L. (1981). *Father-daughter incest*. Harvard University Press.

Lindsay, D. S., & Read, J. D. (1997). *Recollections of trauma: Scientific evidence and clinical practice*. Plenum Press.

Middleton, W. (2023). Beyond death: Enduring incest – The fusion of father with daughter. In M. J . Dorahy, S. N. Gold, & J. A . O'Neil, (Eds.), *Dissociation and the dissociative disorders: Past, present, future* (2nd ed.) (pp. 223–237). Routledge.

Mondragon, N., Miuitus, A., & Txertudi, M. (2022). The breaking of secrecy: Analysis of the hashtag #MeTooInceste regarding testimonies of sexual incest abuse in childhood. *Child Abuse & Neglect, 123*. https://doi.org?19.1016/J.chiabu.2021.105412

Putnam, F. W. (1997). *Dissociation in children and adolescents: A developmental perspective.* Guilford Press.

Russell, D. E. H. (1983). The incidence and prevalence of intrafamilial and extra-familial abuse of female children. *Child Abuse & Neglect, 7*, 133–146.

Russell, D. E. H. (1986). *The secret trauma: Incest in the lives of girls and women*. Basic Books.

Stanton, M. (1997). U-turn on memory lane: Press coverage of recovered memories. *Columbia Journalism Review, 36* (2), 44–46.

Van der Kolk, B. A. (2005). Developmental trauma disorder: Toward a rational diagnosis for children with complex trauma histories. *Psychiatric Annals, 35*(5), 401–408.

World Health Organization. (2018). International Statistical Classification of Diseases and Related Health Problems. Author.

Zhang, S. (March 14, 2024). *DNA test are uncovering the true prevalence of incest.* The Atlantic.

9 To Believe or not Believe

The Assault on the Truth, the Mind, and the Body

Orit Badouk Epstein

> They tried to bury me; they didn't realise I was a seed
>
> Sinead O'Connor (1966–2023)

"Do you believe me; do you really believe me?" asked one of my first clients soon after telling me about the horrific sexual abuse and mind control torture she had endured at the hands of her family and other group members. The year was 2003 and I was still in training to become an Attachment-based Psychoanalytic Psychotherapist at the Bowlby Centre in London. I still remember the wave of shock that travelled through my body when this haunted woman shared her "unbelievable truth". What felt different to other clients though, was the fog and fear that occupied the space between us, leaving me in a state of dissonance and confusion. I trusted nonetheless, the visceral sensation in my body. I believed her.

It took another decade for similar truths from other survivors to appear and take a clearer shape, this time in the public domain. Five days after the children's entertainer Jimmy Savile was buried in November 2011, 35 survivors came forward alleging him as their perpetrator. What followed felt like a pivotal moment in the history of the investigation of child sexual abuse in the UK. In 2012, the British Home Secretary, Theresa May, announced a new police inquiry into allegations of child abuse in north Wales in the 1970s and 1980s, one of eight inquiries launched in the wake of the Jimmy Savile revelation (BBC, July 2012).

Peter Spindler was the first police commander at the Metropolitan Police to initiate a major inquiry, "Operation Yewtree", investigating claims from 450 potential victims of Savile which dated from 1955. This was a watershed moment. It appeared that for at least five decades Savile had perpetrated sexual abuse on hundreds of children and disabled adults ranging from age 5 to 75. The culture of denial at the BBC, National Health Service (NHS), Police, and other major institutions around the UK which Savile had close contact with, were now under scrutiny. The biggest fear of survivors was they would not be believed, but with the big institutions implicated, institutional memory became available, and Britain's biggest public inquiry into childhood sexual abuse now had a hallmark of credibility. Once the veil of disavowal around the credibility of survivors reporting sexual abuse was removed from the gatekeepers of denials, the secure base offered in therapy was

DOI: 10.4324/9781003431466-10

now less fearful for exploration and where shame and dissociation could finally find a safe home.

In her recently published book, *Truth and Repair* (2023), Judith Herman writes:

> Acknowledgment of the survivor's truth, acknowledgment of the harm she has suffered, and full apology, with remorse and without excuses – for many survivors, these are the requisite actions by which perpetrators and bystanders can begin the process of healing, moving from truth to repair.
>
> (p. 109)

Being believed routinely faces challenges from an alternative explanation based on fantasy. When the real is too hard to hear, there is a presumption that it does not afford the truth and fantasy becomes an easy default position. As Masson (1984) makes so clear in *The Assault on Truth*, Freud moved from the reality of child sexual abuse as a causal factor in the development of neurosis, an idea which irked his colleagues, to a theory of childhood sexual fantasies, which won him a favour and a following. In bringing the reality and impact of child sexual abuse back into psychoanalytic consciousness, Masson himself felt the full force of efforts to shut down his message and reinstate the dominance of fantasy (See Masson, Chapter 1).

Like Sandor Ferenczi, Alice Miller, Jeffery Masson, and other psychanalysts, being the outsider within his own psychoanalytic community, John Bowlby (1988) was alone in paying attention to the importance of actual life experiences. He expressed his grave concerns with psychoanalysis's reliance on the client's internal fantasies:

> [T]he concentration in analytic circles on fantasy and the reluctance to examine the impact of real-life events have much to answer for. Ever since Freud made his famous, and in my view disastrous, volte-face in 1897, when he decided that the childhood seductions, he had believed to be etiologically important were nothing more than the products of his patients' imaginations, it has been extremely unfashionable to attribute psychopathology to real-life experiences. It is not an analyst's job, so the conventional wisdom has gone, to consider how the patient's parent may really have treated him or her, let alone to entertain the possibility, even probability, that a particular patient may have been the target for the violent words and violent deeds of one or both parents. To focus attention on such possibilities, I have often been told, is to be seduced by our patient's prejudiced tales, to take sides, to make scapegoats of perfectly decent parents. And in any case, it is asserted, to do so could be of no help to the patient, would in fact be anti-therapeutic. It was indeed largely because the adverse behaviour of parents towards their children was such a taboo subject in analytic circles when I was starting my professional work that I decided to focus my research on the effects on children of real-life event of another sort, namely separation and loss.
>
> (p. 78)

However, Bowlby also admitted his lack of awareness around sexual and physical abuse for most of his career. In his last interview (1990) when asked about domestic and sexual abuse Bowlby replied:

> I've been appalled, frankly, at how ignorant we have been, I have been, about physical abuse and sexual abuse. I mean, I was totally unaware of physical abuse until, I think it was 1960 when Henry Kempe came over here and talked about physical abuse. And I was unaware of sexual abuse until, about ten years ago or fifteen years ago. Most of my professional career has been lived in ignorance of these things, and I think that's terrible.
>
> (p. 149)

So where are we now?

Many early analysts, including Freud, had sexual abuse histories that were ignored or not worked through (Middleton, 2018; Rachman, Chapter 3), so their own subjectivity arguably tilted them away from contemplating the reality of abuse on psychological functioning. Furthermore, two world wars, the Holocaust, Hiroshima, mass displacement, and other events that have global impacts, with millions of people killed, dislocated, and dispossessed from their families, homes, and countries, are traumas too large to miss but often too big to face. In their book *Faces in the Cloud*, Atwood and Storlow (2001) acknowledge that theories such as those offered by Freud, Jung, Reich, and others use subjectivity as a way of limiting their theories. Thus, the aggressive world Freud and his followers lived through may offer an additional explanation about the unconscious process that involved the abandonment of his original ideas on hysteria, and instead, he came up with the death instinct and the pleasure principle.

Traumatic events, just like the shock after a heart attack, leave the body with a reduced sense of time and space, unable to look into the distant future, its spontaneity lambasted with a sense of disorganisation, sometimes replaced by calculated efforts to control the present. Traumatic events also bring rigidity to the self, hinder exploration, and make relationships fraught. It is perhaps not surprising the twentieth-century landscape spawned such interest in aggression and conflict theories. But it doesn't account for the outright denial of aggression in the family and largely towards children and women. In the UK, John Bowlby was alone among his psychoanalyst colleagues in considering the social impact of traumatic events on one's sense of loss and the mobilisation of anger as a defence against that loss.

Like Bowlby, Sándor Ferenczi, Ian Suttie, Alice Miller, and others, have all helped us develop a psychological road map towards expanded empathy in understanding the reality behind mental health problems and one which helps acknowledge and prevent cruelty towards children. Similarly, Jeffery Masson's contribution is a defining marker in understanding one significant historical cause which prevented sexual abuse of children from being exposed in the way it is today, which sadly invited shame and retribution from the psychoanalytic community at the time. In Masson's words: "These were not merely minor squabbles about the history of psychoanalysis. We are talking about the very fundamentals of human society" (Chapter 1). Therefore, Masson's courage confronting Freud's "initial error" deserves acknowledgement and reward rather than ostracisation and exclusion. In addition, attachment theory and the body of the traumatised client, have been steadily integrated into more sophisticated therapeutic models and interventions, that move well beyond the reliance and primacy of interpretation, so central to analytic casework.

Yet, it was not only down to Freud's error in turning away from the seduction theory, other critical human errors were also made by other major thinkers. For example, the influence of the philosophers Descartes and Boyle, who thought that human cognition is separate from our bodies and that just sitting and thinking would provide us with all the answers. In *The Feeling of What Happens*, the neuroscientist Antonio Damasio (1999) tells us that the Cartesian view is no longer viable. It is both mind and body which influence consciousness and are critical to homeostasis. Homeostasis reflects the confluence of a range of possible states that are compatible with life. Additionally, the way we experience thoughts may be linked to physical aspects of attachment experiences that begin in infancy. Since the mind never properly separated from the body, the very nature of thoughts will be influenced by characteristics of primary relationships we have early in life that involve the body and others' engagement with it (Fonagy & Target, 2007).

The studies of trauma, attachment, and the body are all now well accepted by mainstream institutions and organisations, and psychoanalysis is gradually incorporating these experiences into their way of treating patients. Still, traumatic events will always invite a setback in human behaviour. The sudden appearance of the Covid-19 pandemic in 2020 upended our lives and filled our homes with unprecedented fear and disorganisation. In the UK, the high rate of mortality at the beginning of the pandemic left many NHS workers with a moral injury; feeling a pressing dilemma: can I do my job well but stay alive? For therapists, the social distancing imposed upon us by using technology made this moral injury feel less pertinent. The embodied psychological space created in the therapy room was now confined to the size of a small TV screen. The sacredness of our consulting rooms lost their walls and overnight we became digital citizens spending a great amount of time online.

At first the online sessions felt like a safe echo chamber, a container, a cosy bubble where some clients reported feeling safer while talking from the comfort of their sofas, beds, kitchens, cars, and so on. I soon positioned my computer against the window so I could get the best light. Devoid of the lower body, breath, smell, sweat, heartbeat, and touch, my mirror neurons had to adjust to reading the emotional cues of a face and torso. We stare at the screen and away from our physical bodies. The computerised world has encouraged an absence of the body. In his book *The Absent Body* (1990) the philosopher and medical doctor, Drew Leder elaborates on this concept. He distinguishes the terms body disappearance and body dys-appearance. Disappearance is a natural function of the body which includes the process of aging. Dys-appearance is a dysfunction of the body that takes place in moments of breakdown and failure. I find Leder's distinction to be illuminating and timely in understanding how the distance-seeking and increased dependency on technology made us morph, in Leder's way of thinking, to the dys-appearance of our bodies. I notice the loss, the increased efforts attending to the client's facial movement; the speed of which their eyelids flicker, the averted gaze, the clenched lips, the increased yawning, and how whenever they feel understood, their upper body rushes forward, their face almost touching the screen. In this new space formation, our torsos dance, we try to find some mutuality, even if compromised.

During lockdown there were reports of increased child abuse. As a therapist who works regularly with survivors of organised abuse, my thoughts were with those children who were now confined solely to the walls of their abusers. In leverage off Masson's efforts to bring the reality of child abuse into awareness, I now present a case designed to demonstrate advances made in not only acknowledging the reality of child abuse but working with survivors of organised sexual abuse, the assaultive impact virtual life has on the body and future hazards that technology imposes on our body and minds in the twenty-first century.

"My Avatar therapist" – the online relationship

It was during the assaulting days of the pandemic when Alice, a 48-year-old woman contacted me for therapy. Just a face on the screen, she arrived like a beautiful portrait, a metaphor to be adored, her smile had the purity of a child, and nothing she said described the storm inside her.

The following session while zooming in, I found her hiding under a duvet, her whisper repeatedly murmured: "Are you there? Am I here?" The screen was dark, I could barely see or hear her. In trying to adapt to the novelty of this new way of being together, I wasn't sure if our connectivity would turn out to be real. For Alice to feel somewhat grounded, I asked her to touch the floor, the wall, and the screen. Continuously self-harming, Alice lived a multifarious existence with a shattered mind and extensive injuries to her body. It was pain which defined Alice, pain that rendered her to feel powerless, yet which also made her powerful. Later I received a long email where I learnt about the horrendous childhood abuse that she encountered at the hands of her sadistic parents and a group of their friends, among whom was Jimmy Savile.

As a child Alice had to excel at enduring levels of pain that no human being could or should. The torture training she regularly received was designed to supply the sex industry with a sex slave who specialised in sadomasochistic activities; "there was big money there", a part of her revealed. As a survivor of prolific sadistic abuse, Alice often conveyed a lack of agency evident in a helpless child, as well as a capacity to be highly dominating. Her dissociation was structured and meant that she had many segregated parts, each with a story to tell. But Alice's pained body emerged from its dissociative "dys-appearance" and its mastery of pain was how she paid her monthly bills. In her adult life, Alice developed a reputation as a highly skilled Sub (short for submissive) who could take pain like no one. The more pain she endured the less embodied she felt. She told me about the recognition and respect she received from many Doms (short for dominatrix) and how rewarding it felt to her. Her dissociation was profound, devoid of any relational context she could not afford to dwell on embodiment and was concerned with matters of dissociated pain: "Can I master my pain or can pain master me?".

Alice believed that she was born evil and was not in a place to consider that her pain infliction was one way of responding to her traumatic childhood while numbing her chronic but failed grief. Her derealisation and depersonalisation led her to believe even though it (i.e., the pain) occurred within herself, that she could never identify it as herself. As we know "Many patients who extensively utilise dissociation, automatically do so as they experience pain. This can be dangerous, since pain is an innate self-protective mechanism that warns us when something is wrong in the body" (Bloom, 2010, p. 157). It was during lockdown when Alice got sick (not with the coronavirus) that she initially contacted me, feeling like her body was threatening on giving up completely. "I want to live" she said in our first session; her eyelids flickered fast.

For a while, unable to tolerate my gaze, Alice's vanishing self was hiding behind the screen, under the bed, moving around different rooms, eating, staring at her phone, listening to her favourite music, playing with her dog, etc. At other times, she would ask me to switch off the camera, in the hope that her shame would go unnoticed. The boundaries needed revisiting, yet I felt that I had very little say, or she could disappear at the press of a button, and I was learning to listen differently.

In Alice's mind the screen provided a sense of unreachability, which brought her closer to me and she could reveal the secrets that were wielding their power inside her. Alice had a kind of guarded openness about her, she would be overly friendly yet overly vigilant. Her phobia of reliance was in contrast with a desire for contact, such that she wanted more sessions but insisted on seeking proximity via the screen only. I wondered with her, whether it was the privilege of lockdown which gave her the confidence to approach therapy with less embodied shame.

The online sessions during those pandemic months, it seemed, had their own merit, opening new vistas of creativity unknown to the traditions of therapy in person. And so, for a while, as she slowly parted with her secrets, we developed a language that felt appropriate to those strange times of need. She would say: "Where am I?" or "I know nothing about you, you are merely a perception of my thoughts, you are my avatar therapist" and I would say, "I'm here, still with you". She reported it made her feel held, but I could sense the frozenness of a child since internal isolation was Alice's primary coping mechanism. In one of our early sessions, I noticed her nose dripping. I leaned forward and told her that I wished I could offer her a tissue. She leaned backwards; her gaze averted, her shame pushing me away with what for her was a comfortable rejection. Alice was alone and I was alone with her. The extensive sexual abuse she endured was easier to talk about via a screen, yet her pain is made by internal experiences that others can't share. It tended to assert itself through intense aloneness, it hurts in its physical solitude and has a hallucinatory quality to it. Without the proximity of a safe person, a safe body, the virtual seemed to offer a means of further extending the flight from her own body, her mind adrift without connection. To be fully present one needs to incorporate their body in the presence of another. To be present is the opposite of going inwards. The present moment according to Daniel Stern (2004) "involves some sense of self. During the lived present moment, you are the sole experience of your own subjective experience. You know that it is you who is experiencing. It does not simply belong to you, it is you" (p. 39).

Alice's reality was regularly obliterated. She grew up during a time when the culture of denial as described in Masson's writings was highly prevalent. Alice spent years in and out of psychiatric hospitals where she was pathologised, objectified, and dehumanised, her reality was eradicated by the professionals who told her that she was manipulative, borderline, and schizophrenic who was deemed unsuitable for therapy. In all her days in the hospital, there was never a mention of the possibility that her parents were the source of her "illness" nor the purveyors of abuse.

It was Bowlby who first acknowledged that humans were predisposed to seek proximity towards their caregivers even when alarmed by them. Some decades later, the researchers Main and Solomon (1986, 1990) conceptualised and named it the disorganised attachment status; when the parent is both the source of comfort and fear to the infant, leaving them with an insolvable dilemma of fright without a solution. In short, for some like Alice, disorganised attachment involves relationships of proximity with their "scaregivers" (Badouk Epstein, 2015, 2017, 2018). Alice's attachment to her now-deceased parents was still yielding the omnipresence of the living and powerful. Wedded to them for eternity, she was made to believe that she was evil and beyond redemption and that ultimately her subjectivity would be negated by meeting them in the afterlife. Alice's suicidal ideation notified how alone she was, and did not allow for the appearance of hope to free her. Her wish to die ("I am evil") was entwined with her fear of dying ("I am going to reunite with my parents"). Confusing love with subjugation and safety with control, it wasn't pleasuring self and others that Alice sought, but the acceptance of her parents. Paired up with fear, her intense pain was tied up to their objectifying sadism, it was intense pain which also equipped her with an exaggerating sense of specialness as well as a sense of alienation from her body, all of which was the source of her adrenaline-fuelled addiction to self-harm. Alas, the psychiatrist she saw in the hospital at the time told her that her oedipal fantasies were overly erotic and diagnosed her as a schizophrenic nymphomaniac. Later she found that he was part of the organised abusing group her parents belonged to.

From the trauma and dissociation field, I have learnt the role of parts and that the client's self-harming parts have no sense of time, always living in the eye of the storm, and are created to serve as protectors and even imitators of the abusers (Dorahy, Gold, & O'Neil, 2023, Van der Hart, Nijenhuis & Steele, 2006). Alice would report harming the body and describe the extent of injury in a playful manner. Pain was Alice's only understanding of care-seeking. It was through pain infliction that she was rejected and disposable (they told her that she was born evil and sexually dirty), and through pain, she got recognition and reward (they told her how special and good at it she was). The fetishisation of her wounds was normalised, her body as an object was all she knew, and I was not invited to comment or intervene. With very little room to manoeuvre, I too, felt controlled.

Alice's rage was never empathically witnessed and could only be expressed through coercion, self-abuse, and suicidal ideation. What became apparent though, was that the desire to die from Alice's suicidal parts was not her desire to be dead, rather this was her rageful protest, her attachment cries. Attachment cries convey the child's protestations against the backdrop of emotional neglect and abuse, since for the securely attached child, protest is part of their right to express their unassuaged frustration against their caregivers. While with the unattended infant, the one who didn't receive an empathic response and is instead left to fend for his/herself, the inhibition of negative affect in time develops into a cumulative protest, sometimes a frozen cry, a dissociative self-state that is often engaged in hostility towards the self and the other (Badouk Epstein, 2022). Attachment cries usually communicate the client's early suffering and unmet needs in a way that can appear to other people as manipulative, repetitive, overwhelming, demanding, unpredictable, and off-putting.

Be it in person or on the screen, and different from classical neutrality, empathic witnessing is one which means that one person witnesses the feelings of another and can respond to them with available sensitivity. Empathic witnessing always involves affect and movement, such as when we say: I am moved by you. Although I was mostly excluded from Alice's outer and inner worlds, my gaze grew to witness her pain with less fear and more compassion. And while her self-harming parts provided an extension of her own self-reliance, other parts were reaching out desperately asking for my support and help. For individuals who suffered needlessly as children, providing the client with analytic neutrality is ineffective and may even feel cruel to the client.

Slowly as Alice was leaking untold abuse, I was helping her link it. My affirming voice became her translator, telling her that she suffered a horrific childhood of rape and torture, and that her parent's sadistic activities were not only an assault on her body, but a severe crime committed on an innocent child. She glanced from behind the duvet, looking with utter dismay. I was hoping that my soothing voice and validating words would hold the promise of tenderness and curb the threat of her violence. But Alices's account of pain was all she knew and involved a complex relationship to power with her tormentors and she could not exile them.

The work with clients with complex trauma always requires a degree of creativity that may stretch beyond the classical framework passed on by traditional psychoanalysis. Alice loved words; it helped a bit when I told her she was a victim of hate crimes. I went on to explain that victims of hate crimes experience physiological and emotional distress ranging from gut problems, rapid pulse, difficulties in breathing, nightmares, hypertension, reckless behaviour, forms of self-harm and suicidality. Hate crimes assault the bodies of those who are made into objects. In a different session, I wrote on a card in big capital letters: Can a Distressed Body be De-stressed? She liked it. Our left-brain connectivity shifted sides, and our expression landed closer, even if our bodies had yet to meet. In this newly formed "we space" my continuing empathic witnessing and dialoguing with all parts provided emotional validation. Alice's reality slowly returned to sight, and she began to show signs of emerging from the depths of her shame, spending less time under the duvet and sitting upright in front of the screen.

In his book, *The Master and his Emissary*, the philosopher Iain McGilchrist (2009) tells us how language and words are a manifestation of the logical part of the left brain. The right brain gives us intuition and makes encounters with our bodies. The left brain always wants to take over. Logic is not our friend but our servant. Without embodied intuition, words are pure logic and will be devoid of human syntax and connection. Language is a function of the body. With nurturing language, we come closer to the minds of others. Yet language alone in its own form of materiality is absent from the body. Whenever I allowed words to nourish Alice, advocating her, telling her that her skin was a canvas for his razor, his knife, his sadistic delights, not hers, and that she was worthy of a painless life, it was words that failed therapy. Her ambivalence remained defiant, her pernicious logic would take over arguing merely reason. It was during those opponent moments that I began to feel the limitations of language, what can language hold for us when our bodies are merely the vessels to carry words?

Desolate in her presence I noticed my own absence and how my mirror neurons flinched less.

When Alice got Covid, her self-disgust increased, and she rushed back into her hiding place. "Disgust is clearly dependent upon contact: it involves a relationship of touch and proximity between the surface of bodies and objects" (Ahmed, 2004, p. 85). "I am repulsive, just like someone with leprosy" she coughed heavily from under her duvet. The virus had clearly triggered times when she was very sick as a child but got the treatment of a disposed and dirty object. My attempts to soothe her, analyse the meaning of her repulsion, or normalise the virus got us nowhere. She could still not surrender to her own vulnerability.

By the end of the second lockdown, our relationship depended on similes and psychological adjectives. At that time many reported that the augmented reality offered online, had a dream-like quality, dwindling between being and not being. I began feeling a cognitive overload and an online fatigue that informed the sessions with most of my clients. There was a frequent deadness during some sessions. Alice's self-harming parts relented: their tyranny gave way. In this state of global dys-appearance, we had no choice but to continue.

"Was is not is", William Shakespeare

Alice's terror of merging and losing herself in the presence of a non-harming other was profound and overwhelming. She could not consider the passing of time to be real, for her body was always "then". Then and there in a hidden farm or a stately home where they sadistically possessed her body and stripped her of any kind of "I-ness" and "You-ness". Worse, the organised group of criminals and paedophiles she grew up with repeatedly told her she wanted and loved it.

As we finally emerged out of the restrictions of lockdown, and life began resuming some physical contact, it became even harder convincing Alice to leave the confines of her home and come to see me in person. By now, her disembodiment also meant that she was invested in the proximity of the screen as a substitute for any relationship, and her addiction to many online sites of pornography flourished. The lack of space she endured all her life meant that she inhabited a body that was never her own. Using the screen became an illusory space which set her free from her bodily context and she could now declare some agency and control. The added tension between her image-making and self-representation saying, "you don't really know me so what does it matter how my body looks", made it clear that it was still not safe for her to venture out of the familiarity of her dissociation. Furthermore, the virtual had also helped sterilise our relationship from the messiness of her bodily shame.

Empathic attunement means that each client requires a different kind of nearness or a different kind of farness. For a mind to grow, a space must be created, and this space is first created in another body and mind (i.e., between infant and parent), and so for a while longer, our unmuted faces were all that Alice could tolerate. I had to be patient and trust that, for me to be included, I first had to be excluded. "You are my avatar therapist, and I am your avatar client", her adolescent parts would sometimes giggle. Still not knowing whether our Zoom meetings would ever lead to a location for our physical selves to find a safe ground for meeting, and so without much prompting, I kept waiting.

The appearance of a present moment is one which indicates movement, change, and hope. Dissociation is the absence of present moments (Stern, 2004, p. 24). A defining moment is part of a present moment. Such a moment came along when I asked Alice: "Do you have a body or are you a body?" she instantly replied: "Neither. I just follow rules, doing what my parents want me to do, [it] is the only way I can protect myself". Referring to her past while stepping outside her control system felt like Alice's appearing-self for the first time acknowledged her dys-appearing-self.

Over the Christmas break, I decided to send Alice a pocket teddy in the post. In an email, parts expressed their gratitude, reporting that she took it to one of her "pain parties" where she was holding the teddy tight during some sadistic engagement. With the transitional object helping Alice keep me in her mind, I noticed a growing sense of coherence and she was able to remember what had taken place in the previous session. Such flickers of light helped pave the way for more change. After two years and whilst the ambulances were still screaming loudly on our streets, Alice felt less afraid to come and meet me in person.

As our connection grows to be more embodied, Alice is slowly taking in the care that therapy can offer, while learning to understand that seeking pain was her only means of seeking care and that was is and no longer is.

The Wild Web – some implications for the future

In his book *Amusing Ourselves to Death*, Neil Postman (2006) wrote,

> Orwell fears those who would deprive us of information. . . . Huxley feared those who would give us so much that we would be reduced to passivity and egoism. Orwell feared that the truth would be concealed from us, Huxley feared that the truth would be drowned in the sea of irrelevance.
>
> (p. 140, 156)

The internet helped us expose the likes of Jimmy Savile and exposed many untold stories and realities. But with the pace at which technology is moving, it seems already that Huxley's dystopian prediction is the one we are currently facing.

We have entered an age where music and information stream like water, our minds overloaded and suffer the risk of drowning. There are too many writers and not many readers and too many bands and not many fans. Cramped with words and ideas our semiotic communications have been reduced to emojis. Our social dys-appearance is increasingly being noticed. We think we live in a more transparent world where we are more aware, and more exposed, yet our disembodied life puts us at risk of being fully hidden and finding it harder to distinguish truth from fiction. And with it comes the risk of further dissociation (as seen with Alice) and more sophisticated forms of child exploitation.

Here in the UK, one of this summer's news headlines (17.7.2023), was about how illegal AI images of child pornography are currently rife online. Predators around the world are sharing galleries of photo-realistic pictures of child pornography. The potential exists for paedophiles to produce unprecedented quantities of life-like child sexual abuse imagery that will distort reality and put children in danger. These AI-generated images are going to increase these predilections of potential perpetrators, reinforce their deviance on distorted realities, and lead to greater harm and risk to vulnerable children. In a way, if we are unable to distinguish images of real children from virtual children, this form of digital gaslighting can allow the fantasy narrative to repackaged itself, taking us right back to where we were a century ago, but worse.

Social media evoked social awareness like never before, but social awareness without self-awareness can be assaultive and remains a great concern to our humanity. The information overload that floods our minds is difficult to maintain and makes us vulnerable to new forms of exploitations. In Leder's words (1990):

> Our cultural belief in the dissociation of mind and body leads to an increase in dissociative practices; we are encouraged to abandon sensorimotor awareness for abstracted mathematical or linguistic. This in turn intensified the day-to-day experiences of mind as disembodied, confirming the initial cultural premise. As I sit here pursuing our socially sanctioned model of advanced intelligence – typing words on a computer screen – mind does seem like something disembodied indeed.
>
> (pp. 152–153)

Summary

Jeffrey Masson played a significant part in bringing child sexual abuse out of the shadows in psychoanalysis and psychoanalytically oriented psychotherapy. His efforts, in combination with the feminist movement of the 1970s and 1980s, the growth in attachment, trauma, and neuroscience research, and the digital revolution all helped mental health professionals and society at large take the blinkers off denial associated with child abuse from their eyes.

And yet, the reality and impact of more organised forms of child abuse has taken much longer to face and some forms today continue to meet resistance.

The Covid-19 pandemic created a global sense of disorganisation and dysregulation. For us therapists, lockdown and the confinement of our consulting rooms had to change for the screen, and with it came disembodiment and the loss of sensorial creativity. As seen with Alice, to begin with, the online relationship offered a sense of safety and control, something she could never master before. However, the hallucinatory presence within these sessions added a layer of dys-appearance to her already dissociated body which gave the relationship an avatar quality. Since healthy, intersubjective meetings are based on people with embodied minds who can act and react physically and mentally, the in-person therapy of two people in the room, on many levels, offers a more convincing representation of reality.

The largely negative treatment of the body we see with survivors of sexual and physical abuse is what I consider to be a form of dys-appearance: a devaluation of the body in the form of neglect, torture, and outright condemnation. The overload of information and its assaultive quality is leaving us already numb and indifferent to a suffering planet and growing online criminal activities. We need space between words and space between us. We need to learn to breathe again. It is bodies that create movement and space, not language or any form of digital manipulation. Whether on screen or in person our ethical gaze and work is to be-lived and stay presently embodied.

The world is moving as always, as we unbutton ourselves from the strictures of denials around child sexual abuse, we need to be cautious not to get stuck in the combative and binary camps bequeathed to us by the twentieth century. We can perceive Masson's acts of truth-teller as a helpful overture to the reality of childhood sexual abuse. It can be used as scaffolding for the next truth-telling act to bring further enlightenment and change for future generations. I perceive this as the need to concentrate our efforts in the coming century on our embodied life and to be present enough and aware of the new opportunities available to sexual predators online in exploiting vulnerable children and adults through various organised criminal activities and AI distorted reality. The virtualisation of our emotions, our sensorial subjectivity, and our sociability to an extent are all under threat. It has never been more pressing for us to infuse this world with embodied relatedness of meaning and wonder.

References

Ahmed, S. (2004). *The cultural politics of emotion.* Edinburgh University Press.

Atwood, G. E., & Storlow, D. R, (1999). *Faces in the clouds.* Aronson.

Atwood, G. E. & Storlow, R. D., (2001). *Faces in a Cloud: Intersubjectivity in Personality Theory*. Aronson, Inc.

Badouk Epstein, O. (2015). Cross the bridge to redefine the pain. *Attachment: New Directions in Psychotherapy and Relational Psychoanalysis*, 9(30), 290–294.

Badouk Epstein, O. (2017). The occupied body: On chronic fatigue, affect regulation and psycho-neuroimmunology. Attachment: New Direction in Psychotherapy & Relational Psychoanalysis, 11(3), 257–272.

Badouk Epstein, O. (2018). From proximity seeking to relationship seeking: working towards separation from the 'scaregiver". *Frontiers in the Psychotherapy of Trauma & Dissociation*, 1, 290–306.

Badouk Epstein, O. (Ed). (2022). *Shame matters: Attachment and relational perspectives for psychotherapists*. Routledge

Bloom, S. (2010). *Creating sanctuary: Towards the evolution of sane societies*. Routledge.

Bowlby, J. (1988). *A secure base*. Routledge.

Damasio, A. R. (1999). *The feeling of what happens*. Harcourt Brace & Company.

Dorahy, M., Gold, S., & O'Neil, J. (2023). *Dissociation and the dissociative disorders: Past, present, future*. Routledge.

Duchinsky, R., & Foster, S. (2021). *Mentalizing and epistemic trust*. Oxford University Press.

Fonagy, P. & Target, M. (2007). The rooting of the mind in the body: New links between attachment theory and psychoanalytic thought. *Journal of the American Psychoanalytic Association*, 55(2), 411–456.

Herman, J. L. (2023) *Truth and repair: How trauma survivors envision justice*. Basic Books.

Kakutani, M. (2018). *The death of truth*. William Collins.

Leder, D. (1990). *The absent body*. The University of Chicago Press.

Leder, D. (2016). *The distressed body*. The University of Chicago Press.

Main, M., & Solomon, J. (1986). Discovery of an insecure-disorganized/disoriented attachment pattern. In T. B. Brazelton & M. W. Yogman (Eds.), Affective development in infancy (pp. 95–124). Ablex Publishing.

Main, M., & Solomon, J. (1990). Procedures for identifying infants as disorganized/disoriented during the Ainsworth Strange Situation. In M. T. Greenberg, D. Cicchetti, & E. M. Cummings (Eds.), Attachment in the preschool years: Theory, research, and intervention (pp. 121–160). The University of Chicago Press.

Masson, J. (1984). *The assault on truth: Freud's suppression of the seduction theory*. Farrar Straus and Giroux.

McGilchrist, I. (2009). *Master and his emissary*. Yale University Press.

Middleton, W. (2018) Robert Fliess, Wilhelm Fliess, Ernest Jones, Sandor Ferenczi and Sigmund Freud. In W. Middleton, A. Sachs & M. J. Dorahy (Eds.). *The abused and the abuser: Victim – perpetrator dynamics* (pp. 234–250). Routledge.

Oskis, A. (2015). John Bowlby the last interview. *Attachment: New Directions in Psychotherapy*, 9(2), 138–157.

Postman, N. (2006). *Amusing ourselves to death*. Penguin.

Shakespeare, W. (2015). *As you like it*. Penguin Classics.

Stern, D. (2004). *The present moments in psychotherapy and everyday life*. Norton.

Van der Hart, O. Nijenhuis, E., & Steele K. (2006). *The haunted self*. Norton.

10 Grappling with Truth

Psychotherapy and *The Assault on Truth*

Kate McMaugh and Martin J. Dorahy

This chapter explores our experience of reading *The Assault on Truth* (Masson, 1984) and the impact of the book upon psychotherapy. We first situate Freud's seduction theory within its historical context, and within a gendered framework. We explore how Freud's recantation of his seduction theory had consequences that continue to pervade over a century later and arguably underpin specific social phenomena, including the development of 'false memory' rhetoric, ongoing medical and psychological doubt about self-reports of abuse and related symptoms (e.g., dissociation), and the minimisation of child sexual abuse prevalence and sequelae. We explore the contemporary impacts of these, as practising psychological therapists. Further, we explore the professional response to Masson's book and its implications for those who challenge psychological theories, as well as the impact on the contemporary mental health field.

Our experience of reading *The Assault on Truth*

As psychotherapists working primarily with survivors of child abuse, we recall reading *The Assault on Truth*, but some years after publication, when various changes in the field had occurred. We also come from a country lacking a rich tradition in Freudian psychoanalysis, though were taught the broad concepts of Freudian theory as an historical introduction to psychology. The implications of this theory for clinical practice and psychoanalytic techniques were not taught in our academic training as Australian psychologists, although one of us had a more in-depth exposure to Freudian orthodoxy during postgraduate studies in the United Kingdom, where tension between Masson's perspective and the Freudian power of sexual fantasy had not been fully laid to rest. Initially, then, for us *The Assault on Truth* was a fascinating historical account, even a detective story of sorts. Freud's recanting of the 'Seduction Theory' and his replacement theory that child sexual abuse reports were the product of fantasy seemed strange and shocking. At university there was disbelief among our fellow students that people could have believed this (even though there was acknowledgement that fantasy may play an important role in psychological life). Perhaps, with the passage of time, Freud and his colleagues seemed misogynistic and, at the very least, unsupportive bystanders

DOI: 10.4324/9781003431466-11

to those who experienced early child sexual abuse. It was later, as psychologists invested in the study and treatment of early childhood trauma and dissociation, that we began to look at the book, and the characters within it, in a more nuanced manner.

Freud and the history of doubting women

It is not possible to explore the impact of the book upon psychotherapy and reactions to it, without first examining the cultural and historical context within which Freud's theory evolved, and in which the writing of the Masson's book is situated. *The Assault on Truth* tells a story about the denial of female testimony, a story that began, at least in some cultures, thousands of years earlier, and one which, to some extent, is still being played out today. This is a very gendered story.

Doubts as to the veracity of female testimony have their roots in ancient societies that predate Islam, Judaism, and Christianity, although various scholars of these faith traditions throughout history have controversially imposed limitations on accepting a woman's testimony, with females being portrayed as having inferior memory to males, or lacking the self-control and strength necessary to be a good witness (al Alwani, 1996; Franiuk & Shain, 2011; Malka, 2019). Seventeenth- and eighteenth-century medical and legal texts defined rape and outlined investigative procedures in a manner that presumed a woman was likely to make false allegations, and the negative impact of allegations on males was of paramount concern. Genuine sexual abuse of women or children was seen as rare, and doubt was cast as to whether a healthy adult woman could be raped as she would 'fight off' her attacker (Quilter, 2015).

Within this historical context Freud developed his theories about his patients' reports of early sexual abuse. That most patients were female, reporting abuse by males, cannot be diminished in importance, given this long cultural, religious, medical, and legal history. Late nineteenth-century analysts were steeped in this history when confronted with emotional women reporting terrible childhood sexual atrocities. After Freud was challenged about his seduction theory, perhaps it did not seem a radical step to wonder if these distressed, emotional patients were wrong, confused, and having problems that were the creation of their own minds. So, while he initially listened to and believed his female patients, Freud later privileged male opinion and perspective, through discussions with and support from an almost exclusive cohort of male colleagues. Tertiary-matriculated women were rare in nineteenth-century Europe and their influence was minimal on psychological thinking.

Freud's theory of childhood sexual fantasies, his renunciation of the 'Seduction Theory', and the doubts he cast on the veracity of early childhood sexual abuse played a role in the continued suppression of predominantly female reports of sexual abuse and the ongoing mistreatment of survivors. For decades after Freud, scholars and sexologists presented contradictory views on women's sexuality, with women portrayed as both repressed and dangerously seductive. Some writings have argued that women have an unconscious rape wish bought about by a conflict between their natural sexual urges and suppressive social restrictions (Gavey, 2019). Writing about the history of incest in America, Sacco (2009) reports that by the early twentieth century the influence of Freudian thinking about fantasy as the etiological driver in sexual abuse reports replaced Victorian views about the innocence and purity of children and led to health and legal professionals upholding a view that girls and women lie about sexual abuse. She notes a subsequent downturn in criminal convictions for incest in the decades that followed, as forensic and medical experts discredited the reports of women and children, labelling victims as seductive instigators of incest. Sacco (2009) argues that from the 1940s to 1960s the psychoanalytic profession largely viewed father–daughter incest in terms of a daughter's fantasy for her father, and the responsibility for incest was increasingly placed on the daughter.

When females, who are more commonly victims of child sexual abuse (e.g., Mathews et al., 2023), are discredited and disbelieved, this also impacts negatively on male victims. By the 1980s researchers and clinicians were beginning to identify that male survivors were ashamed, taught that vulnerability is incompatible with masculinity, and hampered by a myth that adolescent males fantasised about seduction by an older female, with such events not deemed harmful. Victims of male abusers often feared that they would be accused of homosexuality or that the experience must have meant they were homosexual, in an era when homosexuality was highly stigmatised. Furthermore, victims felt no one would believe them as such events were exceptionally rare, or that physical arousal would be confused with consent (Holmes et al., 1997; Nasjleti, 1980). It is easy to see parallels to some of the earlier myths about female sexual abuse or incest: assumptions about the sexualised fantasy life of children; minimisation of harm; and assumptions of event rarity. These complex issues were compounded for males by a lack of knowledge and skills in responding to male victims of sexual abuse in the feminist-oriented services of the era (Nasjleti, 1980), resulting in less frequent reporting or an unhelpful response to reporting (Holmes et al., 1997).

In the 1990s, just as these notions were being openly challenged, and the prevalence and impact of childhood sexual abuse was bought into the open, we saw the False Memory Syndrome movement unfolding. Here, women coming forward with memories of childhood sexual abuse were openly challenged as liars, fantasists, and creators of false memories that had no reflection on any veridical truth. This movement was in part a 'backlash' against growing awareness of the veracity and impacts of child sexual abuse. The therapist's role in assisting the generation of 'false' sexual abuse memories was a focal point for the false memory syndrome movement and in many ways echoed what Freud came to think about sexual abuse reports when in 1925 he wrote, '*they were only phantasies which my patients had made up or which I myself had perhaps forced on them…*' (Freud, 1925, cited by Masson, 2003, p. 198).

Masson's book fits somewhere towards the end of this history, written in an era when the discussion of violence towards women and children was just unfolding. However, the field of psychoanalysis had trouble hearing the message, perhaps because of how Masson framed it (e.g., questioning the character of Freud) and perhaps because it was too hard to hear. The broader issues of the prevalence and impact of childhood sexual abuse got swamped in the need to defend the integrity of Freud and psychoanalysis itself. This is exemplified in Masson's commenting that reviewers of *The Assault on Truth* attacked him, blaming him for sullying Freud's reputation and bringing psychoanalysis into disrepute (Masson, 2003). The terrible impact Freud's retraction had on women and children for almost 100 years appears to have generated far less dismay, distress, or outrage.

This 'blame the messenger' attack on Masson (see Chapter 1) also has parallels with the attack on therapists that occurred in the 1990s when the False Memory Syndrome Foundation began a well-funded public relations campaign to discredit therapists who worked in the field of child sexual abuse, accusing them of implanting in their clients false memories of non-existent sexual abuse in childhood (Crook, 2022; Salter & Blizard, 2022; see Crook, Chapter 7). The ferocity of the 'blame the messenger' attacks both Masson and these therapists received illustrate the lengths humanity can go to, to avoid facing both the horror of child sexual abuse and the guilt of being a non-protective individual or organisational bystander.

Despite the attacks Masson endured, and his alienation from the therapy world, his book powerfully cast doubt on Freudian theory that women's reports of child sexual abuse were the result of unconscious fantasies. Health professionals began to reconsider Freud's theory, debate it, and listen more closely to what women were recounting (Sacco, 2009). This subsequently opened up more space for men, too, to tell their stories of child sexual abuse. As Masson says at the end of book, 'the time has come to cease hiding from what is, after all, one of the greatest issues in human history' (Masson, 2003, p. 192).

Freud, Masson, and trauma reactions

An initial reading of *The Assault on Truth* may leave one seeing Freud as a misogynist who discredited women, or as a man so concerned with his own social standing that he bowed to peer pressure and became, at the very least, a profoundly non-protective bystander and, at worst, a man who played a part in facilitating the denial and cover up of child sexual abuse that continues in different ways to this day. Furthermore, Masson makes a strong case that some of those opposed to Freud's seduction thesis were in fact abusing children, including his own close friend and colleague Wilhelm Fleiss, who was later accused of abusing by his own son, and his disciple Ernest Jones who was charged with the sexual abuse of several children (Kuhn, 2002; see Middleton, Chapter 2). It has also been suggested that some of the key analysts of Freud's time, including Freud himself, were also victims of sexual abuse (Middleton, 2016), leaving open the possibility that Freud and at least some of his colleagues were denying or dissociating their own childhood horrors (see Rachman, Chapter 3). Masson himself concludes that Freud abandoned the theory because of a 'personal failure of courage' (Masson, 2003, p. 190). Any and all of these perspectives may have some accuracy and other less hostile explanations are also likely to be relevant. Swapping the naïve vantage point which we brought to our initial reading of *The Assault on Truth* over 20 years ago, we are now more seasoned trauma therapists with a more sensitive understanding of the issues Freud was grappling with and wonder about some of the other factors at play.

Freud was a man of enormous curiosity and drive, devoting his prodigious intellect to the great psychological mysteries confronting humanity, including how mental health problems derive. While his seduction theory came to dissatisfy him in terms of its ability, as he saw it, to offer a more universal account of neurotic dysfunction, it also brought him face-to-face with the disturbing reality of a grown man sexually gratifying himself with a small child. There is a very human reaction to hearing about the horrific and unspeakable pain of child sexual abuse, as well as the serious ramifications that this can have on victims. At individual and societal levels, we grapple with the 'knowing and the not knowing' (Solinski, 2017) of such trauma. Even as experienced trauma therapists, we can at times find the reality, prevalence, and impact of child sexual abuse hard to fathom and hard to bear. The truth that Freud initially held with his seduction theory becomes a weight hard to carry because of its ability to puncture the positive illusions, psychological resilience, sense of safety, and just-world beliefs that support psychological well-being. Even in a modern, more accepting era, as therapists we can only hold the reality and impact of child sexual abuse with difficulty, and with the support of like-minded colleagues, something Freud, at the time of his initial theory development, did not have. Freud appears to grapple for a time with the horror of incest before finding a place to put it that did not challenge him or his social connections too greatly. While he accepted it could happen, he believed most reports were fantasy.

We now know that trauma is encountered and then avoided. Herman (1992, p. 1) writes that 'The ordinary response to atrocities is to banish them from consciousness'. To bear witness to trauma is deeply painful. It requires one to face their own deepest fears and vulnerabilities. Herman points out that, in fact, it is easier to side with the perpetrator: 'all the perpetrator asks is that the bystander do nothing. He appeals to the universal desire to see, hear, and speak no evil' (Herman, 1992, p. 1).

Herman recounts historical examples of facing trauma then forgetting it, with Freud and his contemporaries a late nineteenth-century illustration. Around the time Masson published *The Assault on Truth* (1984), childhood sexual abuse was making another foray into the consciousness of mental health professionals and society at large, on the heels of the women's movement. The modern dissociation field was also starting a resurgence around that time. Then in the early 1990s came the seemingly inevitable backlash, in the form of the False Memory Syndrome Foundation, which explicitly sided with male testimony, while dismissing and trivialising the testimony of females. The reports from (mostly) female victims that their (mostly) male relatives were sexually abusing them, often from a very early age, were completely invalidated, not explicitly as 'fantasies' this time, but as 'false memories' implanted by therapists. The blame was not directly inside the alleged victim but due to fantasies (under the guise of false memories) created by therapists or in their work with them. Women were impressionable victims of incompetent or misguided therapists. The testimonies of men denying acts of sexual abuse were accepted and validated, almost without question. The denial of trauma, and particularly the trauma of women and children, was again the dominant discourse.

Key implications for psychotherapy today

The story of Freud and the reactions to Masson exposing how Freud grappled, and ultimately avoided, dealing with the horror of child sexual abuse, provide apt demonstrations of the 'approach and avoid' or 'knowing and not knowing' that this topic matter evokes, which has implications for psychotherapy today.

The importance of critique and evidence

For many years Freud's fantasy theory was accepted and gave support to other movements which have been very damaging to survivors of child abuse. While it would be wrong to assume that the entire psychoanalysis community had a uniform response to reports of child sexual abuse, particularly in more recent decades, it is fair to say that the theory was held as important, sacrosanct even, for far too long. Masson speaks of the drive within the psychoanalytic community to almost completely discard a focus on actual trauma as the cause of psychological distress, and focus therapeutic endeavours on etiological origins in the inner world. He proposes that without discarding Freud's seduction theory psychoanalysis would not have developed, at least in the form that it did. Masson's contemporaries felt that his findings were an attack on both Freud and the field of psychoanalysis.

For modern psychotherapy the implications are obvious: it is important that contemporary clinical practice is built around evidence, not eminence. We must be a field that values critical thinking, a field that is a safe place to challenge ideas and theories, even those held by people in positions of prestige and power. We must be dedicated to not just theory development but the careful testing and evaluation of theories, remaining ready to throw out our most dearly held formulations and practices if the evidence mounts against them, and to sit with the loss and grief that may arise. Essentially, we need to remain dedicated to the tenants of psychologically informed, evidence-based practice, albeit within a framework that allows for flexibility, innovation, and testing of new treatment approaches.

The importance of not working in silos

Masson tells a story of a field (psychoanalysis) that was theoretically and clinically minimising the importance of trauma. Yet, quite separately to the psychoanalytic field, the feminist movement from the 1960s onwards was framing rape as instrumental in patriarchal domination and advocating for victims. Since the early 1970s there has been a rise of feminist-oriented sexual assault services in the United States, the United Kingdom, Australia, Canada, and New Zealand. These services treated and supported women and child victims of violence, including those experiencing historical sexual abuse (Herman, 1992; Loney-Howes, 2020). They did not accept reports of child sexual abuse as fantasy.

The acceptance of child sexual abuse as a traumatic reality with grave long-term consequences was an anchor point for the re-emergence of clinical and theoretical interest in dissociation and the dissociative disorders which took place in the 1970s and 1980s (Van der Hart & Dorahy, 2023). In fact, in 1984, the very year Masson's book was first published, the world's first professional society for the study of traumatic dissociation (the International Society for the Study of Multiple Personality and Dissociation, now the International Society for the Study of Trauma and Dissociation, ISSTD) was established (O'Neil, 2003).

Seemingly, feminist-oriented services for women and child victims of violence, the trauma and dissociation field, and Freudian psychoanalysis, along with the various offshoots, developed quite separately, with little apparent cross-fertilisation. We are prone to working in silos, despite the detrimental consequences. There is comfort in being with like-minded people. Additionally, with the ever-increasing pressures of professional life, it is easy to see how liaising with other services, spending time debating with 'foreigners', educating those who are ambivalent, or mobilising energy towards intersectionality and interservice collaboration can fall by the wayside.

However, important work continues to bring together different fields of thought. Publications such as *The Dissociative Mind in Psychoanalysis* (Howell & Itzkowitz, 2016) explore and build bridges between the psychoanalytic and the dissociative fields. Increasingly, the once-isolated dissociative disorders field is realigning with the mainstream trauma field. However, severe dissociation itself remains in somewhat of a silo, with many of the services dealing with the most traumatised people (such as mainstream mental health services, police, housing services, and medical practitioners) being unaware of or dismissive of the more severe dissociative disorders and their links to child sexual abuse. Additionally, educational textbooks that provide the foundations for learning often provide inadequate information on dissociation, dissociative disorders, and child abuse (e.g., Brand et al., 2019).

Recognising the impacts of denial and invalidation

The female survivors we see in therapy today have come from cultures with long histories of invalidating women's and children's testimony, considering them less robust than that of a male. They may have experienced covert or overt prioritisation of the male perspective. Male survivors enter therapy with both overlapping and different messages of denial which invalidate the severity of their abuse and question their masculinity and strength. Both male and female survivors are likely to have experienced doubt and disbelief when telling of their abuse. They may even disbelieve themselves at times, participating in a dance of 'knowing and the not knowing' (Solinski, 2017). Therapists are wise to acknowledge their own capacity for this dance, which can manifest in subtle and overt ways, like minimising the perceived impact of abuse, disbelieving elements of trauma history that we subjectively determine to be too extreme or focusing on other domains of the person's presentation and isolating them from their trauma history. This does not mean that every element of a client's trauma memory should be believed as reflecting objective truth, but our task is to hold our mind open to the subjective experience of the client, and not foreclose the therapeutic process to facilitate a more 'comfortable' narrative. Other manifestations of our own 'not knowing' may include frustration at the slow pace of change, or annoyance at the ongoing mistrust our most traumatised clients display, and at its worst it can lead us to getting stuck in counter-transferential shaming and blaming, without pause to take stock of the impact of trauma dynamics.

As therapists it is important that we understand the implications of historical disbelief in survivor testimony, and that this is a gendered story. Females are more likely to come to therapy and are more likely to report child sexual abuse. Not only may their story of sexual abuse be disbelieved, but additionally females are also less likely to be 'believed' when they report physical symptoms. Women may be labelled as 'hysterical' (or some variant of it) and medically unexplained symptoms can still be seen, without engaging in necessary alternative investigation, as a sign of psychological disorder (Dusenbury, 2018). Women have disproportionately been given psychological explanations and treatments for disorders now recognised as having significant physical aetiology such as chronic fatigue syndrome, endometriosis, and chronic pain (Dusenbery, 2018; Pettersson & Bertero, 2020; Richman & Jason, 2001). Some of these disorders are more common in sexual abuse survivors so, as trauma therapists, we will be treating women who have been disbelieved or trivialised within both society and the wider health system. Such clients have learnt to doubt the importance or validity of their own emotions and body sensations.

Male survivors also experience doubt in the veracity of their sexual abuse stories, and denial of the negative impacts, although their engagement with mental health services and the wider health system may be tainted in a different way. Male clients experience societal pressure to deny vulnerability and pain, and may feel that acknowledging victimhood is incompatible with masculinity. The very fact that stereotypes portray males as perpetrators of sexual violence and females as victims further alienates the male victim. For males, fear of disbelief and invalidation may manifest through withdrawal from help-seeking or feeling intense shame when help-seeking (Widanaralalage et al., 2022). Furthermore, the disbelief, denial, or minimisation of reports of child sexual abuse extends to reports of adult sexual abuse. Re-victimisation is common for people surviving child sexual abuse. The impacts of both male and female 'rape myths' within the health and legal systems, as well as society as a whole, are also likely to further traumatise our clients, who still experience an adversarial legal system where presumption of the accused's innocence frequently plays out as presumption of dishonesty on behalf of the accuser (Minter et al., 2021; Widanaralalage et al., 2022).

It befalls us as therapists to not just treat trauma symptoms, or just hear a trauma narrative, but to facilitate an environment where the impact of intergenerational cultural doubt and disbelief can be safely explored, as this is often needed before other trauma material comes forward. Therapy must also be a place where a client can safely explore their own internalised self-doubts. As trauma-informed therapists we feel the pull to be supportive and to validate the stories we hear. This is the natural reaction of the empathic, compassionate self. Yet, it is at this point in therapy that a gentle, curious, but somewhat neutral (or shall we say non-opinionated) stand on a client's memories is most powerful. This allows therapy to be a safe and open place for the client to explore their own self-doubt, do the hard work of grappling with memory, and ultimately come to their own conclusions about what happened to them. Yet how we allow this space without seeming so neutral that we mimic the non-protective bystander, or so affirming we close the space for doubt and change, is a difficult balancing act. Van der Hart and Nijenhuis (1999) speak to this dilemma and differentiate a 'reflexive belief', which is emotional and automatic, from a 'reflective' belief, which comes from bearing witness to the client's own struggle with their memories over time. Such a position allows for the development of safety and trust in the therapeutic dyad.

Grappling with avoidance of trauma and dissociation

As authors writing about the trauma-avoidance of early psychoanalysts, we reflect upon the sometimes-horrific nature of our own work, and acknowledge within ourselves that, despite our deep investment in the field, we have also hoped and wished that a particular memory be not true, to be instead a dream, a metaphor, or perhaps both. Even our clients whose bodies have experienced such abuse grapple with the knowing and the not knowing, and we can join them, attuned in the confusion and even denial. Herman's (1992) words often echo: it is easier to disbelieve and feign ignorance than face and hold. Perhaps this is the nature of the field, that it causes us to confront things so horrific that we either become hardened and unempathic, or we sit with the suffering and wrestle with how difficult the work is, which includes our own doubts, frustrations, and desires to 'not know'. Being a trauma-informed therapist is painful, and becoming trauma-informed is an ongoing process involving a regular struggle to be mindful of the impacts of trauma on our clients, ourselves, and on others.

Interestingly, in our own journeys as trauma therapists, we observe inside ourselves occasionally finding a sense of avoidance of dissociation. This manifests for us as sometimes feeling a sense of unreality about dissociative internal worlds or inscapes that are so alive in many people with dissociative identity disorder (DID). Deep in a discussion with a dissociated client in which their internal world is explored we may be suddenly struck with a thought of how incredulous this seems, how 'unreal' in some sense. Our clients will also at times stop and say, 'This sounds crazy!' or 'I can't believe what my own mind is showing me!'. In therapy we can feel a deep dissociative attunement (Hopenwasser, 2008) with our clients in that we resonate with their fluctuating acceptance-disbelief regarding their dissociative self-states and inner 'worlds'. We can feel a momentary disorientation when a client with DID suddenly announces that nothing they have discussed in therapy is true and that they have 'made it all up', or that they don't really have DID, despite consistently displaying all signs of it. It is hard at times not to join their flight into health, when even a momentary reprieve from the horror of the work seems difficult to resist.

When faced with such confusion and avoidance inside ourselves and inside our clients, those less educated about the power of dissociative processes will be tempted to simply dismiss or disbelieve the client. The client may be labelled as malingering, having a factitious disorder, or being psychotic. Even those educated in dissociative and trauma processes can at times wrestle with the mind's capacity to creatively respond to overwhelm. It is all too tempting to deny dissociation. In doing so we enter the comfortable zone of denying one of the most serious psychological impacts of early child sexual abuse.

The necessity for vigilance in trauma- and dissociation-informed practice

This century has seen a turn-around in how we face trauma. We have witnessed stories of the exploitation of children in powerful institutions, including churches, schools, and children's homes. This has culminated in multiple investigations internationally and a growing acceptance that organisations have abused children and covered up abuse. The #MeToo movement exposed the exploitation of vulnerable women by powerful men. Accepting the abuse of children by the most powerful institution of all, the family, has been slower but is increasingly occurring. Many practitioners reading this today will be operating in a clinical environment where the phrase 'trauma-informed' is very familiar, even over-used. Few mental health professionals today outright deny the negative impact of trauma, especially childhood trauma, or consider such reports as largely a product of fantasy. However, there is a need for therapists to be constantly vigilant against 'avoidance' of trauma that Herman (1992) describes so eloquently. It is only a generation ago that we experienced a rapid shift from discussing childhood trauma to the emergence of the false memory syndrome movement.

Ongoing education for professionals about the reality and impact of childhood traumas on mental health is essential. Education about dissociation and the dissociative disorders is essential for all therapists, and ideally this should be done during the pre-registration training process, not as an optional professional development add-on. With this education we are better equipped to recognise these moments of longing for another story, of joining with our clients' confusion, denial, or dissociation, and see them for just what they are, so we can respond therapeutically.

Recognising ongoing blind spots in acceptance

Most health professionals, even trauma professionals, are not adequately dissociation-informed and may not be aware of how this lack of awareness interplays with their own natural tendencies to turn away from the horror of child abuse. The mental health profession still tends to turn away from the most serious sequelae of early child sexual abuse: the identity alteration and dissociative amnesia that form the basis of DID. It is no longer possible, after a generation of exposure of institutional and organisational abuse, to deny the reality of child sexual abuse, but it's still possible to avoid or deny some of the more serious ramifications. We repeatedly see therapists, lawyers, and journalists making statements like 'we never forget trauma', something which flies in the face of evidence (e.g., Saadi et al., 2021; Williams, 1995). Others suggest that a lack of memory of child sexual abuse is a sign that the child did not experience the abuse as traumatic, hence forgot it

(McNally & Geraerts, 2009), an extraordinary explanation for dissociative amnesia which minimises the horror of child sexual abuse. Only recently a scholarly paper reviewing the evidence for recovering false memories (Brewin & Andrews, 2017) met with commentary of such a nature that the authors suggested scientific debate was being suppressed. They felt compelled to point out the

> discrepancy between the extreme hostility of some of the original reviews and the questioning of our motives, coupled with the absence of any coherent scientific critique. It is notable that the objections appear to be more about the implications of the data than the data themselves.
>
> (Andrews & Brewin, 2017, p. 48)

Despite all our progress in recognising trauma, this sounds uncomfortably like the reactions to Masson when he reported his evidence in 1984 and perhaps the reactions Freud got around a century earlier when he first introduced his seduction theory.

Additionally, we still tend to deny the most serious forms of sexual abuse that co-occur with dissociative disorders. This has been seen in the avoidance of health and legal professionals in exploring the issue of incestuous abuse that continues into adulthood (Middleton, 2023); organised abuse (Salter & Richters, 2012); and ritualised abuse (Salter, 2012). As practitioners and researchers, we need to go forward acknowledging the pain of hearing about such extreme abuse, and our natural desires to avoid facing such pain, while also being able to remain present with the story. We are encouraged to be clinically neutral, but that is not the same as overt denial and disbelief. Masson explores the impacts of such outright disbelief when he writes, 'In such an atmosphere treatment could be "successful" only if the patient suppresses her (or his) own knowledge of her past' (Masson, 2003, p. 191). He adds that 'Free and honest retrieval of painful memories cannot occur in the face of scepticism and fear of the truth' (Masson, 2003, p. 192). Originally published in 1984, these sentiments remain pertinent today and are worth a reminder.

Conclusions

The Assault on Truth has undoubtedly played a pivotal role in challenging Freud's theory that psychological distress is more the product of fantasy than actual child sexual abuse. More than that, the book 'shook up' the psychotherapeutic status quo and challenged an entire field to re-think their reactions to their client's self-report of sexual abuse during childhood. This, combined with the growth of the women's movement and the dissociative disorders treatment field, has resulted in a vastly different mental health landscape today. It is tempting to think we have passed through the worst of denial, but it exists in both overt and subtle ways in most health and forensic settings. Additionally, the most serious sequelae of child sexual abuse (dissociative amnesia and identity alterations) are still seen in some quarters as preposterous, fantastical, or signs of malingering. Therefore, denial of the (largely female) self-report has shifted from the event to the consequences. Moreover, despite progress, we still see people who report sexual abuse being doubted or intrusively investigated within a legal system still based on outdated presumptions that women in particular make up stories of abuse (Minter et al., 2021). Women have banded together to name alleged perpetrators through the #MeToo movement, and survivors of child sexual abuse have presented *en masse* to various public enquiries globally, but all too often the individual reporting child sexual abuse will not see justice. Today, even after successful events like the Australian Royal Commission into Institutional Responses to Child Sexual Abuse, survivors needed to present in great numbers to be believed, and even then, they run the risk of being accused of colluding. It is also notable that large-scale national enquiries have not investigated the seemingly unspeakable crime of incest, a crime involving a child and an adult where there are often no witnesses. It is therefore a crime ripe for disbelief in its many and varied forms.

References

al Alwani, T. J. (1996). The testimony of women in Islamic law. *American Journal of Islam and Society, 13*(2), 173–196. https://doi.org/10.35632/ajis.v13i2.2329

Andrews, B., & Brewin, C. R. (2017). False memories and free speech: Is scientific debate being suppressed? *Applied Cognitive Psychology, 31*(1), 45–49. https://doi.org/10.1002/acp.3285

Brand, B. L., Kumar, S. A., & McEwen, L. E. (2019). Coverage of child maltreatment and adult trauma in graduate psychopathology textbooks. *Psychological Trauma: Theory, Research, Practice and Policy, 11*(8), 919–926. https://doi.org/10.1037/tra0000454

Brewin, C. R., & Andrews, B. (2017). Creating memories for false autobiographical events in childhood: A systematic review. *Applied Cognitive Psychology, 31*(1), 2–23. https://doi.org/10.1002/acp.3220

Crook, L. (2022). The power of false memory rhetoric. *Journal of Trauma & Dissociation, 23*(2), 148–151. https://doi.org/10.1080/15299732.2022.2028220

Dusenbury, M. (2018). *Doing harm: How bad medicine and lazy science leave women dismissed, misdiagnosed and sick*. HarperOne.

Franiuk, R., & Shain, E. A. (2011). Beyond Christianity: The status of women and rape myths. *Sex Roles, 65*, 783–791. https://doi.org/10.1007/s11199-011-9974-8

Gavey, N. (2019). *Just sex? The cultural scaffolding of rape* (2nd ed.). Routledge.

Herman, J. L. (1992). *Trauma and recovery*. Basic Books/Hachette Book Group.

Holmes, G. R., Offen, L., & Waller, G. (1997). See no evil, hear no evil, speak no evil: Why do relatively few male victims of childhood sexual abuse receive help for abuse-related issues in adulthood? *Clinical Psychology Review, 17*(1), 69–88. https://doi.org/10.1016/s0272-7358(96)00047-5

Hopenwasser, K. (2008). Being in rhythm: dissociative attunement in therapeutic process. *Journal of Trauma & Dissociation*, 9(3), 349–367. https://doi.org/10.1080/15299730802139212

Howell, E. F., & Itzkowitz, S. (2016). *The dissociative mind in psychoanalysis*. Routledge.

Kuhn, P. (2002) "Romancing with a wealth or detail": Narratives or Ernest Jones's 1906 trial for indecent assault. *Studies in Gender and Sexuality, 3*(4), 344–378. https://doi.org/10.1080/15240650309349207

Loney-Howes, R. (2020). *The Contours and Critiques of Anti-Rape Activism: A Brief History.* Online Anti-Rape Activism: Exploring the Politics of the Personal in the Age of Digital Media (Emerald Studies in Criminology, Feminism and Social Change), Emerald Publishing Limited, Bingley, pp. 17–32. https://doi.org/10.1108/978-1-83867-439-720201004

Malka, O. (2019). Disqualified witnesses between Tannaitic Halakha and Roman Law: The archeology of a legal institution. *Law and History Review, 37*(4), 903–936. www.jstor.org/stable/26828689

Masson, J. (1984). *The assault on truth: Freud's suppression of the seduction theory*. Farrar Straus and Giroux.

Masson, J. M. (2003). *The assault on truth: Freud's suppression of the seduction theory* (5th ed.). Ballantine Books.

Mathews, B., Pacella, R. E., Scott, J. G., Finkelhor, D., Meinck, F., Higgins, D. J., Erskine, H. E., Thomas, H. J., Lawrence, D., Haslam, D. M., Malacova, E., Dunne, M. P. (2023). The prevalence of child maltreatment in Australia: Findings from a national survey. *Medical Journal of Australia, 218*(6 Suppl.), S13–S18. https://doi.org/10.5694.mja2.51873

McNally, R. J., & Geraerts, E. (2009). A new solution to the Recovered Memory Debate. *Perspectives on Psychological Science, 4*(2), 126–134. https://doi.org/10.1111/j.1745-6924.2009.01112.x

Middleton, W. (2016). Wilhelm Fliess, Robert Fliess, Ernest Jones, Sandor Ferenczi and Sigmund Freud. *Journal of Trauma & Dissociation, 17*(1), 1–12. https://doi.org/10.1080/15299732.2015.1064289

Middleton, W. (2023). Beyond death: Enduring incest. The fusion of father with daughter. In M. J. Dorahy, S. N. Gold & J. A. O'Neil (Eds.), *Dissociation and the dissociative disorders: Past, present, future* (pp. 218–232). Routledge.

Minter, K., Carlisle, E., & Coumarelos, C. (2021). "Chuck her on a lie detector"—Investigating Australians' mistrust in women's reports of sexual assault (Research report, 04/2021). ANROWS.

Nasjleti, M. (1980). Suffering in silence: The male incest victim. *Child Welfare, 59*(5), 269–275. www.jstor.org/stable/45393680

O'Neil, J. A. (Ed.) (2003). *From organizational infancy to early adulthood, 1983–2003.* Booklet published by the International Society for the Study of Dissociation.

Pettersson, A., & Berterö, C. M. (2020). How women with endometriosis experience health care encounters. *Women's Health Reports, 1*(1), 529–542. https://doi.org/10.1089/whr.2020.0099

Quilter, J. (2015). Rape trials, medical texts and the threat of female speech: The perverse female rape complainant. *Law Text Culture, 19*, 231–270. http://ro.uow.edu.au/ltc/vol19/iss1/11

Richman, J. A., & Jason, L. A. (2001). Gender biases underlying the social construction of illness states: The case of chronic fatigue syndrome. *Current Sociology, 49*(3), 15–29. https://doi.org/10.1177/0011392101049003003

Saadi, A., Hampton, K., de Assis, M. V., Mishori, R., Habbach, H., & Haar, R. J. (2021). Associations between memory loss and trauma in US asylum seekers: A retrospective review of medico-legal affidavits. *PloS One*, *16*(3), e0247033. https://doi.org/10.1371/journal.pone.0247033

Sacco, L. (2009). *Unspeakable: Father-daughter incest in American history.* The Johns Hopkins University Press.

Salter, M. (2012). The role of ritual in the organised abuse of children. *Child Abuse Review, 21*, 440–451. https://doi.org/10.1002/car.2215

Salter, M., & Blizard, R. (2022). False memories and the science of credibility: Who gets to be heard? *Journal of Trauma & Dissociation, 23*(2), 141–147. https://doi.org/10.1080/15299732.2022.2028219

Salter, M., & Richters, J. (2012). Organised abuse: A neglected category of sexual abuse with significant lifetime mental healthcare sequelae. *Journal of Mental Health, 21(*5), 499–508. https://doi.org/10.3109/09638237.2012.682264

Solinski, S. (2017) Knowing and not knowing: A frequent human arrangement. *Journal of Trauma & Dissociation, 18*(3), 397–408. https://doi.org/10.1080/15299732.2017.1295423

Van der Hart, O. & Dorahy, M.J. (2023). History of the concept of dissociation. In M. J. Dorahy, S. N. Gold & J. A. O'Neil (Eds.), *Dissociation and the dissociative disorders: Past, present, future* (pp. 218–232). Routledge.

Van der Hart, O., & Nijenhuis, E. R. S. (1999). Bearing witness to uncorroborated trauma: The clinician's development of reflective belief. *Professional Psychology: Research and Practice, 30*(1), 37–44. https://doi.org/10.1037/0735-7028.30.1.37

Widanaralalage, B. K., Hine, B. A., Murphy, A. D., & Murji, K. (2022). "I didn't feel I was a victim": A phenomenological analysis of the experiences of male-on-male survivors of rape and sexual abuse, *Victims & Offenders, 17*(8), 1147–1172, https://doi.org/10.1080/15564886.2022.2069898

Williams L. M. (1995). Recovered memories of abuse in women with documented child sexual victimization histories. *Journal of Traumatic Stress*, *8*, 649–673.

11 *The Assault on Truth* in the Academy

Talk Therapy and the Social Control of Women

Bruce M. Z. Cohen

This chapter reflects on some of the major implications of Masson's work for critical scholarship on psychiatry and psychotherapy in the academy. After exploring Freud's denial of the sexual abuse of women in *The Assault on Truth* (1984), Masson went on to develop his abolitionist position in *Against Therapy* (1988). The first half of this discussion outlines the scholarship which has followed Masson in challenging the efficacy of psychotherapeutic interventions, concluding that no good quality research yet exists to prove that 'therapy works.' Drawing on critical feminist writings, the second half of the chapter considers the purposes for the continued proliferation of forms of therapy despite the lack of efficacy. It is argued that what Masson discovered in *The Assault of Truth* and his subsequent works continues to be a patriarchal goal for talk therapy; namely, the silencing and social control of women's emotions, behaviour, and experiences in contemporary society.

Published in 1984, *The Assault on Truth* did more than reveal a 'mistake' in Freud's developing ideas on the aetiology of hysteria, it exposed *the lie* on which psychoanalysis was founded as a new method for understanding and exploring the human mind. As Masson has stated in this volume, Freud's initial acceptance of sexual abuse as a real experience underpinning the distress of his patients and then subsequent denial of this 'seduction theory,' is more than 'merely minor squabbles about the history of psychoanalysis. We are talking about the very fundamentals of human society.' We could even suggest that this is psychotherapy's original sin; the point at which a new, promising form of treatment for mental illness was betrayed by its very founder. However, an overwhelming silence came from the psychiatric and psychotherapeutic communities (Bristow, 1992) in response to *The Assault on Truth.* Other responses veered from denial that Freud ever fully rejected the seduction theory, to acknowledgement that Freud was writing in very different times and that ideas on morality and social mores have progressed along with modern forms of psychoanalysis and psychotherapy in general (see e.g., Jacobsen, 2009; Robinson, 1993; Rudnytsky, 2011). In this way, critiques of Masson's research have muddied the waters enough that what might have initially appeared as an existential crisis for psychotherapy has been easily shrugged off: Masson's analysis was inaccurate, a misrepresentation of Freud, and, anyway, times have changed.

DOI: 10.4324/9781003431466-12

In contrast to the critiques from within the psy-professions, considerations of Masson's work by the academy have been a different story. The purpose of this chapter is to reflect upon the latter, demonstrating that Masson's research has been both directly and indirectly of significance in constructing a more complete picture of what critical scholars have sometimes referred to as the 'issues' or 'problems' with the 'therapy industry' as a whole (see e.g., Moloney, 2013; Morrall, 2008). This discussion then will allow the reader to understand the issues with therapy beyond the specific arguments on Freud and the seduction theory, to frame the discussion within a broader structural analysis where such therapy professionals continue to proliferate despite the potential harms they might cause. While, unfortunately, it is not possible to cover all the directions in critical thought on psychotherapy which have followed Masson's work in the academy, there are two main strands of analysis which have previously been central to his critique and are discussed below: first is the issue of the efficacy of psychotherapy, questioning whether, on the basis of the evidence, any therapeutic practice can be justified as a useful and positive intervention for people; and second, drawing heavily upon critical feminist writers, is the silencing and social control of women by psychiatry and psychotherapy.

Therapy in denial

As he has outlined in this volume, the presentation of Masson's research evidence to his psychoanalytic colleagues was generally greeted with disbelief, hostility, and anger. There is a suggestion in the narrative that Masson himself was naive to expect an open debate on the ethics of psychoanalytic theory from a professional guild much more concerned with maintaining group interests and Freudian dogma. Psychoanalysis along with the many schools of psychotherapy which followed has a history of denial of any problems with their practices and of silencing opposition (Davies, 2009; Epstein, 1999), and that has particularly been the case in acknowledging the elephant in the room—namely, the lack of efficacy for psychotherapeutic practices. Several scholars have drawn upon Masson's work to investigate at some length whether there is any evidence that psychotherapy actually 'works.' And—spoiler alert—in *The Illusion of Therapy*, Epstein (1995, p. 1, italics added) sums up the problem when he states that,

> *there is not one credible study conforming to the basic rules of objective proof that testifies to the effectiveness of any psychotherapeutic treatment.* To the contrary, the manifest biases of the research, as well as systematic inferences of client deterioration, suggest grounds on which to assume the actual ineffectiveness and possible harm of psychotherapy—not just the indeterminacy of its benefits.

This claim has of course been disputed by those researchers seeking to build a case for the validity of psychotherapeutic interventions, and the major contestations are briefly outlined in the discussion here. However, it is of some interest to note upfront that, across the academy, both conservative and critical researchers in the area do tend to agree on three factors which have *no bearing* on positive outcomes in therapy, and they might come as a surprise to the reader: first, the credentials and experience of the therapist; secondly, the type of therapy engaged with; and thirdly, the length of therapy (see e.g., Cummings & O'Donohue, 2008; Dawes, 1994; Feltham, 1999; Moloney, 2013; Smith & Glass, 1977; Smith et al., 1980; Watters & Ofshe, 1999). Thus, whether a new student or a professor with 20 years' experience, whether a psychoanalyst or cognitive behavioural therapy practitioner, whether the client is engaged for a few weeks or a few years, all make no significant difference to the chances of a successful outcome in therapy (this is not to ignore the ongoing publication of research on therapy which will occasionally suggest otherwise on these issues—for a brief summation of the chief criticisms of such studies, see Morrall, 2008; for a more substantial review and critique, see Epstein, 2019).

While there is broad agreement that psychotherapeutic training and what is taught is irrelevant in achieving improvement for clients, it is still assumed that therapy, overall, must do something positive for people in distress who seek help from such an expert. A claim that has persisted from early research on the effectiveness of therapy in the 1930s and 1940s is that it improves two-thirds of people while the other third experiences no change or potentially gets worse (Moloney, 2013; Morrall, 2008). However, studies on 'neurotics' by Eysenck (1963, 1966, 1992) in the 1950s and 1960s disputed this finding, suggesting instead that within two years, two-thirds of patients recovered whether they had received therapy or not (Watters & Ofshe, 1999). Rather than therapy aiding recovery, Eysenck argued it was in fact a case of 'spontaneous remission' within the population, a natural recovery from distress and crisis over time (Moloney, 2013). As covered in Watters and Ofshe's (1999) book, *Therapy's Delusions: The Myth of the Unconscious and the Exploitation of Today's Walking Worried*, three decades later Eysenck asserted that there was still no comprehensive evidence that therapy helped people (for more recent reviews and further discussion of these criticisms, see Wampold & Imel's (2015) argument for the 'absolute efficacy' of psychotherapy, and Epstein's (2019) response which proposes quite the opposite).

As Dawes (1994) highlighted in his book *House of Cards: Psychology and Psychotherapy Built on Myth*, what the research on psychotherapy indicated was that other factors unrelated to psychotherapy could explain the improvement in people's mental states. Similar to spontaneous remission, he noted that the 'regression effect' could also explain the feeling from clients that therapy had been a success (even if it had been a terrible experience), as people who enter therapy tend to be in a more extreme emotional state; therapy or none, people tend to regress to the mean of being in less extreme states of unhappiness (or happiness!) over time (Dawes, 1994, p. 44). '[R]egression effects alone can lead to "improvement",' argued Dawes, 'and an illusion that the improvement is due to psychotherapy' (1994, p. 45).

The 'gold standard' in measuring the efficacy of a medical or therapeutic intervention is the randomised control trial (RCT)—that is, the random assignment of similar cases with similar problems to experimental and control groups. In setting the research benchmark in the field, Smith et al. (1980) performed a meta-analysis of 475 studies which they identified as meeting RCT criteria for investigations of therapeutic practice. Their results noted significant benefits of therapy compared to control groups for up to 85% of people (Epstein, 1995; Moloney, 2013). Subsequent follow-up meta-analyses have shown more modest outcomes (e.g., Roth & Fonagy, 2006), but Moloney (2013, p. 69) notes, 'the general message is the same: talking therapy is a reliable remedy for sadness, fear, worry and a host of other personal ills.' Yet critics including Dawes (1994), Epstein (1995, 1999, 2019), Moloney (2013), and Watters and Ofshe (1999) have detailed a host of serious issues with such research which questions whether *any* of the studies included in such analyses fully meets the necessary standards for an RCT. To briefly summate the main concerns, Epstein (1995) noted that gains in Smith et al.'s (1980) analysis were significantly reduced when studies used a placebo as the control group as opposed to making comparisons with an untreated group. Even when such a control group is used in the research, it is difficult to produce a believable placebo (a 'wait list control' is often operationalised, which typically involves a standard introduction interview with an administrator), thus both clients and therapists are usually aware which group they have been selected to, as opposed to 'blind' randomisation of such groups; selection is often subject to researcher bias, with those more likely to respond well (university students, for instance) assigned to the experimental group; reliance for reporting positive outcomes often remains with the self-reports of subjects or therapists rather than independent evaluators; the studies often utilise very small samples and unreliable instruments; and negative research outcomes are less likely to be reported on and published (Epstein, 1999; Moloney, 2013).

As well as finding a 50% fall in the therapeutic gains reported and no difference in outcomes regardless of duration of intervention, Epstein's (1995) investigation of the evidence also found that studies claiming the largest differences for therapeutic interventions were also those more likely to be subject to research bias (see also, Epstein, 2019). He argues that such reviews by Smith et al. (1980) and the many others which have followed (see e.g., Ehring et al., 2014, Kennedy & Xyrichis, 2017, Palpacuer et al., 2016) amount to 'important ideological statements' for public policy (Epstein, 1995, p. 36); they are 'self-serving' and disingenuous on adequately researching and informing the public on the impact of therapy, including the potential dangers of such interventions (Epstein, 1995, p. 37). As Moloney (2013, p. 92) remarks in his book, *The Therapy Industry: The Irresistible Rise of the Talking Cure, and Why It Doesn't Work*, Smith et al.'s (1980) analysis has since set the standard for accepting 'research trials of doubtful integrity' for psychotherapy. In more recently summarising what we know about the effects of engaging with therapy, Epstein (2019, p. 14, italics added) admits that,

> people do get better during psychotherapy and many patients report satisfaction with treatment. However, *there is little if any credible proof that improvement documented during treatment is due to the therapy itself.* Other considerations rather than the therapy per se may account for the improvement: the seasonality

> of the psychological problem, the maturation and changing circumstances of the patient, bias in measuring symptoms, fortuitously small samples, demand characteristics of the research situation, placebo effects, unrepresentative samples, large attrition, the absence of appropriate controls for the intervention, demonstration effects, and others. …*The field's clinical research has been unable to disprove these alternative explanations for measured improvement in outcomes by way of establishing with scientific credibility the effectiveness of psychotherapeutic treatment.*

Moloney's (2013, p. 93, italics added) conclusion is similarly sobering, when he states,

> There is no consistent, good-quality evidence that any type of therapy can outperform a well-designed placebo, that any approach is reliably superior to another, or that any given set of curative ingredients outdo their competitors. *Only one observation is upheld: that confident and emotionally warm professionals are more appreciated by their clients, and get better results, a statement that applies equally to politicians, salespeople and prostitutes.*

Despite these fundamental issues with psychotherapy, its popularity has remained unaffected, and many different models of talk therapy have continued to flourish (Epstein, 2019; Morrall, 2008). To understand the reasons for this seeming contradiction in light of the evidence presented here, critical scholars in the academy have theorised such professions as serving certain political goals in contemporary society. As will be discussed in the next section, by specifically drawing upon critical feminist writers and the evidence from Masson's research, we can better understand therapy as a site of patriarchal power which continues to medicalise and silence the survivors of sexual abuse (for obvious reasons this discussion focuses on women, but this is certainly not to deny the experiences of the many men who have also been subject to sexual violence and abuse, see e.g., Doyle, 2017, Finkelhor et al., 2014).

Therapy as silencing

The Assault on Truth revealed a salient example of something feminist academics, including Chesler (1972), Penfold and Walker (1983), and Showalter (1980), had already identified in their work, namely, the silencing of women's voices by psychiatry and psychotherapy. Freud's mistake in terms of his own reputation, suggests Herman (2015), was not so much his eventual cover-up of abuse and violence against women, but giving space for women to talk about their experiences in the first place. As Masson (1984) makes clear, what should have been Freud's crowning achievement—identifying 'the source of the Nile' regarding the aetiology of hysteria (Herman, 2015, p. 13)—threatened to curtail the uptake of his ideas among the psychiatric profession, causing a *volte-face* in which women's experiences were recast as fantasies. Consequently, Herman (2015, p. 14) summates,

> Freud stopped listening to his female patients … For close to a century, these patients would again be scorned and silenced. … Out of the ruins of the traumatic theory of hysteria, Freud created psychoanalysis. The dominant psychological theory of the next century was founded in the denial of women's reality.

What critical feminist scholarship has revealed of the theory and practice of psychiatry is the systematic attempt by a branch of medicine to silence and pathologise women's experiences, emotions, and behaviours as signs of madness (Busfield, 1996; Caplan, 1995; Chesler, 1972; Jimenez, 1997; Penfold & Walker, 1983; Showalter, 1980, 1985; Ussher, 2011, 2018). The history of psychiatry is riddled with sex-role ideology in which women have been theorised by a male-dominated profession as slaves of their own biology, threatened by madness, particularly at times of 'the female life cycle—puberty, pregnancy, childbirth, menopause—during which the mind would be weakened and the symptoms of insanity might emerge' (Showalter, 1985, p. 55). In fact, the very idea of insanity has always been associated in the mind of the psychiatrist with women and has dominated ideas on 'femininity' (e.g., Broverman et al., 1981). Ussher (2011, p. 76) notes that such stereotypes 'lead to women being positioned as intrinsically more maladjusted; health professionals expect women to be mad … so are more likely to look for it, and to see it even if it is not there.'

Where women's experiences of sexual abuse and violence were previously medicalised as symptoms of 'hysteria,' scholars have identified the continuation of this silencing through the American Psychiatric Association's construction of 'mental illness' categories across editions of their *Diagnostic and Statistical Manual of Mental Disorders* (DSM). This is despite the significant and ongoing validity problems within psychiatric science in accurately defining, measuring, and explaining the current nosology in the DSM (e.g., Allsopp et al., 2019; Burstow, 2015; Cohen, 2016; Whitaker & Cosgrove, 2015; Whooley, 2019). Critical researchers have identified a plethora of labels which have been used over the past few decades to reinforce the dominant view of female survivors of sexual abuse as mentally unstable (and therefore untrustworthy), including somatisation disorder, masochistic personality disorder, histrionic personality disorder, multiple personality disorder/dissociative identity disorder, battered women's syndrome, dependent personality disorder, borderline personality disorder (BPD), and female sexual interest/arousal disorder (Burstow, 2006; Caplan, 1995; Cohen, 2016; Cohen & Hartmann, 2023; Jimenez, 1997; Herman, 2015; Luhrmann, 2000; Masson, 1986; Spurgas, 2016; Ussher, 2011). Then as now, the concern is that survivors of abuse continue to be labelled with a 'mental disorder,' and their experiences devalued and denied by psy-professionals. Orr (1999) has previously noted that half of psychiatrically institutionalised women have reported sexual abuse during childhood. Herman (2015, p. 122) has recently gone further, suggesting 'many or even most psychiatric patients are survivors of child abuse.'

What Masson's body of work has added to understanding this silencing process is identifying that psychotherapy, both in theory and in practice, is guilty of the same systemic patterns of oppressive behaviour as psychiatry, despite the latter being involved more centrally in clinical practice and biomedical forms of treatment. His intention of following *The Assault on Truth* (1984) with *A Dark Science* (1986) and then *Against Therapy* (1988) was to show a clear linkage between historical and contemporary abuse of women by psychiatry *and* psychotherapy. *Against Therapy* reminds us that the very first cases of the new method of talk as treatment—namely, Breuer's Anna O, Freud's Dora, and Krafft-Ebing's Nina R—were of course all women, oppressed by men and the family, frustrated by their lack of access to public and political life, and sympathetic to the women's suffrage movement (Anna O, real name Bertha Pappenheim, would go on to be a significant advocate for women's rights in Germany). Yet Freud and his colleagues agreed that these women were 'sick, and needed "treatment"' (Masson, 1994, p. 83).

A similar fate befalls women diagnosed by psychiatrists and therapists with a personality disorder, especially hysteria's contemporary successor, BPD (Jimenez, 1997). As with hysteria, women labelled with BPD have often been victims of child sexual abuse (Burstow, 2006; Caplan, 1995; Herman, 2015; Ussher, 2011), though this experience is again silenced by a diagnosis which strongly implies that such women are irrational and should not be trusted. In Luhrmann's (2000, p. 115) study of American psychiatry and psychotherapy, she finds that those labelled with personality disorders are the patients that 'you don't like, don't trust, don't want.' '[F]requently used within the mental health professions as little more than a sophisticated insult' (Herman, 2015, p. 123), being 'borderline' is singled out as a general marker for troublesome female patients who are angry, unreliable, 'attention-seeking,' and occasionally suicidal (Luhrmann, 2000). As with the 'hysteric,' the 'borderline' female has become a regular cliché in the modern therapeutic setting with which to deny women's voices as authentic. The women who receive the label, remarks Herman (2015, p. 123), 'evoke unusually intense reactions in caregivers. Their credibility is often suspect. They are frequently accused of manipulation or malingering … Sometimes they are frankly hated.'

Following Masson's research, feminist writers have suggested that examples like BPD are more than anomalies of mental health practice—they instead signify the political role which therapy has continually undertaken to control women in a patriarchal society. This critical approach to theorising psychotherapy as an institution of social control is discussed further in the following section.

Therapy as social control

The silencing, abuse, and general power dynamics highlighted in Masson's research signify that psychotherapy is fundamentally a political discipline. This has also been recognised by advocates of therapy including Totton (2006a, p. xiv, italics in original), who points out that '[a]ll psychotherapists have a political view of their work; because all psychotherapy rests on a theory—explicit or implicit, conscious or unconscious—of *how people should be*.' Yet most practitioners deny this dimension to their work, framing therapy as apolitical and value-free. Outlined in Chapter 1, Anna Freud's response to Masson is symbolic of this illusion when she states to him that '[p]sychoanalysis is concerned with the inner life so it's not surprising that there is so little written about these topics [i.e., fascism, war, child abuse] that you are interested in.' In line with other forms of therapy, through this claim that psychoanalysis is not concerned with external political and social life, it has in fact served the status quo very well by emphasising that the individual is the one in need of correction and change, the one that must 'adjust' to the attitudes and behaviours expected within wider society. Thus, critical scholars in the academy have drawn upon Masson's research to theorise psychotherapy as a form of social control; that is, an institutional apparatus of moral authority which reproduces and reinforces the dominant norms and values of society through its practices. Indeed Cecchin (cited in Totton, 2006b, p. 83) goes so far as to question whether it is ever possible to 'do effective therapy without becoming an instrument of social control, without participating and contributing, often unknowingly, to the construction or the maintenance of a dominant discourse of oppression.'

As critical feminist scholars have argued, psychiatry and psychotherapy are bastions of patriarchal power, responsible for the policing of gender roles, reproducing sex role stereotypes through their discourse and practices, silencing voices and acts of resistance, and reinforcing male privilege through depoliticising 'treatments' that blame and re-victimise women. This is something Masson himself alludes to with the publication of *A Dark Science* (1986), just a year after the original release of *The Assault on Truth* (1984); women who have been abused by men, have attempted to break away from their expected roles as wives, mothers and homemakers, or have in other ways violated gender norms (e.g., been caught masturbating, suspected of lesbianism, or taken an interest in politics or education) have been pathologised by psy-professionals as 'hysterical' and in need of 'treatment.'

Critical researchers have profiled that this 'gaslighting' (Sweet, 2019) and labelling of problematic women as 'mad' has a long history which continues to inform present psychiatric and psychotherapeutic discourse and practice (e.g., Cohen, 2016; Cohen & Hartmann, 2023; Jimenez, 1997; Ussher, 2011, 2018). It is argued that the sexist ideology embedded within psy-discourse (Ehrenreich & English, 2011) is as clear to see in the current symptomologies for BPD, premenstrual dysphoric disorder, and female sexual arousal disorder (e.g., Cosgrove & Riddle, 2003; Flore, 2016; Jimenez, 1997), as it was in the historical labels of hysteria and nymphomania. As Cosgrove and Riddle (2004, p. 128) have commented on such classifications, they 'do not represent value-free truths—they are socioculturally and sociohistorically specific ways of defining behaviour and their construction involves masculine privilege.' Both historically and currently, women are more often the victims of labelling, incarceration, and violence at the hands of the mental health system than men (Chesler, 1972; Cohen, 2016; Ussher, 2011). Women have also been more likely to receive both electroconvulsive therapy and lobotomies (Burstow, 2006; Busfield, 1996; Chesler, 1972; Ussher, 2011), and they continue to be prescribed psychopharmaceuticals at higher rates than men (Burstow, 2015; Ussher, 2018).

In other words, Freud's denial and silencing of women's experiences of child sexual abuse that Masson originally identified in *The Assault on Truth*

(1984) is understood by critical feminist scholars as only part of a wider system of social control which aids patriarchal society by limiting women's freedom and choices and the struggle for gender equality. *Against Therapy* (1988) more specifically alluded to this situation by demonstrating that, as with biomedical psychiatry, psychotherapy's target of oppression has most often been women. This includes details of the physical, emotional, and sexual abuse of women in therapy, along with the misogynist views of 'eminent' therapists such as Jung, Rosen, and Erikson who berated their female clients on the basis of their physical appearance, having a job, and not staying at home with their children (Masson, 1994). Tosh (2019) has recently argued that the continuance of such masculinised aggression in psychotherapy amounts to a 'therapeutic rape culture.' Vulnerable populations who seek help from therapy, she argues, remain subjected to gender stereotypes which naturalise rape and abuse against women as a part of coercive yet 'normal' heterosexual relations (Tosh, 2019). Therapeutic rape culture both '[i]ncorporates constructions, discourses, and structures from rape culture into therapeutic contexts such as normalising violence, blaming victims, and perpetuating harmful gender "norms",' states Tosh (2019, p. 102), as well as '[i]ndividualises, medicalises, and psychologises health issues and emotional distress, neglecting to consider the role of social contexts, discrimination, oppression, and violence' (2019, p. 103).

A similar point to Tosh's has also been made by Tseris (2018, 2019) as a result of her analysis of 'trauma-informed therapy,' a form of psychotherapy which at first appearance would seem to finally give voice to survivors of gender-related sexual abuse and violence (it should be noted that there are many different versions of this therapy now available, including 'trauma analysis' in psychoanalysis itself, see e.g., Rachman & Klett, 2015). Yet she notes that this acknowledgement is double-edged, as recognition and validation of such emotional distress eventuates in the labelling of (usually) women as 'traumatised' and in need of self-adjustment and change, while consideration of those who carry out such crimes (usually men) are excluded from the therapeutic process. Thus, Tseris (2019) theorises such therapy as potentially depoliticising, again risking what Tosh (2019) has referred to as the 'repathologisation' and 'retraumatisation' of survivors of abuse due to their natural reactions to such situations. As the 'trauma' concept has become more formalised within the psychotherapeutic lexicon over the last 20 years, Tseris (2019, p. 105) argues there is a danger that such distress is again medicalised, pathologised, and silenced by 'simply reinstating conventional understandings of women's mental distress, by acknowledging and yet ultimately covering over experiences of violence, focusing on symptoms, and imposing pre-determined meanings onto women's experiences.' As with previous forms of therapy, trauma-informed interventions can be understood as contributing 'to a patriarchal agenda of invisibilising male violence against women and re-establishing cultural motifs about the madness of women' (Tseris, 2018, p. 256). Thus, while trauma-informed therapy would seem to initially give recognition to survivor experience, these scholars argue that it in fact involves the inherent danger of *re-medicalising* that voice through the individualising discourse and processes of psychotherapy.

Conclusion

This chapter has considered the impact of Masson's research on psychiatry and psychotherapy in the academy. Given his discovery of Freud's silencing of female survivors of child sexual abuse in *The Assault on Truth* (1984), the discussion has particularly focused on critical feminist scholarship in the area. Following the identification of a lack of efficacy for psy-professions, what this body of research has shown is the fundamentally political nature of psychotherapy, as an institution of patriarchal power. The history of psychiatry and psychotherapy is a history of silencing, abusing, and correcting the behaviour of socially deviant women to the dominant social order which currently supports male privilege and reduces women to second-class status. The sad irony of this situation is that the effects of gender inequalities caused by current patriarchal relations encourage women to seek refuge and help from an institution which may further depoliticise and individualise such issues, including cases of sexual violence and abuse. Totten (2006b, p. 89, italics in original) has argued that such '[p]sychotherapy that advocates "adjustment," "realism" or dealing with "the world as it is" arguably damages the client's capacity to tolerate a *difference* between their desire and reality—and to do something about it.' Instead, in line with other abolitionists (see also Epstein, 1995, 2019; Szasz, 1978), Masson suggests a succinct alternative to the ongoing illusions of talk therapy at the conclusion of *Against Therapy* (1994: 319): 'I cannot think of a better therapy than exposing the inadequacies of psychotherapy itself. …Becoming active in the struggle against psychiatry (and other forms of injustice) … is a good alternative to the helplessness that psychiatry encourages in patients.'

References

Allsopp, K., Read, J., Corcoran, R., & Kinderman, P. (2019). Heterogeneity in psychiatric diagnostic classification. *Psychiatry Research, 279*, 15–22. https://doi.org/10.1016/j.psychres.2019.07.005

Bristow, M. F. (1992). The assault on Freud: A critique of the works of Jeffrey Masson. *The British Journal of Psychiatry, 160*(5), 722–724. https://doi.org/10.1192/S0007125000124274

Broverman, I. K., Broverman, D. M., Clarkson, F. E., Rosenkrantz, P. S., & Vogel, S. R. (1981). Sex-role stereotypes and clinical judgements of mental health. In E. Howell & M. Bayes (Eds.), *Women and mental health* (pp. 86–97). Basic Books.

Burstow, B. (2006). Electroshock as a form of violence against women. *Violence Against Women, 12*(4), 372–392. https://doi.org/10.1177/1077801206286

Burstow, B. (2015). *Psychiatry and the business of madness: An ethical and epistemological accounting*. Palgrave Macmillan.

Busfield, J. (1996). *Men, women, and madness*. New York University Press.

Caplan, P. J. (1995). *They say you're crazy: How the world's most powerful psychiatrists decide who's normal*. De Capo Press.

Chesler, P. (1972). *Women and madness*. Avon Books.

Cohen, B. M. Z. (2016). *Psychiatric hegemony: A Marxist theory of mental illness*. Palgrave Macmillan.

Cohen, B. M. Z., & Hartmann, R. (2023). The 'feminisation' of psychiatric discourse: A Marxist analysis of women's roles in neoliberal society. *Journal of Sociology, 59*(2), 349–364. https://doi.org/10.1177/14407833211043570

Cosgrove, L., & Riddle, B. (2003). Constructions of femininity and experiences of menstrual distress. *Women & Health, 38*(3), 37–58. https://doi.org/10.1300/J013v38n03_04

Cosgrove, L., & Riddle, B. (2004). Gender bias and sex distribution of mental disorders in the *DSM-IV-TR*. In P. J. Caplan & L. Cosgrove (Eds.), *Bias in psychiatric diagnosis* (pp. 127–140). Jason Aronson.

Cummings, N. A., & O'Donohue, W. T. (2008). *Eleven blunders that cripple psychotherapy in America: A remedial unblundering*. Taylor & Francis.

Davies, J. (2009). *The making of psychotherapists: An anthropological analysis.* Taylor & Francis.

Dawes, R. M. (1994). *House of cards: Psychology and psychotherapy built on myth.* Free Press.

Doyle, T. P. (2017). The Australian royal commission into institutional responses to child sexual abuse and the Roman Catholic Church. *Child Abuse & Neglect, 74*, 103–106. https://doi.org/10.1016/j.chiabu.2017.09.019

Ehrenreich, B., & English, D. (2011). *Complaints and disorders: The sexual politics of sickness* (2nd ed.). The Feminist Press.

Ehring, T., Welboren, R., Morina, N., Wicherts, J. M., Freitag, J., & Emmelkamp, P. M. (2014). Meta-analysis of psychological treatments for posttraumatic stress disorder in adult survivors of childhood abuse. *Clinical Psychology Review, 34*(8), 645–657. https://doi.org/10.1016/j.cpr.2014.10.004

Epstein, W. M. (1995). *The illusion of psychotherapy*. Routledge.

Epstein, W. M. (1999). The ineffectiveness of psychotherapy. In C. Feltham (Ed.), *Controversies in psychotherapy and counselling* (pp. 64–73). Sage.

Epstein, W. M. (2019). *Psychotherapy and the social clinic in the United States: Soothing fictions*. Palgrave Macmillan.

Eysenck, H. J. (1963). Behaviour therapy, spontaneous remission and transference in neurotics. *American Journal of Psychiatry, 119*(9), 867–871. https://ajp.psychiatryonline.org/doi/abs/10.1176/ajp.119.9.867?journalCode=ajp

Eysenck, H. J. (1966). *The effects of psychotherapy*. International Science Press.

Eysenck, H. J. (1992). The effects of psychotherapy: An evaluation. *Journal of Consulting and Clinical Psychology, 60*(5), 659–663. https://doi.org/10.1037/0022-006X.60.5.659

Feltham, C. (1999). Controversies in psychotherapy and counselling. In C. Feltham (Ed.), *Controversies in psychotherapy and counselling* (pp. 1–5). Sage.

Finkelhor, D., Shattuck, A., Turner, H. A., & Hamby, S. L. (2014). The lifetime prevalence of child sexual abuse and sexual assault assessed in late adolescence. *Journal of Adolescent Health, 55*(3), 329–333. https://doi.org/10.1016/j.jadohealth.2013.12.026

Flore, J. (2016). The problem of sexual imbalance and techniques of the self in the *diagnostic and statistical manual of mental disorders*. *History of Psychiatry, 27*(3), 320–335. https://doi.org/10.1177/0957154X16644391

Herman, J. L. (2015). *Trauma and recovery: The aftermath of violence—From domestic abuse to political terror* (Rev. Ed.). Basic Books.

Jacobsen, K. (2009). *Freud's foes: Psychoanalysis, science, and resistance*. Rowman & Littlefield.

Jimenez, M. A. (1997). Gender and psychiatry: Psychiatric conceptions of mental disorders in women, 1960–1994. *Affilia, 12*(2), 154–175. https://doi.org/10.1177/0886109997012002

Kennedy, L., & Xyrichis, A. (2017). Cognitive behavioral therapy compared with non-specialized therapy for alleviating the effect of auditory hallucinations in people with reoccurring schizophrenia: A systematic review and meta-analysis. *Community Mental Health Journal, 53,* 127–133. https://doi.org/10.1007/s10597-016-0030-6

Luhrmann, T. M. (2000). *Of two minds: An anthropologist looks at American psychiatry*. Vintage Books.

Masson, J. M. (1984). *The Assault on truth: Freud's suppression of the seduction theory*. Penguin.

Masson, J. M. (1986). *A dark science: Women, sexuality, and psychiatry in the nineteenth century*. Farrar, Straus and Giroux.

Masson, J. M. (1994). *Against therapy* (Rev. Ed.). Fontana.

Moloney, P. (2013). *The therapy industry: The irresistible rise of the talking cure, and why it doesn't work*. Pluto Press.

Morrall, P. (2008). *The trouble with therapy: Sociology and psychotherapy*. McGraw Hill/Open University Press.

Orr, M. (1999). Believing patients. In Feltham, C. (Ed.), *Controversies in psychotherapy and counselling* (pp. 53–63). Sage.

Palpacuer, C., Gallet, L., Drapier, D., Reymann, J., Falissard, B., & Naudet, F. (2016). Specific and non-specific effects of psychotherapeutic interventions for depression: Results from a meta-analysis of 84 Studies. *Journal of Psychiatric Research, 87,* 95–104. https://doi.org/10.1016/j.jpsychires.2016.12.015

Penfold, P. S., & Walker, G. A. (1983). *Women and the psychiatric paradox*. Eden Press.

Rachman, A. W., & Klett, S. (2015). *Analysis of the incest trauma: Retrieval, recovery, renewal*. Karnac Books.

Robinson, P. (1993). *Freud and his critics*. University of California Press.

Roth, A., & Fonagy, P. (2006). *What works for whom? A critical review of psychotherapy research* (2nd ed.). The Guilford Press.

Rudnytsky, P. L. (2011). *Rescuing psychoanalysis from Freud and other essays in re-vision*. Karnac books.

Showalter, E. (1980). Victorian women and insanity. *Victorian Studies, 23*(2), 157–181. www.jstor.org/stable/3827084

Showalter, E. (1985). *The female malady: Women, madness, and English culture, 1830–1980*. Penguin.

Smith, M. L., & Glass, G. V. (1977). Meta-analysis of psychotherapy outcome studies. *American Psychologist, 32*(9), 752–760. https://doi.org/10.1037/0003-066X.32.9.752

Smith, M. L., Glass, G. V., & Miller, T. I. (1980). *The benefits of psychotherapy*. Johns Hopkins Press.

Spurgas, A. K. (2016). Low desire, trauma and femininity in the DSM-5: A case for sequelae. *Psychology & Sexuality, 7*(1), 48–67. https://doi.org/10.1080/19419899.2015.1024471

Sweet, P. L. (2019). The sociology of gaslighting. *American Sociological Review, 84*(5), 851–875. https://doi.org/10.1177/0003122419874843

Szasz, T. (1978). *Myth of psychotherapy: Mental healing as religion, rhetoric and repression*. Doubleday.

Tosh, J. (2019). *The body and consent in psychology, psychiatry, and medicine: A therapeutic rape culture*. Routledge.

Totton, N. (2006a). Introduction. In N. Totton (Ed.), *The politics of psychotherapy: New perspectives* (pp. xiii–xx). McGraw-Hill Education.

Totton, N. (2006b). Power in the therapeutic relationship. In N. Totton (Ed.), *The politics of psychotherapy: New perspectives* (pp. 83–93). McGraw-Hill Education.

Tseris, E. (2018). A feminist critique of trauma therapy. In B. M. Z. Cohen (Ed.), *Routledge international handbook of critical mental health* (pp. 251–257). Routledge.

Tseris, E. (2019). *Trauma, women's mental health, and social justice: Pitfalls and possibilities*. Routledge.

Ussher, J. M. (2011). *The madness of women: Myth and experience*. Routledge.

Ussher, J. M. (2018). A critical feminist analysis of madness: Pathologising femininity through psychiatric discourse. In B. M. Z. Cohen (Ed.), *Routledge international handbook of critical mental health* (pp. 72–78). Routledge.

Wampold, B. E., & Imel, Z. E. (2015). *The great psychotherapy debate: The evidence for what makes psychotherapy work* (2nd ed.). Routledge.

Watters, E., & Ofshe, R. (1999). *Therapy's delusions: The myth of the unconscious and the exploitation of today's walking worried*. Scribner.

Whitaker, R., & Cosgrove, L. (2015). *Psychiatry under the Influence: Institutional corruption, social injury, and prescriptions for reform*. Palgrave Macmillan.

Whooley, O. (2019). *On the heels of ignorance: Psychiatry and the politics of not knowing*. University of Chicago.

12 Has '*The Assault on Truth*' Had any Influence on Today's Mental Health Services?

John Read

In *The Assault on Truth* Jeffrey Masson concludes:

> by shifting the emphasis from an actual world of sadness, misery and cruelty to an internal stage on which actors performed invented dramas for an invisible audience of their own creation, Freud began a trend away from the real world that, it seems to me, is at the root of the present-day sterility of psychoanalysis and psychiatry throughout the world.
>
> (Masson, 1984/1992, p. 144)

This chapter discusses whether things have improved since Masson's historic intervention; whether mental health services remain sterile today when it comes to addressing sadness, misery and cruelty.

Some possible biases

I begin with three things that may have influenced my thoughts. First, Jeffrey is a good friend. We met about 20 years ago while both living in Auckland, New Zealand. My partner and I, and sometimes our kids, enjoyed sunny days at his house, on the beach of the exquisite Karaka Bay, with Jeff's partner (Leila), two sons, and Benjy, the star of *The Dog Who Couldn't Stop Loving*, one of Jeff's best-seller animal books. Jeff and Leila hosted my 60th birthday party in that house on the beach.

We have all moved on now, but not before many sun-drenched conversations about the dire state of psychiatry and the world in general. I remember sitting behind Jeff watching the enthralled faces of several hundred of my psychology undergraduates as he unfurled the story of his life, contained in *My Father's Guru* (1993) and *Final Analysis* (1990), culminating in *The Assault on Truth*. I don't know if they realized just how lucky they were. Jeff speaks at least as engagingly as he writes, always with a natural sense of humor. For example, 'How on earth did I think I could become a psychoanalyst? I can't keep quiet for five minutes and would be sure to tell them my problems before they had finished telling me theirs'!

DOI: 10.4324/9781003431466-13

He and I would stage an annual debate for the students on the motion 'Psychotherapy is a complete waste of time'. I would try to counter his withering arguments, from another of his books, *Against Therapy* (1988). Somewhere in these shared New Zealand years (2002–2014) we were at a Melbourne conference, where we were both speaking, along with John Briere, one of the most brilliant lecturers in the sexual abuse field. Determined not to be outdone, Jeff gave a wonderful after-dinner speech, culminating in a true story about how, despite all his animal-loving skills, he had failed to talk a wild elephant out of charging him. 'How was I to know the elephant was antisemitic'?

Second, I was sexually abused by my headmaster. I say this because it seems silly not to, given the topic of this book; and because I hope that the more people talk about their experience of sexual abuse the easier it becomes for others. Freud's public refutation of his belief that sexual abuse is a cause of mental health problems made it harder for several generations of abuse survivors to talk about it and, perhaps, for mental health professionals to ask about, and to believe, it. I mention it also because it may influence my opinions on the issues discussed here. I would certainly have been unimpressed if I had summoned the courage to tell a therapist what happened to me only to discover that s/he thought it was a fantasy based on my childhood sexual desires.

Third, I have always believed that human 'sadness and misery' and, for that matter, 'cruelty' are primarily caused by bad things happening (Read & Dillon, 2013; Read & Sanders, 2022). My shortest ever university lecture lasts 10 seconds. It goes: 'Today we are going to talk about Depression. It is caused by depressing things happening' (I would come back after a brief pause of course; but you have to do weird stuff to keep the attention of 18-year-olds). Recently, a journalist asked me when I developed my belief that mental health problems are caused by life events and circumstances, as if it was unusual and intriguing. I pointed out that the public, in almost every survey conducted anywhere (except the USA), believe that mental health problems, from depression to psychosis, are primarily caused by stressful life events (Read, Magliano & Beavan, 2013b). So, perhaps a better question is, 'what leads a minority to believe something other than that'? Freud's blunder might have been a partial answer to that question throughout the twentieth century. I did tell the journalist, however, how my shared, common-sense psychosocial perspective was repeatedly reinforced by the patients I worked with. Here is an example, from my first job, as a nursing aide in New York, 50 years ago:

> I was 'specialing' a teenage girl. This meant being locked in with her in the 'quiet room' (usually the noisiest place on the ward) to make sure she didn't try to harm herself. She hadn't spoken for weeks. A 'catatonic schizophrenic'. Having had no training, I tried: 'It's OK if you don't want to talk, but if you want to, I will listen.' Nothing. The next day she said one word: 'My'. The next day she said 'father'. The next day she didn't speak. The next day she said 'me'. The missing word, I learned later, was raped.
>
> (Read, 2013a, p. xx)

The Assault on Truth

So, with all that in mind, I believe *The Assault on Truth* is one of the most important books of the twentieth century. It is so important partly because of the specific, previously suppressed, information revealed by Masson's detective work about why Freud changed his mind about child sexual abuse being an important cause of mental health problems. Masson argues that '… without the abandonment of this theory, the development of psychoanalysis would not have been possible' (Masson, 1992, p. 12). Indeed, Anna Freud wrote the following to Masson, in 1981:

> Keeping up the seduction theory would mean to abandon the Oedipus complex, and with it the whole importance of phantasy life, conscious or unconscious phantasy. In fact, I think there would have been no psychoanalysis afterwards.
> (p. 113)

We will never know whether psychoanalysis would have existed today if Freud had not abandoned his belief in the role of child sexual abuse. Perhaps it would exist but in a very different, more reality-based, form. Either way, *The Assault on Truth* is such an important book because of the potential broader importance of psychoanalysis. If psychoanalysis had not had the potential to answer so many of our most pressing individual, societal and international problems, it would matter less how and why it went so badly off the rails at such an early stage of its development. As Masson states:

> The purpose of this book is to make public, evidence hitherto unknown, ignored or discounted, that would point to a more illuminating explanation for the single most important step Freud took, one that helped shape the world we live in.
> (pp. 12–13)

I therefore concur with the accolades, from newspapers on both sides of the Atlantic, on the cover of the 1992 edition:

> 'His findings … have drawn attention to a huge gap at the heart of twentieth-century thought'. (Observer)
>
> 'His scholarship is impeccable.' (Los Angeles Times)
>
> 'Intriguing and thought-provoking… a fascinating detective-like story.'
> (Sunday Times)

The first half of my chapter highlights two themes running through *The Assault on Truth*, from Freud's time in Paris in 1885 through to his 1896 announcement and then retraction of his theory about child sexual abuse, and the rebellion and denouncement of Sándor Ferenczi in 1932. I will then discuss how those two themes are playing out today. The first, obvious, issue is that of resistance to acknowledging and addressing child abuse. The second is the promulgation of genetic, and other biological, theories as alternative explanations for mental health problems. I will argue that the first of these issues is not only central to the history of psychoanalysis but is also a partial explanation for psychiatry's ongoing promotion of unsubstantiated bio-genetic accounts of human distress at the expense of psycho-social factors and for the dysfunctional mental health services that follow from that fundamental error.

'Freud at the Paris Morgue' – 1885 (chapter 2)

In his discoveries of early influences which sensitized Freud to the reality of child abuse in general, and incest in particular, Masson is a scholar, detective and investigative journalist rolled into one. He first painstakingly documents the comprehensive reports of abuse by nineteenth-century French medico-legal experts. He then describes the riveting lectures with their heart-breaking examples of child abuse, and the child autopsies Freud attended in Paris. Had Freud not retracted, he and others could have cited these reports and autopsies in order to start breaking the silence around child abuse early in the twentieth century.

Masson also, however, reports a parallel, competing theme of denial in nineteenth-century France, which is perhaps the first example of the backlash that has repeatedly greeted progress in the acknowledgment of childhood sexual abuse (Herman, 1992), including the reaction to Freud's (1896) paper and lecture:

> But early on there developed a current within the literature which, in the long run, exercised an enduring influence, and in my opinion a sinister one. This is the literature which concerns itself with simulations and the supposed lies of children. There existed a whole series of authors interested in the *pseudologica phantastica* of children.
>
> (Masson, 1992, p. 40)

Masson documents this literature and offers distressing examples of the misrepresentation by the experts at the time (all men) of abuse cases as lies and fantasies. So, Chapter 2 simultaneously provides not only the basis for Freud's discovery of sexual abuse in *The Aetiology of Hysteria* (Freud, 1986), but also the rationale for changing his mind later.

What about my second theme, genetic and other biological explanations for mental health problems? The predominant causal model for 'hysteria' and other disturbances at the end of the nineteenth century in Europe was the 'medical model', with a strong emphasis on inherited or constitutional characteristics. In 1892 Emil Kraepelin invented 'dementia praecox', the precursor of 'schizophrenia', which (with no supporting evidence) he argued was a biologically based, genetically inherited brain disease (Read, 2013b).

Masson gives examples of how the almost exclusively female ailment 'hysteria', which Freud was soon to explain in terms of child abuse, was often used as an explanation for the supposed lies and fantasies. The true causes of the disorder were transformed into imaginary claims which simultaneously became symptoms of the disorder. It seems that, like 'dementia praecox' and other psychiatric diagnoses of the time, either the disorder of 'hysteria' itself, or the specific symptoms of lying or imagining abuse were inherited. Masson asked, 'Who are these victims with a psychology so special that they create their own aggressors'? Brouardel (1837–1906), who had written a book on the rape of children, answers: 'In general it is a question of women who are predisposed, and this is why one must carefully study the hereditary and personal antecedents of these people' (Masson, 1992, pp. 46, 47). Freud's theory that child abuse, not genetics, was the primary cause of human distress was unlikely to be popular with European advocates of bio-genetics at the end of the nineteenth century.

'Freud, Fliess and Emma Eckstein' – 1894–1900 (chapter 3)

Thanks to Masson's translation of unpublished letters (Masson, 1985), we learn of a fascinating and distressing account of a scarily botched operation and Freud's loyalty to the doctor involved, his best friend, Wilhelm Fliess. We see another form of resistance to acknowledging abuse on the basis of ludicrous male theories about female sexuality. This time the maltreatment is not child sexual abuse but physical abuse of an adult. Fliess mutilated the nose of Freud's patient, Emma, in a bizarre attempt to cure her of masturbation, which both Freud and Fliess believed to be causing her 'hysteria'. When he leaves half a meter of gauze in the cavity the hemorrhaging nearly kills Emma. The resistance to seeing the reality of abuse resides, this time, in Freud, who convinces himself that the hemorrhaging is the result of Emma's 'hysterical' conflicts and desires, not Fliess's mad theory and medical ineptitude.

In terms of our second theme, bio-genetic ideology, this tragic episode is another example of the endless array, over centuries and continuing today, of well-intentioned but ineffective and/or dangerous biological, medical solutions to psychological/emotional problems. In this case the 'treatment' was based partly on a biological theory about the supposed connection between the vagina and the nose.

Fliess had another, equally bizarre theory. He thought that the dates of emotionally important events, and even death, were determined by his 'theory of periodicity', based on the 'biologically determined' period of 28 days for females and 23 days for men. This must be a contender for the top ten weirdest biological explanations for human distress, and there have been some doozies, before and since Freud.

In this chapter we also see confirmed the dominance of genetic theories about mental health problems, which Freud's theory temporarily threatened. Jean-Martin Charcot, whom Freud went to study under in Paris, is described by Masson, with good reason, as 'Frances's most illustrious neurologist' (p. 14). Masson informs us that:

> Charcot had been a great defender of *la famille névropathique,* the constitutionally tainted family, and of the unique importance of heredity in the etiology of neuroses.
>
> (p. 90)

Charcot's faith in genetics applied to both female 'hysterics' themselves and their tendency to fantasize and lie. The latter was supposedly a symptom of the former. Again, both the occurrence of abuse and its role in causing emotional problems are simultaneously denied and replaced by unproven male genetic fantasies.

'The Aetiology of Hysteria' – 1896 (chapter 1)

In 1896 Freud presented his theory based on 18 cases (6 men and 12 women) who had been sexually abused as children. Masson reports:

> On the evening of April 21, 1986, Sigmund Freud gave a paper before his colleagues at the Society for Psychiatry and Neurology in Vienna, entitled 'The Aetiology of Hysteria'. Freud realized that in giving this paper he would become 'one of those who disturbed the sleep of the world'. The address presented a revolutionary theory that the origin of neurosis lay in early sexual traumas ... This is what later came to be called the 'seduction theory' – namely the belief that these early experiences were real, not fantasies, and had a damaging and lasting effect on the later lives of the children.
>
> (p. 3)

The backlash started the second Freud opened his mouth. Masson discovered an unpublished letter from Freud to Fliess. We learn that Freud's lecture had received 'an icy reception'. The head of Psychiatry at Vienna University, Baron von Krafft-Ebing, had dismissed Freud's theory as 'a scientific fairy tale'. Freud added, in his letter: 'And this after one has demonstrated to them a solution to a more-than-thousand-year-old problem, a "source of the Nile"! They can all go to hell' (p. 9).

Masson also discovered that a medical journal covered the two other papers given that day in detail but reported only the title of Freud's paper. Masson further reveals that in a letter to Fliess two weeks later, also omitted from the original published edition, Freud had written 'The word has been given out to abandon me, and a void is forming around me' (p. 10).

Freud's paper reveals that he was fully aware of the strength and nature of resistance he would encounter. Among the objections he anticipated, and rebutted, were (i) that childhood sexual abuse is so rare that it could not possibly explain 'such a common neurosis' and (ii) that many people who were sexually abused do not develop problems (p. 275). These arguments were used throughout the twentieth century and beyond to minimize the importance of child abuse.

Another anticipated objection relates to my second theme, about bio-genetic theories drowning out abuse. Freud predicted that his theory would be resisted by those 'unwilling to give up the hope that someday it will be possible' to explain all symptoms in terms of 'anatomical changes' (p. 274). He added:

> If this [his theory] is so, the prospect is opened up that what has hitherto had to be laid at the door of a still unexplained hereditary predisposition may be accounted for as having been acquired at an early age.
>
> (p. 270)

'Freud's Renunciation of the Theory of Seduction' – 1897–1914 (chapter 4)

Chapter 4 illustrates my first, rather obvious theme about resistance to acknowledging child abuse. It is the remarkable story of how one of the first people to highlight child abuse came to discredit his own work. But one of the most important of Masson's findings, some would say *the* most important, is that Freud's rejection of his own theory was far more tentative and nuanced than historians of psychoanalysis would have us believe.

On September 21, 1897, Freud wrote to Fliess expressing doubts about his 'seduction theory'. Masson documents how Anna Freud and other prominent psychoanalysts, then and since, portrayed the letter as a full and permanent retraction. Masson reveals, however, that three months later Freud described a case that led him to write 'My confidence in the father-etiology has risen greatly' (p. 114). A week later he describes a particularly violent case involving a three-year-old girl which 'speaks for the intrinsic genuineness of infantile trauma'. Freud goes so far as to suggest a new motto for psychoanalysis: 'What have they done to you, my poor child?' (p. 117). This, Masson stresses, shows the importance Freud still attached to child sexual abuse even after his 1897 letter to Fliess where he cast doubt on it.

All this was omitted from the published letters and, thereby, from the official history of psychoanalysis. Masson's point is to have us understand the collective desire of prominent psychoanalysts to deny the importance of child abuse and its impacts, and their willingness to edit history to accomplish that goal.

In this chapter we also learn that Masson sees Freud's theory as a direct threat to genetic beliefs:

> The acceptance of external trauma from such an unexpected source (the family) also cast doubts on yet another bulwark of traditional medicine: the primacy of constitutional factors. Indeed, as long as Freud believed in seduction, he would have to reject the conventional explanations in terms of heredity.
>
> (p. 137)

In that momentous letter to Fliess of September 21, 1897, in which he first expressed doubts about his 'seduction theory', Freud comments: '… and with this the factor of a hereditary disposition regains a sphere of influence from which I had made it my task to dislodge it – in the interest of illuminating neurosis' (p. 109).

So, Freud was not only aware of the conflict between the two theories, he believed, as Masson and I do, that the genetic position tends to sweep the real causes of human distress under the carpet. (Epigenetics, meanwhile, offers a more nuanced approach, by focusing on how our inherited genetic makeup can be switched on and off by our environment; Read et al., 2009).

'The Strange Case of Ferenczi's Last Paper' – 1932 (chapter 5)

One psychoanalyst was not prepared to collude with his profession's denial of child abuse and its consequences. In 1932 Sándor Ferenczi (1873–1933), Freud's close friend and nominated successor, presented his truly remarkable paper, 'Confusion of Tongues', at the International Psycho-Analytic Congress in Vienna. He insisted Freud had been right in 1896. Masson documents how the leading psychoanalysts, including Freud, blocked publication of the paper and discredited Ferenczi's attempt to steer psychoanalysis back to reality, as a symptom of his supposed madness.

Masson's righteous anger oozes off the page:

> Faced with his colleague's hostility to his discoveries, Freud sacrificed his major insight. When Ferenczi, a generation later, was led by his patients to the same discovery, he met with a similar response, only this time Freud played the role that forty years earlier had been Krafft-Ebbing's ... The time has come to cease hiding from one of the greatest issues in human history. For it is unforgiveable that those entrusted with the lives of people who come to them in emotional pain having suffered real wounds in childhood, should use their blind reliance on Freud's fearful abandonment of the seduction theory to continue the abuse their patients once suffered as children.
>
> (pp. 192–193)

Masson might have added that psychoanalysis could, and should, have played a crucial role in understanding *why* we humans, including mental health professionals, have such difficulty taking in the reality of child abuse. Instead, it has, for decades, colluded with and actively facilitated our blindness.

Mental health services today

I don't know how many psychoanalysts still assume clients are fantasizing when they talk about child abuse. I suspect they hold a range of positions on the conflicting views of Freud and Ferenczi. Clearly many have moved on from Freud's retraction. For example, the year 2008 saw the publication of a book called 'Psychoanalytic psychotherapy after child abuse: The treatment of adults and children who have experienced sexual abuse, violence and neglect in childhood' (McQueen et al., 2008). (I can hear Jeffrey muttering 'why would anyone seek help from a profession whose founder says the thing they need help for didn't happen?'.) In my own field, psychosis, several prominent psychoanalysts have made major contributions to understanding the relationship between traumas and psychosis (Koehler et al., 2013). In 2014, however, a review found that there were no robust studies of psychoanalytic psychotherapy for sexually abused children and adolescents (Parker & Turner, 2014).

About 20 years ago the Sándor Ferenczi Society in Hungary (his country of birth) invited me to give a seminar on my research about child abuse and psychosis (2005). After my lecture one of the members informed me that it didn't matter whether child abuse had actually occurred or whether it was a fantasy, because the effect on the personality was the same (I don't know how representative she was). My efforts to explain that it matters to a client whether their therapist believes them, and that one of the two circumstances was a serious crime, fell on deaf ears. It seemed that even a society dedicated to celebrating and promoting Ferenczi's views had some conference attendees actually promoting Freud's position on the crucial difference between the two men. As Masson (1992) reports, Freud had ended up, by 1916, believing that '…we have not succeeded in pointing to any difference in the consequences, whether phantasy or reality has the greater share in these events of childhood' (p. 133).

I share Jeffrey's protests:

> To tell someone who has suffered the effects of a childhood filled with sexual violence that it does not matter whether his memories are anchored in reality or not is to do further violence to that person and is bound to have a pernicious effect. A real memory demands some form of validation from the outside world – denial of those memories by others can lead to a break with reality, and a psychosis.
>
> (p. 133)

I had done some detective work of my own. Knowing nothing about Ferenczi when I accepted the invitation to Budapest, I tried to read up while flying from New Zealand to Hungary. All I could find was his correspondence with Freud (Brabant, 1993). Here I learned how Ferenczi was psychoanalyzing Elma, the daughter of his common-law wife, when he fell in love with Elma and started a relationship with her. He wrote to Freud to inform him, adding 'I recognized my strong interest in young pretty creatures'. He said, of Elma, that 'She falls in love compulsively with doctors, i.e., with persons who see her naked, physically, and now mentally'. When Elma's mental health, unsurprisingly, deteriorated, Ferenczi stopped analyzing her and referred her to Freud for further treatment. The two men then regularly wrote to each other about Elma, and Freud's treatment of her. She continued to deteriorate. When Elma's father got 'somewhat upset' about these events, Sándor advised Sigmund: 'don't be influenced by his remarks'. To cut a bizarre story short, Ferenczi proposes marriage to his step-daughter. She declines. Ferenczi blames Freud!

Are we still denying or minimizing child abuse?

In 1975 a prominent Psychiatry textbook announced that the incidence of incest in the general population was 'one per million' (Henderson, 1975, p. 1533). In my work in mental health services in the USA, New Zealand and England (1973–1994) I was often surprised how few of my colleagues were interested in patients' life events and circumstances. Most staff (not all) seemed more interested in making diagnoses and prescribing pills.

When I entered academia, therefore, I decided to research the relationship between child abuse and psychosis. I still remember the hostility from psychiatrists, with their accusations of 'family blaming', and the angry explanations that schizophrenia is a genetically inherited brain disease which has nothing to do with adverse childhood events, or, indeed, any events.

The only study, to my knowledge, which has asked mental health professionals whether they believe patients when they disclose childhood sexual abuse found, 20 years ago, that 85 New Zealand professionals believed, on average, that 84% of disclosures were true, 7% were psychotic delusions, 6% were imagined and 3% were deliberate false allegations (Cavanagh et al., 2004). None of these professionals were psychoanalysts.

Our 2018 review of 21 studies, from six countries, found that only 0%–22% of mental health service users are asked about child abuse or neglect (Read et al., 2018a). Only 28% of abuse or neglect cases identified by researchers are found in patients' files. The good news was that some improvement over time was found (from 1987 to 2017).

A parallel review (Read et al., 2018b) of 13 studies about how staff respond when they do hear about child abuse or neglect from their patients, found that rates of inclusion of abuse or neglect in treatment plans ranged from 12% to 44%. Rates of referral to abuse-related therapy ranged from 8% to 23%. Less than 2% were referred to legal authorities.

Our most recent study (Neill & Read, 2022) does not indicate progress in terms of asking about abuse. Only 13% of the files of 400 people using community mental health services in England contained documentation of any adverse experiences. Just 1% showed evidence that clients had been asked about adversities. On a more positive note, rates of *responses* to the few adversities of which staff *were* aware were high. Ninety percent of records indicated some appropriate support following disclosure.

I will leave the reader to gauge, from these studies, how far we have come from Freud's announcement that child abuse is not a cause of mental health problems and that people who talk about being abused as children should not be believed.

Are we still using unevidenced bio-genetic ideologies?

Freud's retraction removed a major challenge to the genetic theories that were simultaneously being promoted about, for example, 'dementia praecox'/'schizophrenia' (Read, 2013b). We will never know whether, had Freud held his nerve, the stranglehold of genetics on psychiatric thinking might have been weaker and more evidence-based.

Unsubstantiated claims about chemical imbalances (Moncrieff et al., 2022; Read & Moncrieff, 2023) and genetic predispositions (Joseph, 2003, 2023) continue to dominate psychiatry and drug companies.

The evidence for a genetic basis to depression, anxiety, schizophrenia etc. is extremely weak (Joseph, 2003, 2023). Even if there had turned out to be a genetic basis to various mental health problems, what would we have done about it? Professor Richard Bentall once asked some genetic researchers, at a conference, to identify a single person that genetic research into mental health problems had ever helped, in any way. The silence was deafening.

Jeffrey and I have written about one grotesque example (around the time of Freud's death) of how unsubstantiated genetic ideology can be violently misused, in a paper we called 'Biological Psychiatry and the Mass Murder of "Schizophrenics" ':

> This article documents the murder, by psychiatrists, of a quarter of a million patients, mostly diagnosed as 'schizophrenic,' in Europe during the second world war; and the sterilization of hundreds of thousands more internationally, including in the USA and Scandinavia. These sterilizations and murders were justified by biological psychiatry's unsubstantiated hypothesis that the conditions involved are genetically determined. Gas chambers in the six psychiatric hospitals involved, in Germany, were subsequently dismantled and moved, along with the psychiatrists and their staff, to help establish some of the Holocaust's concentration camps, in Poland. The avoidance of these facts and their profound implications, by the profession of psychiatry, internationally, over subsequent decades, is discussed.
>
> (Read & Masson, 2022, p. 69)

The majority (73%) of Germans diagnosed with the supposedly genetically based mental illness 'schizophrenia' were killed or sterilized. If the theory used to justify the atrocities were true, the incidence of 'schizophrenia' in Germany would have plummeted in subsequent generations. It did not. Apart from demonstrating, albeit with an extreme example, the dangers of genetic theories, these hideous events confirm that the theories were, and are, bogus.

Women

There is a third theme to mention. It would be silly to think that the fathers of psychoanalysis were likely to advance our understanding of the mental health of women. The story of how Freud and Ferenczi 'treated' Elma is illustrative. Instead, Freud and his followers generated bizarre, blatantly misogynistic notions, about orgasms that required clitoral stimulation being neurotic, and about penis envy.

Masson points out that while psychoanalysts, and other mental health professionals, were ignoring, or actively denying, child abuse, feminists such as Florence Rush, Alice Miller, Judith Herman, Louis Armstrong and Diana Russell were drawing attention to the high incidence of child sexual abuse, after a century of near silence that followed those nineteenth-century French medico-legal experts to whom Freud was exposed in the Paris Morgue. Herman wrote about the processes involved in seeing child abuse: '… the active process of bearing witness [to child abuse] gives way to the active process of forgetting. Repression, dissociation, and denial are phenomena of social as well as individual consciousness' (Herman, 1992, p. 32).

Another of Masson's undervalued books (compared to his animal books) is *A Dark Science; Women, Sexuality and Psychiatry in the Nineteenth Century* (1986). Its title speaks for itself.

In the 21st century women are still diagnosed with most 'mental health problems' at higher rates than men and are prescribed antidepressants, benzodiazepines (Public Health England, 2019) and electroconvulsive therapy (Read et al., 2021) roughly twice as often as men. Perhaps the 'hysteria' of Freud's time has been replaced by 'borderline personality disorder' (aka 'emotionally unstable personality disorder') in the current era. Seventy-one percent of people with this diagnosis report one or more traumatic childhood experiences (Porter et al., 2020). Women are *three* times more likely than men to get this diagnosis.

Conclusion

Child abuse is still often ignored, minimized or denied by mental health services. This is facilitated by the simplistic 'medical model' that still dominates psychiatric services, keenly promoted by drug companies and psychiatry.

There are, however, clear signs that a paradigm shift may be approaching. Both the World Health Organization (Funk, 2021) and the United Nations (Puras, 2020) are demanding a shift away from medical understandings and solutions toward psycho-social, community-based approaches which respect human rights (W.H.O. and U.N., 2023). Many examples already exist, including Trauma-Informed Services (Sweeney et al., 2016), the Power Threat Meaning Framework (Johnstone & Boyle, 2018), Open Dialogue (Bergström et al., 2023), the Hearing Voices Network (Romme et al., 2009) and Soteria Houses (Friedlander, 2022; Mosher et al., 2004).

There is no objective way to evaluate whether Freud's lack of courage helped strengthen the 'medical model' that has wreaked such havoc on mental health services and the lives of millions of people around the world. We don't know whether Freud significantly exacerbated the mental health field's denial of child abuse or its exaggeration of bio-genetic factors. He certainly did not help.

Did Masson's *The Assault on Truth* nudge psychoanalysis and mental health professionals in general back toward reality? Again, it is hard to know. The book was completely shunned by psychoanalysis, which to this day has failed to respond meaningfully to Masson's questions. It is hard to see how anyone who did read it, with anything other than a completely closed mind, could fail to be persuaded. But one of the many things that Freud did get right is that denial is a very powerful defense mechanism against painful facts and feelings. Sadly, he did not apply the construct to himself or his colleagues when it came to the sexual abuse of children.

Prior to publication of *The Assault on Truth*, a reporter (Malcolm, 1983) wrote a critique of it, which was essentially a character assassination of Jeffrey (leading to years of litigation). He replied:

> I [do not] believe that the driving force of this hostile response lies in any personal animus against me. One cannot escape the feeling that most men (and

> some women) have terrible difficulty when it comes to even hearing about the miseries of childhood, and about the suffering many girls undergo in their early years, first at the hands of a trusted adult (generally a close male relative) and later at the hands of a therapist (generally male) who does not believe their memories and will not take seriously what has really happened to them in childhood.
>
> (Masson, 1992, p. xvi)

Rather than helping us understand why we so readily deny child abuse, Freud and his blind followers, perpetuated the denial. Masson tried to make us see how, and why, this tragic and disastrous blunder came about.

References

Bergström, T., Seikkula, J., Köngäs-Saviaro, P., Taskila, J., & Aaltonen, J. (2023). Need adapted use of medication in the open dialogue approach for psychosis. *Psychosis, 15*(2), 134–144. https://doi.org/10.1016/j.psychres.2018.09.039

Brabant, E. (Ed.) (1993). *The correspondence of Sigmund Freud and Sándor Ferenczi, Vol.1: 1908–1914.* Harvard University Press.

Cavanagh, M., Read, J., & New, B. (2004). Sexual abuse inquiry and response: A New Zealand training programme. *New Zealand Journal of Psychology, 33*, 137–144.

Freud, S. (1986). The aetiology of hysteria. In *The standard edition of the complete psychological works of Sigmund Freud* (vol. 3 , pp. 187–221). Hogarth.

Friedlander, A., Bitan, D., & Lichtenberg, P. (2022). The Soteria model: Implementing an alternative to acute psychiatric hospitalization in Israel. *Psychosis, 14*, 99–108. https://doi.org/10.1080/17522439.2022.2057578

Funk, M. (2021). *Guidance on community mental health services: Promoting person-centred and rights-based approaches.* World Health Organisation.

Henderson, D. J. (1975). Incest. In A. Freedman, H. Kaplan, & B. Sadock (Eds.), *Comprehensive textbook of psychiatry* (2nd ed., pp. 1530–1539). Williams & Wilkins.

Herman, J. (1992). *Trauma and recovery.* Basic Books.

Johnstone, L., & Boyle, M. (2018). *The power threat meaning framework.* British Psychological Society.

Joseph, J. (2003). *The gene illusion*: PCCS Books.

Joseph, J. (2023). *Schizophrenia and genetics: The end of an illusion.* Routledge.

Koehler, B., Silver, A-L, & Karon, B. (2013). Psychodynamic approaches to understanding psychosis: Defenses against terror. In J. Read & J. Dillon (Eds.), *Models of madness* (pp. 238–248). Routledge.

Malcolm, J. (1983). Trouble in the archives. *The New Yorker*, December 5.

Masson, J. (1985). *The complete letters of Sigmund Freud to Wilhelm Fliess, 1887–1904.* Harvard University Press.

Masson, J. (1986). *A dark science: Women, sexuality and psychiatry in the nineteenth century.* Farrar, Straus and Giroux.

Masson, J. (1988). *Against therapy: Emotional tyranny and the myth of psychological healing.* Common Courage Press.

Masson, J. (1990). *Final analysis: The making and unmaking of a psychoanalyst.* Addison-Wesley.

Masson, J. (1992). *The assault on truth: Freud and child sexual abuse.* Harper Collins.

Masson, J. (1993). *My father's guru: A journey through spirituality and disillusion.* Addison-Wesley.

McQueen, D., Itzin, C., Kennedy, R., Sinason, V., & Maxted, F. (Eds.) (2008). *Psychoanalytic psychotherapy after child abuse.* Routledge.

Moncrieff, J., Cooper, R., Stockmann, T., Amendola, S., Hengartner, M., & Horowitz, M. (2022, July 20). The serotonin theory of depression: A systematic umbrella review of the evidence. *Molecular Psychiatry.* https://doi.org/10.1038/s41380-022-01661-0

Mosher, L., Hendrix, V., & Fort, C. (2004). *Soteria; through madness to deliverance.* Xlibris.

Neill, C., & Read, J. (2022). Adequacy of inquiry about, documentation of, and treatment of trauma and adversities. *Community Mental Health Journal, 58,* 1076–1087. https://doi.org/10.1007/s10597-021-00916-4

Parker, B., & Turner, W. (2014). Psychoanalytic/psychodynamic psychotherapy for sexually abused children and adolescents: a systematic review. *Research on Social Work Practice, 24,* 389–399. https://doi.org/10.1177/1049731514525477

Porter, C., Palmier-Claus, J., Branitsky, A., Mansell, W., Warwick, H., & Varese, F. (2020). Childhood adversity and borderline personality disorder: A meta-analysis. *Acta Psychiatrica Scandinavica, 141,* 6–20. https://doi.org/10.1111/acps.13118

Public Health England. (2019). *Dependence and withdrawal associated with some prescribed Medicines: An evidence review.* P.H.E.

Pūras, D. (2020). *On the right of everyone to the enjoyment of the highest attainable standard of physical and mental health.* United Nations Human Rights Office of the High Commissioner.

Read, J. (2013a). Preface to the first edition. In J. Read & J. Dillon (Eds.), *Models of madness* (pp. xviii–xx). Routledge.

Read, J. (2013b). The invention of 'schizophrenia'. In J. Read & J. Dillon (Eds.), *Models of madness* (pp. 20–32). Routledge.

Read, J., Bentall, R., & Fosse, R. (2009). Time to abandon the bio-bio-bio model of psychosis. *Epidemiology and Psychiatric Sciences, 18,* 299–310. https://doi.org/10.1017/S1121189X00000257

Read, J., & Dillon, J. (Eds.) (2013). *Models of madness: Psychological, social and biological approaches to psychosis.* Routledge.

Read, J., Harper, D., Tucker, I., & Kennedy, A. (2018a). Do mental health services identify child abuse and neglect? A systematic review. *International Journal of Mental Health Nursing, 27,* 7–19. https://doi.org/10.1111/inm.12369

Read, J., Harper, D., Tucker, I. & Kennedy, A. (2018b). How do mental health services respond when child abuse or neglect become known? A literature review. *International Journal of Mental Health Nursing, 27,* 1606–1617. https://doi.org/org/10.1111/inm.12498

Read, J., Harrop, C., Geekie, J., Renton, J., & Cunliffe, S. (2021). A second independent audit of ECT in England. *Psychology and Psychotherapy: Theory, Research and Practice, 94,* 603–619. https://doi.org/10.1111/papt.12335

Read, J., Magliano, L., & Beavan, V. (2013). Public beliefs about the causes of 'schizophrenia'. In J. Read & J. Dillon (Eds.), *Models of madness* (pp. 143–156). Routledge.

Read, J., & Masson, J. (2022). Biological psychiatry and the mass murder of 'schizophrenics'. *Ethical Human Psychology and Psychiatry, 24,* 69–85. https://doi.org/10.1891/EHPP-2021-0006

Read, J., & Moncrieff, J. (2023). Depression: why drugs and electricity are not the answer. *Psychological Medicine 52,* 1401–1410.

Read, J., & Sanders, P. (2022). *A straight talking introduction to the causes of mental health problems.* PCCS Books.

Read, J., Van Os, J., Morrison, A., & Ross, C. (2005). Childhood trauma, psychosis and schizophrenia: A literature review with theoretical and clinical implications. *Acta Psychiatrica Scandinavica, 112*, 330–350. https://doi.org/10.1111/j.1600-0447.2005.00634.x

Romme, M., Escher, S., Dillon, J., Corstens, D., & Morris, M. (Eds.) (2009). *Living with voices: 50 stories of recovery*. PCCS Books.

Sweeney, A., Clement, S., Filson, B., & Kennedy, A. (2016). Trauma-informed mental healthcare in the UK. *Mental Health Review, 21*, 174–192. https://doi.org/10.1108/MHRJ-01-2015-0006

World Health Organization and the United Nation. (2023). *Mental health, human rights and legislation: Guidance and practice*. Geneva: W.H.O

Afterword

Martin J. Dorahy and Warwick Middleton

In the Hollywood motion picture, *A Few Good Men*, the character played by Jack Nicholson, ruffled in the courtroom from questions levelled at him by Tom Cruise's protagonist, unleashes his now famous tirade, 'You want the truth … you can't handle the truth'! The truth in the course of human history has often been too hot to handle, with efforts made to bypass, dismiss, undermine or attack it. One need not look very far for examples, even in the present era, with the reality of global warming still debated and denied not just around lunchroom tables but at the level of international policy and politics. Whistle-blowers, like Daniel Ellsberg and Edward Snowden, those exposing secrets in religious, voluntary or statutory institutions, along with many of those who less dramatically and less publicly come forward with sexual abuse disclosures, are typically fated with vilification, character assassination and efforts to evoke mortification, in an effort to keep hidden the intolerable truth their courage has exposed.

As many of the chapters in this book eloquently note, the existence, prevalence and impact of childhood sexual abuse have piqued curiosity and investigation in medical and psychological circles, and even hooved into the view of society at large, only to be met with the sort of resistance that combats truths too confronting and uncomfortable to tolerate. The example from psychoanalysis that Masson provides also demonstrates various facets of the complexity of resistance. Those challenging the existence or impact of child sexual abuse may be motivated by a desire to keep their own abuse history or their history of violation away from their own awareness or the awareness of others. Several chapters observed the boundary violations and abuses of at least some psychoanalysts closely connected with Freud (see Middleton, Chapter 2; Rachman, Chapter 3) and Middleton (2018; see also Rachman, Chapter 3) has pointed out the abuse histories in many famed analysts, including Freud himself. Yet, there are other personal motives that may also help explain the nature of resistance that Masson faced when the reputation of Freud was at stake.

Freud and his followers: The man and his ideas as a foundation of identity

A young upstart (Masson) attacking the very fabric of psychoanalysis from within would inevitably lead to misgivings and strong feelings, including anger,

DOI: 10.4324/9781003431466-14

resentment, righteous indignation and envy-fuelled hostility. Powerful projective and parallel processes would follow, including showing the same disrespect to the 'perpetrator' Masson that he was accused of showing to the 'master' Freud, and publicly rejecting (shaming) him and attacking his character flaws in the same way he publicly 'outed' and attacked the character of Freud. But the visceral response to Masson, the hostile ostracisation and vitriol may speak to processes deeper in the psyche of those who take such exception to empirically informed ideas that contrast with their own well-held beliefs. Such alternative ideas seem to rattle the very core of the person's existence to the point they are not just ideas to be mulled over and with consideration accepted or rejected, but threats to the self so potent they need to be discarded or neutralised quickly and reactively.

The concept of 'the self' is highly debated in psychology and psychoanalysis (Hood, 2012; Kirshner, 1991), with Stolorow and Atwood (2012) pointing out the conceptual and clinical challenges in conceiving of 'the self' as an object or thing separate from the contexts it exists within. Rather, the experiencing of selfhood is always dependent on context and is relational. The development of selfhood is generally understood (e.g., in object-relations, self-psychological and attachment theories) to involve the internalisation of key developmental figures in the person's life and as development progresses through adolescence and adult life on the identification with other objects that give the experience of one's selfhood meaning and shape. Kohut's construct of the selfobjects is of interest here (e.g., Kohut & Wolf, 1978), where external objects (both animate and inanimate) are needed for the development of self and become part of the self; not distinct or independent from one's view of self, but a core part of it. The internalisation of these objects as part of one's view of their self, or self-concept, happens throughout life, as new people, ideas, activities and inanimate objects are internalised into a more rigid or more supple representation (or representations) of self. Thus, developing a representation of the self as a psychotherapist or psychoanalyst requires taking in and merging with one's self-concept the ideas and figures of those being absorbed. In the myriad of content, some will be identified with more profoundly (e.g., Freud vs Klein, Lacan vs Bowlby) in terms of resonance for one's sense of self as a talk therapist (i.e., they will be integrated into the self-concept associated with being a psychotherapist/analyst).

Freud's side-lining of the psychological impact of incestuous abuse for the development of psychopathology allowed him to develop his theory that mental anguish primarily has its origins in fantasies and a failure to satisfactorily resolve them. There is no doubt that the ontological, clinical and theoretical value of fantasy (and phantasy – unconscious fantasies) for understanding mental life (including distress) has been enormous. Yet, as with all good ideas, they can be taken too far or interpreted in too insular a manner. When Masson suggested that Freud turned his back on the truth that childhood sexual abuse by a parental figure was a central aetiological driver for neurotic adaptation, he would have challenged Freud's followers to the core. Their professional identities were built on a strong identification with the man of Freud, and his theories, and to have his legacy sullied would have felt like a personal and professional affront. Masson's attack on Freud was very deeply personal and not levelled at a figure who died 45 years before the book's publication, but (perhaps unwittingly) at a man whose representation was not independent or separate from some contemporary analysts' sense of self. Therefore, Masson's thesis was a direct shot into the heart of who they were and how they functioned. As American novelist James Baldwin (1961) so eloquently stated, 'Nothing is more desirable than to be released from an affliction, but nothing is more frightening than to be divested of a crutch' (p. xii). Masson (1984) was doing both with *The Assault on Truth*, where the affliction of fantasy dominating reality could be remedied to free up thinking and technique but this also knocked out a crutch that supported the analysts' identity.

Additionally, Masson cast doubt on the courage and integrity that Freud's followers experienced him as having or imagined him to have. Like Freud himself, when presented with major challenges to his ideas, his followers in the face of Masson's accusations fought off the threat with great vigour. This was done in an effort to not only preserve the reputation of Freud as a tireless pursuer of truth no matter what the cost but also to preserve their own identities that were built on him and his ideas. Not only had they internalised Freud's ideas, but they also seemed to have replicated his way of dealing with any challenges to these ideas. Kluft (Chapter 4) notes that Freud's followers learned from his playbook when dealing with threats to his theorising. Similar to Jung, Ferenczi and Adler, who were all attacked and ostracised by Freud for questioning his orthodoxy, Masson fell to the same fate for the same heretical crime at the hands of Freud's exponents. Masson's courage, brashness, impiety, impertinence and desire to be heard in a very public manner may have made him an easier target for attack and offered both conscious and unconscious justifications for those impelled to not only point the gun but pull the trigger. It is likely however that even without these qualities, Masson was already well in the firing line.

One would expect that the harshest critics were those whose professional self-identities were tied up with Freud the man. Consistent with this, Masson's introductory chapter in this book notes the experience of being told by a former friend that 'Our friendship was based on a mutual respect for Sigmund Freud'. Here the preservation of self and selfobjects (i.e., Freud the Man, his ideas and his movement) needed to trump a long-term friendship. The ideas and person who challenged the selfobjects (i.e., Masson) needed to be dismissed, minimised and at times attacked to disarm his threat. In short, for those whose professional identity was built on Freud, his ideas and his character were not abstract concepts that could be entertained with a degree of distance and subjective curiosity, but rather they were and are foundation stones for their identity. Here self-identification becomes based on (1) Freud the man, (2) his ideas and (3) the movement and profession he generated: psychoanalysis. Thus, attacks on Freud are felt with crippling force to various pillars of psychological existence.

The same principle may be at work in religious settings, where the church, its leader/s and its underpinning ideas are so important to the sense of self for people who identify with them, that an abusive member of the clergy is seen as a victim of scurrilous rumour and personal attack rather than the perpetrator of a heinous crime. The selfobject (e.g., the church, its leader/s) so central to the person's sense of self then remains protected and the self is buoyed against threatening attack.

Kluft (Chapter 4) offers an examination of the character of Freud, from his doubts about his ideas and capacities to his determination to be solely revered and remembered. Drawing on Freud's own selfobject tendencies to have around him people who shone him in a positive light and venerated him, while cutting out competitors and those who might challenge openly what he had to offer, he was able to build and maintain his theoretical and clinical empire. This empire like that of all others has brought the world some treasures and some trash, with the latter the cause of much harm. In our Preface we showed the framing of Freud by disciples like Ernest Jones as honest and trustworthy beyond reproach, failed to convey the complexity of Freud the man, who was not above human fallibility and could ignore truths or interfere in the affairs of others to feather his own nest. Kluft (Chapter 4) notes the imprimatur of Freud and the ways he ruthlessly and determinedly maintained his ideas and approaches meant that close scrutiny has not been imposed upon aspects of his work, with psychoanalysis being historically phobic of self-reflection and very late to the party of empirical investigation. Freud jettisoned ideas and techniques that might challenge psychoanalysis and Kluft argued that (beyond moving away from the core impact of child sexual abuse) his treatment of hypnosis was amongst his most egregious actions.

'Whack-a-mole'

The impact of sexual abuse in childhood that Masson was again bringing to light was also innately activating because of how it confronts personal beliefs about the world, including human capacities for cruelty, the satisfaction of one's own needs at the cost of others and the failure to protect the innocent and vulnerable (Herman, 1992). Knowing such things challenges the comfort that ignorance and silence may bring. Several chapters in this book examine to varying degrees the difficulty child abuse has had coming into full public consciousness for any length of time. Like the unwitting target in a game of whack-a-mole, its head pops up, typically courtesy of the courage of those mobilised to make its agonising silence audible, before it is quickly clobbered back down. Jennifer Freyd's concept of DARVO (Deny, Attack, Reverse Victim and Offender) and the application of her own Betrayal Trauma theory to institutions in which there is a capacity to be blind to their own betrayals (Chapter 6), speaks to ways and means the mole can be whacked. DARVO allows the alleged perpetrator to protect their own reputation by attacking the reputation of the alleged victim. It is an active strategy needed if the 'threat' cannot be neutralised in more passive or indirect ways. Institutional betrayal is less active in nature as it turns a blind eye to truths, visible but too inconvenient to see. This sort of motivated ignorance operates in individuals and society at large (Freyd, 1996; Freyd & Birrell, 2013), and renders DARVO unnecessary if the truth can be expunged before it forcefully enters one's own awareness or that of others.

Several chapters provide a sobering message of the reality of different manifestations of denial associated with child sexual abuse and the impact of child abuse and neglect more broadly on psychiatric distress. We now have dedicated journals devoted to studying the impact of childhood maltreatment. Large epidemiological studies exist on the prevalence and impact of childhood abuse. Professional societies have been set up for those studying and treating individuals impacted by relational trauma exposure in childhood and its impact throughout the lifespan. Yet, as Read (Chapter 12) points out, the dominant theories associated with the aetiology and maintenance of psychopathology are biological and genetic. He persuasively argues that environmental theories associated with abuse are drowned out or even inhibited by biological accounts fuelled by pharmaceutical company interests.

Additionally, mental health professionals are often still reluctant to see human cruelty and the narcissistic use of children as objects for self-satisfaction as viable dominant accounts of psychological misery. Genetics and biology remain more savoury in explaining psychiatric distress than the chronic impact of children being mistreated by those entrusted with their care. Those around Freud found the idea that hysteria was caused by adults sexually abusing children unacceptable, but the theory that children want to be seduced or have phantasies of being seduced by their opposite-sex parent was a more palatable account. Biology and genetics currently offer more tolerable (and profitable) alternatives to child abuse as an explanation for the development of psychiatric disorders. Yet research findings, the advent of trauma-informed care and efforts to integrate real-life experience with biological accounts (see the rich literature on the biology of posttraumatic stress disorder and dissociative disorders – e.g., Schiavone & Lanius, 2023; Nijenhuis, 2023) have created enough of an impact to hold some cautious optimism that the next backlash against child abuse will not lead to wholesale denial of its existence and may limit forces operating to undermine the nature and extent of its impact on psychological function in children, adolescents and adults.

Still backlash against the existence, prevalence or impact of child abuse which follows interest and progression in understanding can be pernicious. Seemingly when the implications of the topic get too much to handle, the natural tendency is to attack the reality of child abuse rather than face the implications of it. Drawing on *The Assault on Truth*, Read also reminds us that one way this was done in Freud's time was by coming to see those who disclosed incidents of sexual abuse as liars and fantasists. This seemed to represent an early example of professional DARVO, where the denial from doctors was facilitated by blaming children for creating stories that tarnished the reputation of adults.

In the modern era, Crook (Chapter 7) shows that one way this reactive denial, with its retreat away from the existence, prevalence and impact of childhood sexual abuse, played out was in the so-called recovered memory wars. This had as its precursor the growing acceptance and acknowledgement of childhood sexual abuse in the 1980s and began to galvanise in 1991. Accusations of sexual abuse in childhood by a family member were promoted as false memories via the creation of a catchy nomenclature designed to capture a non-existent psychological condition that provided an active defence against the existence of incest (or other forms of sexual abuse): false memory syndrome. This rhetoric gave the general population an easy-to-understand and very accessible narrative to distance from the reality of childhood sexual abuse. They could believe that the disclosures of those affected were the result of false memories rather than the explication of actual events. Those accused also had a ready legal defence, which in the 1990s and early 21st century, was highly effective courtesy of shrewd marketing and the well-resourced coffers fed by those accused of abuse. A willing media also played its part, lapping up and distributing unfounded claims of widespread 'false memory' production of child sexual abuse memories by unwitting or even malevolent therapists. Therapists were framed as the enemy that needed to be stopped by any means, which included picketing, intimidating, suing, shaming and getting the false memory message out to the public. Textbooks for students training to be mental health professionals were also part of this 'campaign'. The False Memory Syndrome Foundation was the group behind this active movement to silence by force victims of childhood sexual abuse and protect those allegedly perpetrating the abuse. DARVO was their primary operating strategy. It would be ill-advised to think that people can't have memories that are distorted, inaccurate or even at times created, but there is no evidence that wholesale creation of a memory that did not reflect autobiographical experience in some form is the primary reason adults disclose experiences of sexual abuse in their childhood. But this 'assault on truth' does offer a very effective means of arming oneself against the reality of child molestation by those in caring roles. With the false memory message, the public and media 'were sold a pup', but the human tendencies to find ways to distance from the existence and outcome of childhood sexual abuse meant this particular pup was very cute and too alluring to step back from and see that it was not what it seemed.

Courtois (Chapter 8) tracks the history of the modern study and treatment of incest, which began to come out of the shadows courtesy of the feminist movement in the 1960s and 1970s. It led to some social acceptance of the reality of incest around the time, and immediately after, Masson's work in the mid-1980s, until what she described as the predicted backlash arrived. Enter the memory wars and the rise of influence in 'false memory syndrome' in the early 1990s to squash the reality and impact of family members sexually violating their own kin. Courtois notes the ongoing efforts through 'language muting' to suppress the term 'incest' by encapsulating it under more tolerable terms (e.g., childhood maltreatment). She also argues that a contemporary form of ignorance and denial of incest and its effects comes in the form of recent laws in the US restricting or denying women their reproductive rights, including terminating pregnancy resulting from incest or rape. Such experiences and their real-life repercussions are seen as less important than forcing a woman to have no choice in how she deals with her pregnancy and the circumstance that brought it about; again suppressing the reality and impact of sexual abuse, but with 'new clothing' via a different rhetoric to promote the denial and suppression.

Childhood sexual trauma need not be denied to have a pernicious impact on one's functioning and thinking, it can have the same outcome if it's acknowledged but ignored. The costs have been all too real in the field of psychoanalysis, the tradition Masson was schooled in and then critiqued. Rachman (Chapter 3) captures the immense consequences of both denial and ignorance in comparing the psychological journeys of Freud and Ferenczi regarding their own personal experiences of child molestation and its impact on their theorising. He argues that Freud's failure to face his sexual abuse at the hands of his nursemaid impeded his ability to see the true impact of such mistreatment on psychological distress. The aetiological dominance of fantasy offered a more attractive and less emotionally evocative starting place. His oedipal theory was centrally organised around sex in childhood, so the topic matter was not far away from his own experience, but with the child's fantasies as the driver not their actual experience at the hands of an adult. Rachman outlines how this failure to address his personal abuse history limited Freud as a therapist not just a theorist, such that he could not go to places where victims of sexual abuse needed him to go. Ferenczi felt the force of this when Freud analysed him, and Ferenczi's abuse history remained off the table. Yet, his work with Elizabeth Severn allowed Ferenczi to not only know what had occurred to him but also the impact of it. It was acknowledged, faced and processed. Ferenczi then came to see and accept the immense value in Freud's seduction theory, but his efforts to revive and expand on child sexual abuse as a primary driver for psychiatric disorders were ridiculed and he was excoriated and rejected from the psychoanalytic community; another victim of bravely speaking about the impact of childhood molestation. Middleton (Chapter 2) shows how others have fallen to the same fate when they have tried to reintroduce childhood sexual abuse into analytic theory as a competitor to fantasy; Robert Fliess and Jeffrey Masson are among them.

Even Freud himself fell foul of not keeping silent when he first introduced his seduction theory and experienced the same initial fate (ridicule and ostracisation). Yet, Lothane (Chapter 5) counters the claim that Freud abandoned his seduction theory. He makes the case that Freud himself has become the victim of denial where his persistent acceptance of the aetiological importance of seduction for psychopathology is evident throughout his body of work, but this has been denied and dismissed by Masson and others. Lothane argues that neither seduction nor phantasy in isolation offers an adequate psychological formulation of the drivers of psychiatric distress, positing that both need to be considered: real experience and imagination. For Lothane, Masson overstated the 'real' while orthodox Freudians, unlike Freud himself, largely ignored it.

Brave new world

A lot has changed in the domain of psychotherapy since 1984, and the world into which *The Assault on Truth* was born is different to the one in which this current volume takes its first breath of life, some 40 years on. Psychotherapeutically and socially the reality and impact of childhood sexual abuse is a widely accepted fact, even if there are some vocal pockets that dispute or ignore one or both of these factors (see McMaugh & Dorahy, Chapter 10). Arguably more so than ever, the consulting room has become a space open to discussions of the personal cost of child abuse in its various forms. McMaugh and Dorahy (Chapter 10) note that along with *The Assault on Truth*, the women's movement and the dissociative disorders field have had a role to play in widening and deepening acceptance of child abuse and its consequences. They discuss the 'gendering' of the child abuse narrative, where in medical and mental health settings women have been the primary disclosers of child abuse. Yet, women have generally been seen as poor reporters of their own history, prone to fantasy, fabrication and hysterical exaggeration. McMaugh and Dorahy point out that disbelief, victim blaming and dilution of the impact of abuse may all present themselves in the minds of both the client and therapist, to create some psychological space from the impacts of child abuse. Acknowledgement of these is an important part of the therapeutic journey, and they need to be 'held lightly' and not acted upon.

Epstein (Chapter 9) outlines the rise in attachment theory, trauma-informed practitioners and body-mind integration that now characterises much of the trauma therapy field. Her case of Mary captures these themes in modern-day therapy, including technological advances that allowed for, and created the challenges of, working online during Covid lockdowns. Such an environment is an anathema to the sanctity of physical intimacy and face-to-face contact in psychotherapy but became a necessity to maintain connectedness while social distancing was required. Advances in technology raise opportunities and challenges for trauma therapy and society more broadly. They also allow another unsavoury reality of child sexual abuse to be exposed in an accessible way to anyone who has an internet connection; that it can be well organised, sadistic and perpetrated by groups of offenders, including those leading 'double lives' in the public spotlight. These are all key features of Epstein's case of Mary and a reality grappled with increasingly in the clinical literature (see Middleton, 2023).

Despite advances made in the recognition and treatment of trauma disorders and the manner in which symptoms arise from various forms of child abuse, the whole enterprise of psychological therapy has not gone unchallenged. Cohen's thesis draws on Masson's critique that psychotherapy is a failed enterprise and a tool of oppression especially for women and children. It provides sober and challenging reading that rattles the cage of those at the coal face doing therapy with vulnerable individuals, giving them pause for thought. *The Assault on Truth* was about challenging understanding, confronting idealisation and attempting to bring into focus the abysmal treatment of victimised children, women and men in psychiatric and psychological thinking. It behoves all of us to challenge our perceptions, see the filters we have over our own eyes and acknowledge the limitations of our work and the forces operating in our professions. We (the two editors) found Cohen's chapter confronting and difficult to grapple with, seeing ourselves as so-called trauma therapists. We also appreciate what it forces us to do in terms of looking carefully at what we engage in and how we are part of a bigger system. Rather than succumb to the temptation to defensively retreat into the comfort of what we each find familiar we must look carefully at what we do and how we do it. We need to acknowledge how the forces of oppression may operate in subtle and overt ways within our chosen professions and within ourselves. Such reflections may expose painful and unwanted truths that via our own actions and/or beliefs we have passively or actively initiated or perpetuated harm.

Becoming aware of the harm created by holding onto views that a client's sexual abuse history reflected what they imagined rather than what they experienced may have been too painful for some analysts confronted with Masson's thesis, and attack offered the best form of defence. We are challenged to notice how our efforts to assist our clients may not always be helpful for personal, systemic and/or structural reasons. Cohen's brave chapter in a book of this nature follows the work of Masson in asking us to examine the lenses that may have us distorting or denying what is real.

What do we take away

As we come to the end of this collective enterprise, which set out to (1) commemorate the publication of *The Assault on Truth* and (2) examine how the reality and impact of child abuse have fared in the 40 years since its publication, several salient points can be distilled from the chapters. These points have implications for society at large, professions within the mental health and health sectors and each person reading this book. We conclude with them and hope they, and the chapters of this book, may carry sway as the intolerability of child sexual abuse and abuse of all kinds becomes again too hard to face and efforts are made to attack the victim with ignorance or blame, lambast those trying to help or protect those engaged in mistreatment.

- Empathy towards children has been an uneven, late historical achievement and Lloyd de Mause (2002) notes 'the world is now in a race between our slowly improving child rearing and our rapidly evolving destructive technology' (p. viii).
- The most pathogenic factor in human 'dis-ease' is not deficits in neurotransmitters associated with inherited brain malfunctions that cause problems with psychological structure (Salmon, 2004) but mankind itself.
- There is a congruence in multiple published studies which indicate that around two-thirds of mental health patients seen in either inpatient or outpatient settings will have a childhood history of sexual and/or physical abuse (e.g., Read et al., 2004).
- Young people (e.g., aged 16–24 years) are much more likely to have mental health disorders if they have experienced childhood maltreatment (Mathews et al., 2023).
- The existence, prevalence and impact of child sexual abuse have always sat uncomfortably in the human psyche and data regarding them are profoundly susceptible to being distorted, avoided or expunged.
- A sense of safety underpinned by ideas like the world is safe, fair and just is severely threatened by the reality and impact of child abuse. It can evoke less fear, powerlessness and shame maintaining such ideas over the realities which threaten them.
- Systems and individuals resistant to the impact of child abuse are more likely to pathologise the victim by focusing on what is wrong with them than understand

the victim by focusing on what has happened to them and how they have adapted.

- The next potent backlash against the biopsychosocial impact of child abuse is most reasonably assessed, based on past experience, as not being too far away, if it can be even argued that the last one has passed (e.g., 'false memory syndrome').
- The world is filled with notable citizens who lead exemplary public lives, yet at home are abusers and tyrants. Their activities and behaviours are offered camouflage by the position in social and civil life they hold.
- Mankind can organise through its churches, sporting bodies, scouting groups, online groupings and various other institutions (including 'the family'), the abuse of children in industrial numbers. Here like-minded individuals may find each other and foster their secret activities, often for years and in some cases decades.
- When we make a hero out of anyone, we tend to diminish ourselves. Our ability to think for ourselves is stifled as we create and give over to a 'greater power'.
- Freud's desire to be recognised and his attitude and behaviour towards dissenters sat alongside his genius and his abiding contribution to social and psychological life. These complex attributes made him more 'man' than 'god'. While admiration is warranted, worship is mistaken.
- When publishing *The Assault on Truth*, Masson was not only dealing with analysts trying to preserve the reputation of Freud and his ideas but also those trying to protect their own identity, and the selfobjects which underpinned their professional sense of self.
- In surveying the landscape we have covered with this volume, we are reminded of an observation (sometimes attributed to Albert Einstein, and perhaps a unifying observation of those who find themselves in the role of whistle-blower): 'Blind belief in authority is the greatest enemy of truth'.
- The mental health professions, specifically psychiatry and psychology, have been at the centre of attempts to deny the impact and prevalence of child sexual abuse and child abuse of all forms for over a century, even when society has been open to hearing about such realities. In light of the evidence afforded by years of clinical, phenomenological, neurobiological and psychosocial research, each mental health professional can now judge whether they themselves perpetuate this denial or acknowledge the painful reality of many of those who seek their assistance.

References

Baldwin, J. (1961). *Nobody knows my name*. Penguin

De Mause, L. (2002). *The emotional life of nations*. Karnac.

Freyd, J. J. (1996). *Betrayal trauma: The logic of forgetting childhood abuse*. Harvard University Press.

Freyd, J. J., & Birrell, P. J. (2013). *Blind to betrayal: Why we fool ourselves we aren't being fooled.* Wiley.

Herman, J. L. (1992). *Trauma and recovery.* Basic Books/Hachette Book Group.
Hood, B. (2012). *The self illusion: How the social brain creates identity.* Oxford University Press.
Kirshner, L. A. (1991). The concept of the self in psychoanalytic theory and its philosophical foundations. *Journal of the American Psychoanalytic Association, 39*(1), 157–182. https://doi.org/10.1177/000306519103900108
Kohut, H., & Wolf, E. S. (1978). The disorders of the self and their treatment: An outline. *The International Journal of Psychoanalysis*, *59*, 413–425.
Masson, J. (1984). *The assault on truth: Freud's suppression of the seduction theory.* Farrar, Straus, & Giroux.
Mathews, B., Pacella, R., Scott, J. G., Finkelhor, D., Meinck, F., Higgins, D. J., Erskine, H. E., Thomas, H. J., Lawrence, D. M., Haslam, D. M., Malacova, E., & Dunne, M. P. (2023). The prevalence of child maltreatment in Australia: Findings from a national survey. *The Medical Journal of Australia, 218*(Suppl 6), S13–S18. https://doi.org/10.5694/mja2.51873
Middleton, W. (2018.) Robert Fliess, Wilhelm Fliess, Ernest Jones, Sandor Ferenczi and Sigmund Freud. In *The abused and the abuser: Victim–perpetrator dynamics* (pp. 234–250). Routledge.
Middleton, W. (2023). Beyond death: Enduring Incest – The fusion of father with daughter. In M. J. Dorahy, S. N. Gold, & J. A. O'Neil, (Eds.), *Dissociation and the dissociative disorders: Past, present, future* (2nd ed.) (pp. 223–237). Routledge.
Nijenhuis, E. R. S. (2023). Towards an ecology of dissociation in the context of trauma: Implications for the psychobiological study of dissociative disorders. In M. J. Dorahy, S. N. Gold, & J. A. O'Neil, (Eds.), *Dissociation and the dissociative disorders: Past, present, future* (2nd ed.) (pp. 602–633). Routledge.
Read, J., Goodman, L., Morrison, A. P., Ross, C. A., & Aderhold, V. (2004). Childhood trauma, loss and stress. In J. Read, L. R. Mosher, & R. Bentall (Eds.), *Models of madness* (pp. 223–252). Brunner-Routledge.
Salmon, P. (2004). The schizococcus: An interpersonal perspective. *Personal Construct Theory & Practice, 1,* 76–81.
Schiavone, F. L., & Lanius, R. A. (2023). The neurobiology of dissociation in chronic PTSD. In M. J. Dorahy, S. N. Gold, & J. A. O'Neil, (Eds.), *Dissociation and the dissociative disorders: Past, present, future* (2nd ed.) (pp. 634–642). Routledge.
Stolorow, R. D., & Atwood, G. E. (2012) Deconstructing "the self" of self psychology. *International Journal of Psychoanalytic Self Psychology, 7*(4), 573–576. https://doi.org/10.1080/15551024.2012.710930

Postscript

Preliminary Notes Toward a New Psychoanalysis and Facilitating Psychoanalysts' Work with Dissociative Disorder Patients

Richard P. Kluft

The editors of this volume presented me with an intimidating challenge – to envision a modern psychoanalysis both attentive to the concerns raised by Masson and others and able to embrace and reintegrate concepts and observations exiled from mainstream psychoanalytic interest and attention for over 125 years. I will attempt to do so by offering preliminary notes toward a new psychoanalysis, and a pragmatic introduction to psychoanalytic/psychodynamic work with dissociative disorders. These overlap somewhat.

Two introductory remarks are necessary. First, rather than repeating subject matter covered in my earlier chapter, I will refer the reader to that source (see Chapter 4). Second, although Freud began to develop his "psycho-analysis" from the study of severe hysterics (who today would be diagnosed as suffering dissociative disorders and complex posttraumatic stress disorder [PTSD]), his focus shifted as he moved toward what became the psychoanalysis of today (Berman, 1981; Brenner, 2009; Kluft, 1995a, 2018a, 2018b, 2018c, 2018d). Viewed objectively, Freud's early hypnosis-based work with this group of patients was rather effective, but in developing his new approach, he developed both theories and techniques that may actually have been his greatest contribution to patient care. Freud was the first to develop an effective treatment for those who were not amenable to treatment with hypnosis (Kluft, 2018c, 2018d).

Over the years, "hysteric" gradually became a synonym for patients with Oedipal issues, good subjects for psychoanalysis, and the "grand hysterics" of Freud's early efforts were subsumed under emergent psychotic diagnoses (Rosenbaum, 1980). Freud's clinical work moved toward what we now would consider character neuroses, with his efforts more directed toward conflictual dynamics than exploring severe symptoms. Many years would pass before the dissociative disorders would be extricated from a tangle of misdiagnoses and receive serious attention in their own right. The grand hysterics of the past and the dissociatives of the present have always been with us, their existence often obscured by changes in theory and diagnostic fashion.

Preliminary notes toward a new psychoanalysis

Implicit in the editors' challenge was the need to address problematic considerations in psychoanalytic thinking, and acknowledge their deleterious impacts,

DOI: 10.4324/9781003431466-15

many left largely unexamined for generations. This would necessitate placing external and psychological reality on an equal plane, removing obstacles to a revision and expansion of traditional psychoanalysis in order to both create a more trauma-sensitive approach and build an enabling array of pragmatic clinical bridges between classical techniques and the interventions helpful in work with patient populations Freud had marginalized (Berman, 1981; Brenner, 2009; Kluft, 1995a, 2000, Chapter 4). These remarks can do no more than begin the exploration of these complex and potentially controversial difficulties and propose preliminary steps toward their resolution (see Kluft, 2018a, 2018b, 2018c, 2018d; Chapter 4). Notwithstanding his marginalizing the importance of exogenous trauma as his theories evolved, Freud was an astute traumatologist. His 1914 "Remembering, Repeating, and Working Through" remains a landmark among trauma studies.

Revisiting ideas long revered but remaining suppositional

Psychoanalysis is rife with individual and institutional beliefs or countertransferences that conflate loyalty to Freud and Freud's metapsychology with the defense of scientific psychoanalytic truth. However, several of Freud's long-held concepts and ideas remain unproven (Ratner, 2019). These include his ideas about abuse, dissociation, and hypnosis (see Chapter 4).

Freud wrote that the abstractions in his theories were dispensable (see Waelder, 1962) and then acted as if they were beyond question. Eisogesis (see Chapter 4) is a form of inquiry designed to find and demonstrate what the person formulating the mode of inquiry already believes is the case. Freud's eisogetic style has instructed generations of analysts to search for and emphasize apparent expressions of his theories in their clinical practices and theory-building, independent of their validity or relevance in a given case. Should we not reconsider the wise guidance offered in Freud's more balanced recommendation; however, often it was contradicted by his behavior?

Democratized theorization and theory-free assessment of data

It is unrealistic to believe that efforts to demonstrate/explore/confirm valued abstract notions with other abstractions, however tightly reasoned, will bring psychoanalysis increased validation and respect in the eyes of non-psychoanalysts, academics, scientists, consumers, and third parties. Demonstrations that psychoanalysis reduces distressing symptoms and improves subjective well-being, metrics far from mainstream psychoanalytic considerations, would provide more compelling arguments.

It is essential to consider all data as worthy of study and exploration. Studying basic data without *a priori* assumptions that they convey or imply particular unconscious meanings or bear implications of particular configurations actually facilitates understanding the transference. A dynamic may be, or may be believed to be, universal, but this does not mean that it speaks to the crucial concerns in a given case. Luborsky and his colleagues have demonstrated (e.g., Luborsky, 1996; Luborsky

& Crits-Christoph, 1998) that patients' configurations of unconscious conflicts and transferential concerns are always in the process of declaring themselves. Why leap to "off-the-rack" top-down eisogetic models of understanding when customized individualized bottom-up understandings are there for the taking?

When clinicians approach patients with minds dedicated to discovering manifestations of (presumedly) universal dynamics, they risk privileging preconceptions above the pursuit of the deeper understanding of those particular individuals. They risk implicitly and explicitly suggesting, and then interpreting, dynamics that may never have been either true or pre-eminently salient but now always will be. When interpretations are made on the basis of assumptions rather than actual clinical data, treatment may go awry or become hopelessly intellectualized. Granted, if treatment is influenced or even dominated by eisogetic understandings shared by analyst and analysand alike, a healing ritual may occur independent of the accuracy or veracity of that frame of reference (see Ellenberger, 1970; Frank, 1973). Problems may arise when the patient cannot/does not/will not work within the frame supported by the analyst (see Kluft, 1992).

The joint acceptance of unwanted realities

Marginalizing the significance of unwanted reality events in the etiology of psychological suffering ranks among the most toxic residua of Freud's moving from a trauma-based understanding of mental distress to a model focused on psychological reality.

Gubrich-Simitis (1984) described the importance of the joint acceptance, by analyst and patient alike, of the reality and importance of the patient's traumatic experiences. She and Oliner (1996) explored reality issues in the treatment of Holocaust victims and second-generation Holocaust survivors. Shengold (1989) dealt with acknowledging the issues of dissociation and reality events in the traumatized. Kogan (2003) considered the importance of both past trauma and contemporary stressors in the analyses of second-generation Holocaust survivors. Leuzinger-Bohleber (2008) analyzed the many layers of pain overlying unresolved childhood medical traumata.

These analysts approached the treatment of the traumatized by creating an atmosphere of shared acceptance and understanding of the reality of trauma in their patients' lives. They argued that without an acknowledgment of the reality of trauma in an individual's life as a baseline, the impacts of reality and manifestations of transference phenomena may become confused with one another. This makes it difficult to work within the as-if, ludic world of transference, compromising a major aspect of analytic treatment.

Analysts as a group seem to deal more readily with traumata not obscured by traditions of long-standing denial or displacement into abstract and hermeneutic realms. However, less publicly expressed forms of trauma long discounted in analysis, such as the abuse of individual women and children, often continue both to receive less vocal advocacy and to receive less sensitive handling in analytic settings. At several recent psychoanalytic meetings, I have gone from presentations that discussed the traumatization of minorities with profound sensitivity to presentations in which allegations of childhood mistreatment by an individual woman were greeted with queries as to whether these might be fantasies.

Psychoanalysis erred in failing to acknowledge the prevalence of these commonplace indignities and atrocities (Simon, 1992). When such events are reported by patients, they are likely to be true in whole or in part (see Brown, Scheflin, & Hammond, 1998; Kluft, 1995b). Absent denial, the world stands revealed as a meaner and more dangerous place. Many of our analysands and psychotherapy patients must contend with the impact of harm deliberately inflicted upon them by others. Given that, therapeutic approaches that fail to acknowledge unwanted realities risk adding insult to the injuries of those already traumatized (Kluft, 2016).

The persistence of these long-standing and often vigorously defended errors remains a discourtesy to patients and a cancer on the credibility and integrity of psychoanalysis as a profession and paradigm of thought. My experience and findings suggest that distortions (often inadvertently) built into the framework of psychoanalysis as a model and profession often have rendered it insensitive to injustices of many sorts, especially to those it has repeatedly overlooked or inflicted as a matter of course (Masson, 1984; Kluft, Chapter 4).

Undoing Freud's mischaracterizations of hypnosis

Sigmund Freud's mischaracterizations of hypnosis have long been misunderstood as accurate critiques of its shortcomings and dangers. This has been addressed in detail elsewhere (Kluft, 2018a, b, c, d, Chapter 4; O'Neil, 2018) and need not be repeated here.

Dissociative identity disorder (DID) patients constitute the most highly hypnotizable clinical population (Frischholz, Lipman, Braun, & Sachs, 1992). Even if no effort is made to induce hypnosis, autohypnotic and spontaneous trance episodes are inevitable in their treatments. Instances of trance logic, the simultaneous acceptance of incompatible perceptions, opinions, and similar distortions abound. They do not necessarily indicate psychotic or borderline psychopathology in the highly hypnotizable. Further, instances of strong emotion that might raise concerns about loss of reality testing usually respond to more frequent therapist interventions, which provide grounding and orientation. When patients seem stuck in altered states, usually gentle observation of that fact, increasing the frequency and length of therapist interventions, and requesting a reconfiguration of the executive aspects of the alter system prove helpful. That is, after commenting on what seems to be causing the current difficulty, asking upset parts of the mind to step back and calmer elements to assist in supporting stability is often helpful. These are appeals to the unintegrated components of the patient's observing ego in support of safety and the therapeutic alliance, akin to intervening with any upset patient in treatment. Whenever possible, a patient should not be allowed to leave the session in a dysfunctional state, and advised against resuming usual activities until settled.

Dissociative patients may have very vivid visual imagery and other intense sensory experiences. It is often possible to facilitate the treatment not only by enlisting the participation of various alters as noted above, but also by asking about visual, auditory, and physical sensations (including haptics) associated with topics under discussion. I often inquire about gustatory and olfactory elements, which often open up powerfully withheld shame aspects of abuse experiences.

Please note the minimal role of suggestion in the above discussion. Freud's emphasis on this element alone mischaracterizes hypnosis. In dealing with dissociative patients in psychoanalytic/psychodynamic therapies, attention to modularity and altered states are important foci, although the use of gentle suggestion in the service of stability may be useful (e.g., Brenner, 2018; Kluft, 2000, 2022a, 2022b).

Interpretation in a new key

Heinz Kohut (1970, 1977; Kohut & Wolf, 1978) observed the intrusive, invasive, potentially aggressive, guilt-, and shame-provoking aspects of interpretation along classical lines. Interpretation within a self-psychological framework (Kohut & Wolf, 1978; Lessem, 2005) leads with empathic understanding. Some models in object-relations theory and relational thinking are perceptively sensitive within their paradigms to the impact of what transpires within the therapist/patient dyad (e.g., Bromberg, 2006, 2011; Caligor, Diamond, Yeomans, & Kernberg, 2009).

However, these approaches do not address adequately certain problems encountered in working with the severely traumatized, especially the traumatized dissociative patient. A revised psychoanalysis must be sensitive to the fact that the traumatized, or those who may prove to have been traumatized, will usually respond to any observation that concerns a potential weakness, failure, erotic, aggressive, or other anxiety-ridden subject as proof that the analyst is finally saying what they feared the analyst had been thinking all along (i.e., that they caused the abuses that were visited upon them). What the analyst understands as careful exploration in the service of understanding may be experienced by the patient as implying or stating the analyst's feared, but previously unstated, condemnations.

Early in my career, a fellow analytic candidate covered my inpatient practice in my absence. A brutalized and trafficked DID patient from a paradoxically abusive but rigidly Roman Catholic family became infatuated with him. My colleague made superficially accurate (but unfortunate) observations about her feelings. That night she attempted to hang herself.

Upon my return, she said nothing for a week. Then, she "confessed" that my colleague understood her far better than I. He had found the core of evil, unbridled lust that she had tried to hide. She now presented a revised version of her history in which her evil inclinations and mortal sins had brought others' sexual advances upon her. Of course, she was incested and prostituted by her parents! They knew she "wanted it," etc.

Actually, afraid and feeling rejected in my absence, some parts regressed to a defensive posture of anticipating sexual subjugation to those she feared would hurt or abandon her. Her "erotic feelings" were defensive, expressed with strong feelings, but with only minimal elements of actual sexual interest.

While this example is extreme in degree, it is not unusual in kind. Approaching traumatized patients with a scheme of understanding that brings with it the risk of imputing dangerously inaccurate, incomplete, or easily misconstrued meanings is best avoided.

Interpretations ideally should focus primarily on helping the patient understand the patient's mind and experience of circumstances. This newer stance would actually encourage less constraint in making extra-analytic interpretations. While classical analytic training still focuses primarily on psychoanalysis, it neglects the fact that most psychoanalysts spend only a fraction of their time doing classic psychoanalysis. This strongly suggests that many treatments by analysts cannot focus primarily on matters of classical transference, as if a classical transference neurosis were in place. Many patients will talk primarily about their problems and relationships with others. It is worth wondering whether judicious occasional extra-analytic observations may not only help patients in the here and now but may also help them learn more about the transference concept "at a safe distance," which may in turn enable them to better address traditional transferences as their treatments progress.

Facilitating psychoanalytic/psychodynamic work with dissociative disorder patients

Freud marginalized dissociation and treated the dissociative disorders dismissively (e.g., Berman, 1981). The world of dissociation is not the world of the Freudian unconscious and has received minimal acknowledgment from mainstream psychoanalysis (Brenner, 2001, 2009; Kluft, 2000, 2022a, 2022b). No current psychoanalytic (or non-psychoanalytic) model successfully encompasses the complete range of phenomena within the dissociative domain (see Cardeña, 1994; Kluft, 2022a, 2022b). Normal forms of dissociation such as meditation, intense prayer, reveries, day-dreaming, and mild spontaneous trance (see Butler, 2006) should be understood, lest all dissociative phenomena be misunderstood as pathological.

When colleagues oriented toward relational, intersubjective, and attachment-oriented perspectives returned "dissociation" to psychoanalytic discourse, they defined this term narrowly within their paradigms. Analysts more aware of (1) normative forms of dissociation, (2) dissociative hypnotic and trance phenomena, and (3) stress trauma-related dissociation appreciated the need for more comprehensive and inclusive models (see Kluft, 2022a, 2022b).

That is, relational analytically oriented models have focused primarily on the dissociative defenses as sequelae of relational hurts *per se*, without according importance to dissociation-proneness and the DSM-5 Dissociative Disorders, the primary focus of those in the dissociative disorders field. It is not uncommon for those focused on relational dissociation to omit mention of dissociative disorders from their work (Kluft, 2022b).

The late Philip Bromberg and I (Kluft, 2022a, 2022b) discussed these matters in depth. We concluded that in regarding dissociation as defined by relational/interpersonal/intersubjective approaches, which are amenable to hermeneutic understandings (Stolorow, Brandshaft, & Atwood, 1987), there is a failure to encompass the elements of posttraumatic stress and the major trauma-related dissociative phenomena as encountered in the posttraumatic and dissociative disorders.

To conceptualize these two models as competitive, or to privilege one over the other, is realistic only in the minds of their loyalists. In clinical practice, these models address two different types and realms of phenomena. Both may afflict the same patient. Relational dissociation is often found in the absence of traumatic dissociation (Kluft 2022a, 2022b). Posttraumatic dissociation is more likely to afflict traumatized individuals already rendered vulnerable due to relational dissociation.

The major dissociative disorders, especially DID, are dissociative self-pathologies. Their self-states are centers of initiative and experience, sensitive to rebuffs to their particular senses of self (Kohut, 1970, 1977; Kohut & Wolf, 1978). The notion that one part is or should be considered "the core" or "the real patient," and that the entire treatment should work through that alter, is developmentally absurd, subscribing to wishful myths on the parts of patient and therapist alike. Such myths invite therapeutic misadventure.

DID was previously known as Multiple Personality Disorder. As Coons (1980, 1984) observed, the personality of a patient with multiple personalities is to have multiple personalities. Assuming that dissociative identities that are not obviously active and present are not participants in the therapeutic process at any given moment repeats early relational trauma and is generally injudicious. Failing to consider and understand dissociative identities' wished-for initiatives suggests indirectly that they must act them out to be noticed. Kluft's "Invitational Inclusionism" makes all identities welcome stakeholders in the treatment (Kluft, 2006, 2017). Inviting inclusion is more helpful than distancing, and risking identities' feeling (and being) neglected and/or becoming (or remaining) adversarial.

Accordingly, the approximation of a unified observing ego and optimization of the therapeutic alliance is best promoted by inviting all parts of the mind to understand that the therapy is for all of them, and by the therapist's making that invitation "real" by encouraging their input and participation. The therapist's good relationship across all identities is a potent force for enhancing the therapeutic relationship and for integration. It supports the stance that every issue raised in treatment can be explored for its potential to promote greater insight, deeper empathy, an enhanced therapeutic alliance, and greater inter-identity communication on the way to integration. The therapist can hear what a patient says about a dream, dream element, or any subject at all from the self-state in executive control and follow up by asking if any other parts have something to offer. If a second speaks, one can invite still others. At times it may be useful to actively request additional input from particular identities (Kluft, 2000). Management of the process of working with the patient's system of identities, a matter too complex for exploration here, is discussed in Kluft (2006).

Classic interpretations are designed to render the unconscious conscious. As noted earlier, certain types of interpretation are usually problematic in the traumatized. Currently unavailable traumatic scenarios and deep hurts sequestered in identities and/or shrouded by amnesia are likely dissociated, not repressed (Kluft, 2000, 2006, 2022a; Brenner, 2001, 2004, 2009, 2014). They may be quite familiar to, and known in that moment by, other aspects of mind. The analyst cannot assume that comments on matters apparently out of awareness will not generate powerful reactions within other centers of self-experience.

Shame and narcissistic injury are crucial concerns. Long-dissociated traumatic material often emerges or is shared after shame reduction. Such material may become accessible once shame and fear have been addressed in the context of a safe relationship, and rapport established with those concerned identities who are cooperative and accessible (Kluft, 2000, 2006, Chapter 4). An affect-focused approach to understanding dissociative structures based on Nathanson's (1991) "Compass of Shame" is available (Kluft, 2007).

In instances involving posttraumatic dissociation, it is likely that relational failures have also inflicted powerful foundational hurts. An optimal therapeutic stance will be both warm and more active (Dalenberg, 2000; Kluft, 2000). Too often, classic neutrality will be interpreted as uncaring, hostile, and rejecting. Silence invites the creation and projection of negative fantasies that may undermine the safety of the treatment. Parental neglect, silence, and withdrawal were often routine forms of psychological abuse and/or punishment for many DID patients. Taking a less-than-welcoming stance risks retraumatization (Dalenberg, 2000; Kluft, 2000, see Chapter 4).

The treating clinician is likely to be perceived as an abuser by some or all aspects of the mind, requiring much work in a variety of negative transferences. Further, many transference phenomena that become apparent prove related to fear of the repetition of traumatic scenarios rather than to full or split object relationships with those involved in perpetrating abuse and/or neglect. These traumatic transferences or scenario-based reactions may become manifest abruptly, often in a manner discrepant with the conscious content of the ongoing dialog and/or in conjunction with another identity assuming control of the body and mind. Conversely, they may often be withheld and denied for long periods of time. Unless an acute negative reaction is endangering the treatment, it is often more effective and less threatening to comment on the resemblance of a traumatic scenario to a concern in the present and wonder how it impacted and impacts the patient (perhaps asking for thoughts about that) before commenting directly on how this scenario depicts the therapist. The former allows the traumatic expectation to be discussed from a position of relative safety, while the latter risks the patient feeling the relationship to the therapist is imperiled, which may trigger enactments/reenactments. Often DID patients' dissociating traumatic material involves protecting themselves from appreciating the overall nature of their relationships with those with whom they yearn for safe attachment. Transference interpretations which refer to classic unconscious dynamics are at the core of classical psychoanalysis, but less useful here; transference interpretations which refer to unconscious or dissociated material still far beyond the awareness of an alter in executive control may damage the patient's ability to feel safe and understood, as if the therapist is "making stuff up" or "making them feel crazy."

While modern analysts are generally familiar with models of dissociation discussed in connection with relational failures and relational trauma (e.g., neglect), neither stress-related dissociation (e.g., sexual abuse) nor an understanding of the high-hypnotizable individual are commonly explored in the analytic literature. Contemporary analysts should become familiar with how to assess a patient's proclivity for absorption and range of normal dissociation (Butler, 2006) and ask mental status questions likely to ferret out dissociative symptoms. Grossly apparent dissociative symptoms are often withheld or volunteered tentatively and/or ambiguously. When clinicians do not recognize them as such, and fail to follow them further, valuable therapeutic opportunities are forfeit. Loewenstein's (1991) mental status for the diagnosis of complex, chronic, dissociative disorders is a valuable resource, modeling useful lines of inquiry.

Much as the patient may become disconcerted in dealing with switches between identities, events, feelings, or with information not shared in common across all identities, so may the therapist feel deskilled and overwhelmed until becoming familiar with these clinical phenomena. Further, many therapists, especially those with histories of personal trauma, may suffer painful counteridentifications. In addition, those therapists with high dissociative/hypnotic talent may become swept up in the dissociative patient's dissociative defenses, leading to what Loewenstein (1993) described as the dissociative countertransference.

The limitations of available knowledge and certainty can become agonizing matters to patient and therapist alike. Limitations of scientific knowledge about dissociative conditions and their treatment are difficult for both patient and therapist. More painful still is sincere distress over the often-uncertain accuracy of recollections of the past, especially those of abuse. Historical documentation is rarely available. Different self-states may seem committed to different autobiographical scenarios, or divergent interpretations thereof. Patients may be torn by indecision, often fearful of not being believed on the one hand, but fearing they may be tarnishing the reputation of an innocent person on the other. It becomes important to validate the core concepts that hurt has been experienced and harm has been suffered, and to hear all statements with compassion and sensitivity, no matter what the various and often conflicting narratives state. In many instances, the historical truth will never become clear, let alone completely clear.

Few patients are satisfied by references to matters of fantasy and psychological truth when important decisions must be made. Treatment moves along with much remaining painfully uncertain. While I often have been able to document aspects of abuse histories, I rarely have had such information until the treatment was either well-advanced or concluded (Kluft, 1995b). Waiting to be sure before addressing a patient's suffering is not a viable strategy. It may condemn the patient to prolonged distress, indefinite uncertainty, and confusing agony. Whatever material is causing pain and/or disruption must be addressed. It cries out for therapeutic attention, independent of the historical completeness or verification of memories available. To expect otherwise defies what is known about traumatic memory, which is often fragmented and incomplete initially, and may remain so. Treatment must be respectful of the patient's pain and the need to have it heard and addressed in the manner in which it is expressed.

Flexibility is crucial. No approach is acceptable to all patients or will be helpful to all who try to work with it. One frequent query from analysts concerns whether the patient is best served by using the couch or sitting in a chair. The analytic couch is the direct descendant of the nineteenth-century hypnotist's couch. Freud's hypnosis couch became the first analytic couch. Its use is dissociogenic (i.e., facilitates dissociation). While I have conducted classic analyses of such patients on the couch, I rarely do so. Too many associate the supine position with experiences of sexual assault, and too much valuable information conveyed in non-verbal expressions of unvoiced affects and covert switch processes can go unnoticed (Kluft, 1987). Regressions on the couch may lead to disoriented crises, actions, and panics. If psychoanalytic/psychodynamic treatment *per se* does not provide sufficient support and structure, a more controlled, supportive, and structured psychodynamically informed process may prove preferable. The use of a chair is usually safest.

Those inexperienced in the treatment of posttraumatic forms of dissociation would do well to consult with a more experienced colleague. Should the treatment not progress well, consultation and/or a trial of another modality or augmentation with same is preferable to stalemate.

Summary

These are very preliminary and incomplete observations on matters of great complexity. For some readers, they will raise more questions than provide answers. They are meant to initiate rather than complete the consideration of these topics of importance.

Psychoanalytic/psychodynamic psychotherapy provides an excellent foundation for the treatment of dissociative disorders, even if augmentation with other modalities proves necessary, advisable, or simply expeditious. Moving beyond questionable abstractions, acknowledging the importance of traumatic realities and the importance of hypnotizability for understanding psychopathology, particularly dissociative psychopathology, and introducing several minor modifications can render this approach a far more safe, welcoming, encouraging, and better accepted setting for the successful treatment of traumatized and dissociative patients.

Masson provided courageous and persistent advocacy for more respectful and effective recognition of the role of abuse in the etiology of many forms of psychopathology. In doing so, he became a major force in promoting the improvement of the treatment of the traumatized and helped reawaken attention to and improve treatment of the dissociative disorders by psychoanalytic/psychodynamic clinicians.

References

Berman, E. (1981). Multiple personality: Psychoanalytic perspectives. *International Journal of Psychoanalysis*, *62*, 283–300.

Brenner, I. (2001). *Dissociation of trauma: Theory, phenomenology, and technique*. International Universities Press.

Brenner, I. (2004). *Psychic trauma: Dynamics, symptoms, and treatment*. Aronson.
Brenner, I. (2009). A new view from the Acropolis: Dissociative identity disorder. *The Psychoanalytic Quarterly*, *78*(1), 57–105. https://doi.org/10.1080/00029157.2018.1400843
Brenner, I. (2014). *Dark matters: Exploring the realm of psychic devastation*. Karnac.
Brenner, I. (2018). Catching a wave: The hypnosis-sensitive transference-based treatment of Dissociative Identity Disorder (DID). *American Journal of Clinical Hypnosis*, *60*(3), 279–295. https://doi.org/10.1080/00029157.2018.1400843
Bromberg, P. M. (2006). *Awakening the dreamer*. Routledge.
Bromberg, P. M. (2011). *The shadow of the tsunami and the growth of the relational mind*. Routledge.
Brown, D., Scheflin, A., & Hammond, D. C. (1988). *Memory, trauma treatment, and the law*. Norton.
Butler, L. (2006). Normative dissociation. *The Psychiatric Clinics of North America*, *29*(1), 45–62.
Caligor, E., Diamond, D., Yeomans, F., & Kernberg, O. (2009). The interpretive process in the psychoanalytic psychotherapy of borderline personality pathology. *Journal of the American Psychoanalytic Association*, *57*, 271–298. https://doi.org/10.1177/0003065109336183
Cardeña, E. (1994). The domain of dissociation. In S. J. Lynn & J. W. Rhue (Eds.), *Dissociation: Clinical and theoretical perspectives* (pp. 15–31). The Guilford Press.
Coons, P. (1980). Multiple personality: Diagnostic considerations. *The Journal of Clinical Psychiatry*, *41*(10), 330–336.
Coons, P. (1984). The differential diagnosis of multiple personality. A comprehensive review. *Psychiatric Clinics of North America*, *7*(1), 51–67.
Dalenberg, C. J. (2000). The argument for highlighting, examining, and disclosing countertransference in trauma therapy. In C. J. Dalenberg (Ed.), *Countertransference in the treatment of trauma* (pp. 23–56). American Psychological Association.
Ellenberger, H. (1970). *The discovery of the unconscious*. Basic Books.
Frank, J. (1973). *Persuasion and healing: A comparative study of psychotherapy*, 2nd Edition. Johns Hopkins University Press.
Frischholz, E., Lipman, L., Braun, B., & Sachs, R. (1992). Psychopathology, hypnotizability, and dissociation. *American Journal of Psychiatry*, *149*(11), 1521–1525. https://doi.org/10.1176/ajp.149.11.1521
Gubrich-Simitis, I. (1984). From concretism to metaphor—Thoughts on some theoretical and technical aspects of the psychoanalytic work with children of Holocaust survivors. *The Psychoanalytic Study of the Child*, *39*, 301–319. https://doi.org/10.1176/ajp.149.11.1521
Kluft, R. P. (1987). Unsuspected multiple personality disorder: An uncommon source of protracted resistance, interruption, and failure in psychoanalysis. *Hillside Journal of Clinical Psychiatry*, *9*, 104–115.
Kluft, R. P. (1992). Paradigm exhaustion and paradigm shift and thinking through the therapeutic impasse. *Psychiatric Annals*, *22*, 502–508. https://doi.org/10.3928/0048-5713-19921001-06
Kluft, R. P. (1995a). Treatment of dissociative disorders. In J. Barber & P. Crits-Christoph (Eds.), *Dynamic therapies for psychiatric disorders (Axis I)* (pp. 332–385). Basic Books.
Kluft, R. P. (1995b). The confirmation and discontinuation of memories of abuse in dissociative identity disorder patients: A naturalistic clinical study. *Dissociation*, 8, 253–258.

Kluft, R. P. (2000). The psychoanalytic psychotherapy of dissociative identity disorder in the context of trauma therapy. *Psychoanalytic Inquiry*, *20*, 259–286. https://doi.org/10.1080/07351692009348887

Kluft, R. P. (2006). Dealing with alters: A pragmatic clinical perspective. *The Psychiatric Clinics of North America*, *29*(1), 281–304. https://doi.org/10.1016/j.psc.2005.10.010

Kluft, R. P. (2007). Applications of innate affect theory to the understanding and treatment of dissociative identity disorder. In E. Vermetten, M. Dorahy, & D. Spiegel (Eds.), *Traumatic dissociation: Neurobiology and treatment* (pp. 301–316). American Psychiatric Press.

Kluft, R. P. (2016). You have to be carefully taught: Dignity considerations in clinical practice, scholarship, and trauma treatment. In S. Levine (Ed.), *Dignity matters: Psychoanalytic and psychosocial perspectives* (pp. 141–158). Karnac.

Kluft, R. P. (2017). Trying to keep it real: My experience in developing clinical approaches to the treatment of DID. *Frontiers in the Psychotherapy of Trauma and Dissociation*, *1*(1), 18–44.

Kluft, R. P. (2018a) Reconsidering hypnosis and psychoanalysis: Toward creating a context for understanding. *American Journal of Clinical Hypnosis*, *60*(3), 201–215. https://doi.org/10.1080/00029157.2018.1400810

Kluft, R. P. (2018b). Freud's rejection of hypnosis: Part I: – The genesis of a rift. *American Journal of Clinical Hypnosis, 60*(4), 307–323. https://doi.org/10.1080/00029157.2018.1426321

Kluft, R. P. (2018c). Freud's rejection of hypnosis: Part II: – The genesis of a rift. *American Journal of Clinical Hypnosis*, *60*(4), 324–347. https://doi.org/10.1080/00029157.2018.1426326

Kluft, R. P. (2018d). Freud's rejection of hypnosis: Perspectives old and new: Part III of III—Toward healing the rift. *American Journal of Clinical Hypnosis*, *61*(3), 208–226. https://doi.org/10.1080/00029157.2018.1544432

Kluft, R. P. (2022a). Toward the effective treatment of dissociative symptoms and dissociative disorders. *Psychoanalytic Social Work*, *30*, 3–31. https://doi.org/10.1080/15228878.2022.2095876

Kogan, I. (2003). On being a dead, beloved child. *The Psychoanalytic Quarterly*, *72*(3), 727–804. https://doi.org/10.1002/j.2167-4086.2003.tb00650.x

Kohut, H. (1970). *The analysis of the self.* University of Chicago Press.

Kohut, H. (1977). *The restoration of the self.* International Universities Press.

Kohut, H., & Wolf, E. (1978). The disorders of the self and their treatment: An outline. International *Journal of Psycho-Analysis*, *59*, 413–425.

Lessem, P. (2005). *Self psychology: An introduction*. Aronson.

Leuzinger-Bohleber, M. (2008). Biographical truths and their clinical consequences: Understanding 'embodied memories' in a third psychoanalysis with a traumatized patient recovered from severe poliomyelitis. *International Journal of Psychoanalysis*, *89*, 1165–1187.

Loewenstein, R. (1993). Posttraumatic and dissociative aspects of transference and countertransference in the treatment of multiple personality disorder. In R. P. Kluft & C. G. Fine (Eds.), *Clinical perspectives on multiple personality disorder* (pp. 51–86). American Psychiatric Press.

Loewenstein, R. J. (1991). An office mental status examination for complex chronic dissociative symptoms and multiple personality disorder. *Psychiatric Clinics of North America*, *14*(3), 567–604.

Luborsky, L. (1996). *The symptom context method: Symptoms as opportunities in psychotherapy*. American Psychological Association.

Luborsky, L., & Crits-Christoph, P. (1998). *Understanding transference: The core conflictual relationship method*, 2nd Edition. American Psychological Association.

Masson, J. M. (1984). *The assault on Truth: Freud's suppression of the seduction theory.* Farrar, Straus, & Giroux.

Nathanson, D. (1991). *Shame and pride*. Norton.

Oliner, M. (1996). External reality: The elusive dimension of psychoanalysis. *Psychoanalytic Quarterly*, *65*, 267–300. https://doi.org/10.1080/21674086.1996.11927491

O'Neil, J. (2018). Hypnosis and psychoanalysis: Toward undoing Freud's primal category mistake. *American Journal of Clinical Hypnosis*, *60*(3), 262–278. https://doi.org/10.1080/00029157.2018.1400841

Ratner, A. (2019). *The psychoanalyst's aversion to proof.* International Psychoanalytic Books.

Rosenbaum, M. (1980). The role of the term schizophrenia in the decline of diagnoses of multiple personality. *Archives of General Psychiatry*, *37*(12), 1383–1385. https://doi.org/10.1001/archpsyc.1980.01780250069008

Shengold, L. (1989). *Soul murder: The effect of childhood abuse and deprivation.* Yale University Press.

Simon, B. (1992). "Incest—See under Oedipus Complex": The history of an error in psychoanalysis. *Journal of the American Psychoanalytic Association*, *40*, 955–988. https://doi.org/10.1177/000306519204000401

Stolorow, R., Brandschaft, B., & Atwood, G. (1987). *Psychoanalytic treatment: An intersubjective approach.* Routledge.

Waelder, R. (1962). Psychoanalysis, scientific method, and philosophy. *Journal of the American Psychoanalytic Association*, *10*, 617–637. https://doi.org/10.1177/000306516201000310

Index

Note: Endnotes are indicated by the page number followed by "n" and the note number e.g., 136n2 refers to note 2 on page 136.

9781032555225